CONVERSION TABLES

Measurements for weights, lengths, and liquids have been rounded for convenience.

OVEN TEMPERATURES

FAHRENHEIT	225°	250°	275°	300°	325°	350°	375°	400°	425°	450°
CELSIUS	110°	120°	140°	150°	160°	180°	190°	200°	220°	230°

WEIGHTS

IMPERIAL	METRIC
½ oz	15 g
1 oz	30 g
4 oz (¼ lb)	125 g
6 oz	185 g
8 oz (½ lb)	250 g
12 oz (¾ lb)	375 g
14 oz	440 g
1 pound (16 oz)	500 g
1½ lb	750 g

LENGTHS

IMPERIAL	METRIC
¼ in	5 mm
½ in	1 cm
1 in	2.5 cm
6 in	12 cm
12 in	30 cm

SPOON MEASURES

IMPERIAL	METRIC
¼ tsp	1.125 ml
½ tsp	2.5 ml
1 tsp	5 ml
1 tbsp	15 ml

BODY TEMPERATURE

°F	°C	
104	40	high fever
103	39.5	
102	39	moderate fever
101	38.5	
100	38	low fever
99	37.5	normal (rectal)
98	37	normal (oral)
97	36.5	
96	36	
	35.5	

SPEED

IMPERIAL	METRIC
30 mph	50 km/h
40 mph	60 km/h
50 mph	80 km/h
55 mph	90 km/h
60 mph	100 km/h

LIQUIDS

IMPERIAL	METRIC
¼ cup	60 ml
⅓ cup	80 ml
½ cup	125 ml
⅔ cup	160 ml
¾ cup	180 ml
1 cup	250 ml

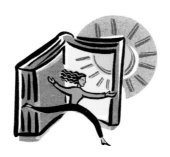

LOOKING
AFTER
YOUR
BODY

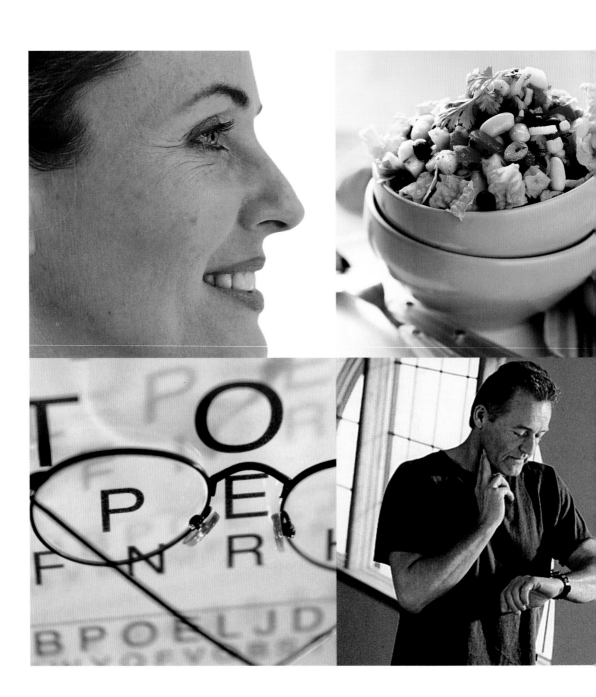

LOOKING AFTER YOUR BODY

▶ An Owner's Guide to Successful Aging

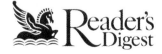
Reader's Digest

The Reader's Digest Association (Canada) Ltd., Montreal

LOOKING AFTER YOUR BODY

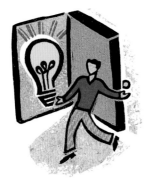

Reader's Digest Canadian Staff

PROJECT EDITOR
Anita Winterberg

DESIGNER
Cécile Germain

PRODUCTION MANAGER
Holger Lorenzen

PRODUCTION COORDINATOR
Susan Wong

EDITORIAL ADMINISTRATOR
Elizabeth Eastman

Contributors

PHARMACEUTICAL CONSULTANT
Gerald Rotenberg

RESEARCHER
Martha Plaine

COPY EDITOR
Judy Yelon

Books and Home Entertainment

VICE PRESIDENT
Deirdre Gilbert

MANAGING EDITOR
Philomena Rutherford

ART DIRECTOR
John McGuffie

Reader's Digest US Staff

EDITOR
Marianne Wait

SENIOR DESIGNER
Susan Welt

PRODUCTION TECHNOLOGY MANAGER
Douglas A. Croll

EDITORIAL MANAGER
Christine R. Guido

CONTRIBUTING EDITORS
Susan Carleton, Kimberly Ruderman

Note to Readers
The information in this book should not be substituted for, or used to alter, medical therapy without your doctor's advice. For a specific health problem, consult your physician for guidance.

Address any comments about LOOKING AFTER YOUR BODY to Editor, Books and Home Entertainment, c/o Customer Service, Reader's Digest, 1125 Stanley Street, Montreal, Quebec H3B 5H5.

For information about this and other Reader's Digest products or to request a catalogue, please call our 24-hour Customer Service hotline at 1-800-465-0780.

You can also visit us on the World Wide Web at www.readersdigest.ca

Printed in the United States of America.
01 02 03 / 5 4 3 2 1

National Library of Canada Cataloguing in Publication Data

Main entry under title:
    Looking after your body: an owner's guide to successful aging
  Includes index.
  ISBN 0-88850-741-0
    1. Longevity. 2. Aging—Prevention. 3. Health. I. Title

RA776.75.L67 2001   613   C2001-900417-6

Produced by The Philip Lief Group, Inc.

EDITORIAL DIRECTOR
Maryanne Wagner

EXECUTIVE EDITORS
Rhonda Heisler, Heidi Hough

ASSOCIATE EDITOR
Rose Foltz

ASSISTANT EDITOR
Lynne Kirk

EDITORIAL ASSISTANT
Marybeth Fedele

Contributors

WRITERS AND EDITORS
Marylou Ambrose, Bryan Aubrey,
Robert A. Barnett, Jeanine Barone, Linda
Benson, Diana Benzaia, Sheryl Birsky,
Jan Bresnick, Sheila Buff, Hilary Macht
Felgran, Michael Fillon, Joan Friedrich,
Ph.D., CCN, CDN, Blythe Hamer, Harriet
Harvey, Francine Hornberger, Janis
Jibrin, Valerie Latona, Jane Leder, Lynn
Madsen, Michele Meyer, Kristin Robie,
M.D., Deborah S. Romaine, E. Manning
Rubin, Cindy Spitzer, Nancy Stedman,
Jane Summer, Kathleen Thompson,
Bibi Wein, Lyn Yonack

RECIPE DEVELOPMENT
Susan McQuillan, M.S., R.D.

COPY EDITOR
Nora Reichard

INDEXER
Felice Levy

Art Direction
Lemonides Design
ART DIRECTOR
Diane Lemonides

DESIGN ASSISTANT
Sharon Wienckoski

PICTURE RESEARCH
Carousel Research, Inc.
Laurie Platt Winfrey, Van Bucher,
Matthew Connors

ILLUSTRATORS
Calef Brown, John Edwards, Joel Harris,
Sharon Harris, Becky Heavner

PHOTOGRAPHERS
Beth Bischoff, Rich Dunoff,
Susan Goldman, Mark Thomas

Editorial Board of Advisors

CHIEF MEDICAL ADVISOR
Richard W. Besdine, M.D., F.A.C.P.
Director, Center for Gerontology
and Health Care Research, Division
of Geriatrics, and Greer Professor of
Geriatric Medicine, Brown University
School of Medicine

ADVISORS
Elizabeth Barrett-Connor, M.D.
Professor and Chief, Division of
Epidemiology, Department of Family and
Preventive Medicine, University of Cali-
fornia at San Diego School of Medicine

Johanna T. Dwyer, D.Sc., R.D.
Professor of Medicine and Community
Health (Nutrition), Schools of Medicine
and Nutrition Science and Policy;
Director, Frances Stern Nutrition Center,
New England Medical Center Hospital

Salvatore Fichera, M.S.
American Council on Exercise Certified
Strength and Conditioning Specialist

Sanford I. Finkel, M.D.
Medical Director, Leonard Schanfield
Research Institute and Geriatric
Institute, Council for Jewish Elderly

Joyce Frye, D.O., F.A.C.O.G.
Instructor, Obstetrics and Gynecology,
Jefferson Medical College

Charlyn Marcusen, Ph.D., C.C.R.C.

Tedd Mitchell, M.D.
Medical Director, Wellness Program,
Cooper Clinic at the Cooper Aerobics
Institute

Marion Nestle, Ph.D.
Professor and Chair, Department of
Nutrition and Food Studies, New York
University

Harry Preuss, M.D., F.A.C.N., C.N.S.
Professor of Physiology, Medicine,
and Pathology, Georgetown University
Medical Center

Curt Woolford, M.A., R.Y.T.
Kripalu Certified Yoga Instructor

Contents

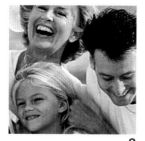
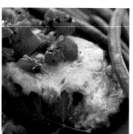
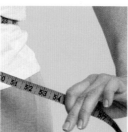
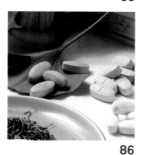
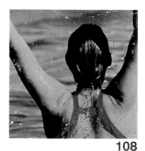
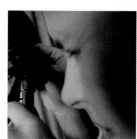
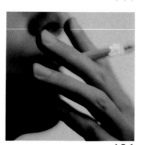
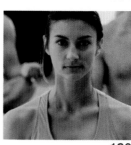

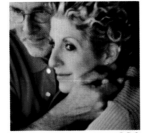
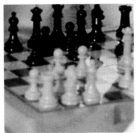
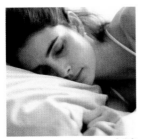
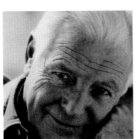

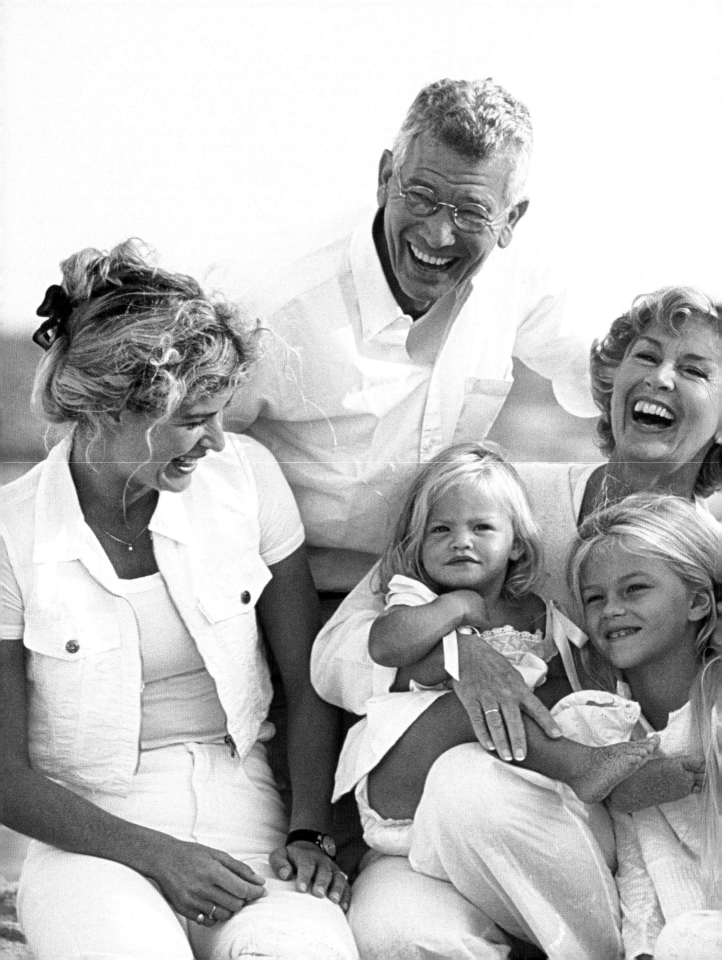

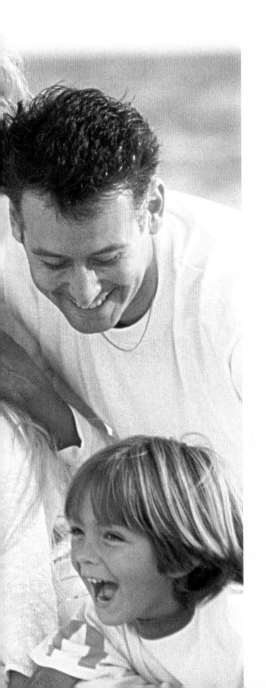

INTRODUCTION

SLOWING THE CLOCK

A New Perspective on Aging

Aging isn't what it used to be. If you picture yourself becoming frail or sickly, erase that image. New research tells us the keys to living longer and staying healthier are in our hands.

If our grandparents had only known what we know now about health and aging, they might have lived longer and stayed more active later in life. They couldn't reap the benefits of the extraordinary research that's turned the concept of aging on its ear—but you can.

Start with the revolutionary idea that *you don't have to get sicker as you get older*. Sound too good to be true? It's not. By taking small steps to protect your health right now, you can lead a vibrant life into your eighties, nineties, and perhaps beyond.

Consider what the research is telling us. Back in 1958 the Baltimore Longitudinal Study of Aging started monitoring the health of more than a thousand people. The results have been amazing. Despite our conceptions of what it means to get older, the study has found that the physical changes caused by aging alone— rather than disease—are *almost insignificant*. In other words, aging is not an illness. As long as you're not struck by major trauma or disease, you can remain healthy and robust throughout your life.

Maybe you think your fate has already been sealed by your genes. If so, think again. In 1984, a major new research endeavor was launched called the MacArthur Foundation Study of Aging in America. Across the U.S., medical scientists—cell biologists, sociologists, geneticists, neuropsychologists, and others— studied different aspects of how we age, and how we might stay younger longer. Their most dramatic discov-

ery was that lifestyle plays a considerably larger role in determining our health than genes do. For example, the study's research on twins who were raised apart has shown that only about 30 percent of physical aging can be blamed on genes. The rest involves factors such as the way you eat, the health risks you take, how active you are, and how often you get medical checkups.

The Secrets of Aging Well

Have you ever wondered why some people seem to age so much better than others? Researchers are now learning the secrets to their success. "Successful agers" appear to:

- stay physically and mentally active
- take preventive measures to avoid major diseases
- stay engaged in life by keeping a positive attitude and staying connected socially.

Successful agers may even get better as they get older. In another MacArthur Foundation study, scientists followed the progress of 4,000 people age 70 to 79. They were periodically tested on both mental and physical performance. Physical tests assessed their ability to use their hands, trunk, and legs, as well as their balance and gait. During the eight-year study, more than half maintained their level of functioning and almost 25 percent improved it. The ones who were most likely to improve had a high measure of mental and physical fitness and exercised at least moderately. The study reinforced the notion that your functional age is up to you.

An Owner's Guide

In hindsight, the research makes perfect sense. Think about it this way: If you were to liken your body to an automobile, what would it look like? A peppy sportscar? A sturdy-bodied sedan that's just starting to show its age? Or an old gas-guzzling clunker that's on its way to the junkyard? Whatever comes to mind, you're probably realizing that the amount of care you've put into your body *shows.*

The best way to keep your car running smoothly is a little routine maintenance. The same goes for your body. Think of this book as an owner's manual—your guide to keeping your body in prime condition for years to come. Part I, *Your Game Plan for Good Health,* gets right down to the nuts and bolts of what you can do for your body now—small steps you can take to feel better, look better, and live longer. For example, in the first chapter, *Eating to Age Well,* you'll find out that eating a few walnuts every day might reduce your risk of a heart attack by as much as 40 percent. You'll take tests to see if your current diet is aging you, and learn how to choose foods the easy way—by their color. In other chapters, you'll discover:

- that simply taking a multivitamin every day can help you live longer (Chapter 3)
- easy exercises that are great for your back (Chapter 4)
- simple screening tests that could save your life (Chapter 5)
- a six-weeks-to-success plan to stop smoking (Chapter 6)

Are you in need of some body work? A little care and maintenance can keep your body looking younger and running smoother so you can get more mileage from life.

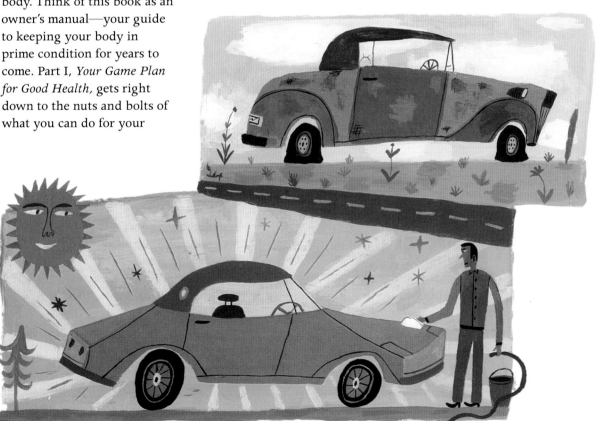

"You're just getting older" is no longer an acceptable excuse from your doctor, so don't use it yourself. Aging is not a disease.

- proven de-stressors that can actually boost your immune system (Chapter 7)
- the surprising emotional link to staying well in middle age and beyond (Chapter 8)
- natural solutions for enhancing your sex life (Chapter 9)
- easy ways to exercise your brain and maintain your mental edge (Chapter 10)
- secrets to getting a better night's sleep (Chapter 11)
- wrinkle treatments that actually make a difference (Chapter 12).

Part II, *Ailments A to Z,* is your troubleshooting guide. You'll learn about common disorders associated with age and red flags to watch for. To-the-point prevention plans help you avoid the conditions you're most at risk for. Did you know that drinking two to three glasses of milk a day may help lower your blood pressure? That soy may protect against prostate enlargement? That aspirin therapy may guard against colon cancer? If you can avoid or reverse the ailments described in this section, you'll be on your way to staying healthy for life.

Redefining Your Age

If Sean Connery at 62 could be voted one of the world's sexiest men and John Glenn could return to orbit at age 77, the term "old" needs a new definition. Update your image of what your later years might be like.

Don't expect disability. In a Stanford University study, people who exercised, controlled their weight, and avoided smoking lived longer than those who didn't. They also had fewer disabilities and developed them later in life, so they had fewer unhealthy years overall.

Don't expect to be frail. Whatever your age, exercise can make you stronger. In one study, people age 60 to 70 who started an exercise program improved their oxygen-using capacity by a remarkable 38 percent. Twelve weeks after starting a strength-training program, men between the ages of 60 and 72 improved their muscle strength by up to 227 percent. And a study from the Harvard School of Public Health recently found that vigorous activity significantly decreased the risk of dying prematurely from any cause.

Don't expect your brain to fail. There's no need to panic just because you tend to lose your car keys or forget names; your mind is probably holding up better than you think. Why? Mental function has not been found to decline significantly with age, only with disease. The Seattle Longitudinal Study (SLS), a large study on how aging affects mental

Beating the Olympians

Did you know that in recent Senior Olympic Games, several winners actually beat some of the regular Olympic gold medal times? For example, Keefe Lodwig, 53, swam the 100-meter freestyle in 57.93 seconds, beating Johnny Weissmuller's 1928 medal win at 58.6 seconds. Other winners achieved their personal best, such as Bob Bailey, who swam the 100-yard freestyle in 52.62 seconds when he was 53. His previous best, which he achieved as a college student, was 52.7 seconds.

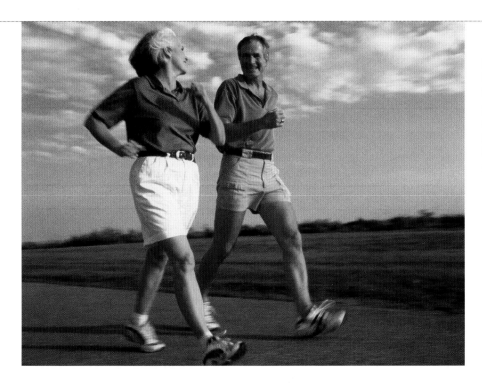

Some gerontologists believe you could add two years to your life if you start a vigorous aerobic exercise program—at least three 30-minute sessions a week—at age 40.

function, has been observing more than 3,000 mentally healthy adults since 1956. To date, the SLS has discovered that performance in the areas of verbal meaning, spatial orientation, inductive reasoning, number skills, and word fluency begins to decline only slightly by about the age of 74. However, most participants in the study have maintained or *increased* their level of performance in at least one area.

Don't expect your sex life to stall. According to Health Canada, on average, approximately 70 percent of healthy 70-year-olds continue to have regular sexual intercourse. More than 25 percent of healthy men and women age 80 and older are still sexually active—having intercourse four times a month. What's more, older persons consistently report more satisfaction with their sex lives than young people. Writing in *Passionate Marriage*, David Schnarch, Ph.D., suggested that the love lives of 60-year-olds can be better than those of 20-year-olds. "This is a time when people have the best sex in their lives, and it all has to do with maturity."

You're in Control

As you picture yourself getting older, remember this: You can remain active and productive. You might not run a marathon—but then again, you might. You wouldn't be the first person to astonish the world with physical feats once considered the province of youth alone. Of course, it won't happen by accident. Today it's clearer than ever before that we have to "use it or lose it." Activity of all kinds—physical, mental, social, and spiritual—can slow or even reverse the aging process. So can simple acts like eating what's good for you and getting the medical screening tests you need. When it comes to turning back the clock, research proves that it's never too late to start. So begin one step at a time, and begin now.

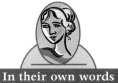

In their own words

Approach your future with a sense that anything is possible. Kay Thomas, a woman in her fifties, says, "My parents always talked about 'when we retire' as though it were 'when we grow up.' They considered living on a houseboat or teaching abroad. When they did retire, they designed a house and did most of the building themselves. In their seventies, they added a room and a garage, getting help from the neighbors only for putting on the roof. They gave me the sense that life is a continuum of opportunities. When I'm finished with one thing, I'll just go on to the next."

15 Ways to Slow the Clock

Making small changes in your daily routine is all it takes to slow the hands of time. Focus on these 15 ways to stay well.

1 Eat your medicine. Did you know that eating fish once a week could cut your risk of sudden cardiac death? Good nutrition is more than consuming less fat. It's knowing the difference between good and bad fats, paying more attention to the variety and proportions of the foods you eat, and making good nutritional choices a *habit* (the hard part for most people). For example, even though eating five or more fruit and vegetable servings a day may cut overall cancer risk by 20 percent, less than 40 percent of older people do this. If you've had poor nutritional habits for a long time, you won't be able to change overnight, but you can succeed if you improve your diet gradually.

2 Get a move on. Physical inactivity is the most prevalent risk factor for premature death and disability for Canadians of all ages. According to the Canadian Fitness and Lifestyle Research Institute, two-thirds of all Canadians have dangerously inactive lifestyles. However, even modest amounts of exercise (20 minutes a day) can do a world of good, especially if you are faithful to a regular routine and get the various forms of exercise you need to build your endurance, strength, balance, and flexibility.

3 Supplement your diet. You may know that getting enough of the antioxidant vitamins C and E and beta carotene is one of the best ways to slow the clock. But if you're serious about staying young, there are other supplements you should know about too. Vitamin B_{12} is one of them, since deficiencies of this nutrient—common in people over 60—can result in dementia and memory loss. So is calcium, which not only guards against osteoporosis but may also help prevent the most common type of stroke.

4 Watch your weight. We all know that obesity can lead to serious health problems and shorten your life. But even 10 or 20 pounds of extra weight can pose an unnecessary risk, especially if it's sitting mostly around your middle. Your metabolism slows with age, so you're not burning the calories you once did. That means you should be cutting down on how much you eat or stepping up your exercise, or both.

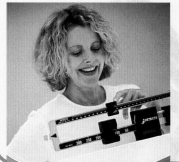

5 Be good to your bones.

If you're a woman, don't wait until after menopause to address your risk of osteoporosis. You start losing bone density at least a decade before menopause, so you need to get enough calcium and vitamin D every day, stop smoking, and get regular weight-bearing exercise right now. When you approach menopause, discuss hormone replacement therapy with your doctor. And men, don't think you're immune to osteoporosis. Your risk is increasing more slowly than a woman's, but by your seventies or eighties, it can be just as great. According to the Osteoporosis Society of Canada, there are some 25,000 hip fractures each year. Seventy percent of these are osteoporosis-related.

6 Get checked.

Many people hate to see the doctor, but he or she can be your best friend when it comes to preventing health problems. Getting your blood pressure checked annually, for example, can help prevent serious cardiovascular and kidney problems. You can easily avoid 23 strains of pneumonia (a leading killer of older Canadians) by getting a pneumococcal vaccine, and yearly flu shots can ward off not only the flu but also the complications that can come with it. And you'll never regret detecting cancer or diabetes early on, when there's still time to do something about it. Find out what tests you should have at what age (see page 149 and post the list on your refrigerator).

7 Limit the liquor.

It's true that one or two drinks a day may lower your risk of heart disease and stroke, but you shouldn't start drinking to gain these benefits. Exercise and diet can help you achieve the same results. Also, the older you get, the more alcohol affects you. Drinking a glass of sherry, then a glass of wine with dinner might be one thing for a 40- to 50-year-old, but quite another for a 70-year-old, who metabolizes alcohol more slowly and may be more prone to falls. And overdoing alcohol increases a woman's risk of breast cancer.

8 Say no to smoking—and to smoke.

Heart disease, cancer, and stroke account for at least one out of every two deaths today, and smoking is clearly behind them all. If you still have this habit and you want to live, then quit before you think of doing anything else. It doesn't matter how many times you've tried to quit before; the next time can work, if you get all the help you need. See page 168 on how to start. If you're an older smoker, take heart: Your chances of staying smoke-free if you quit are greatest if you're over 65. As for passive smoking, realize that sitting in smoke-filled rooms may shorten your life. Dr. Michael Roizen of the University of Chicago estimates that breathing in smoke for one hour equals smoking four cigarettes yourself.

9 Mind your medications. Like a lot of people, you might find yourself taking a host of different drugs as you get older. The biggest problem with "polypharmacy," as it's called, is the increased risk of interactions among drugs and with food, alcohol, and herbs. Did you know that drinking alcohol when taking Tylenol can cause liver damage? That one out of four cases of impotence may result from drug side effects? That as you age, you become more sensitive to drugs and may need lower doses? You can't afford not to be savvy about drugs.

10 Sidestep stress. As you get older, you tend to experience new types of stress. You may have more responsibility than ever on the job, or aging parents to look after. Perhaps retirement isn't what you thought it would be, or you're lonely after the death of your spouse. Chronic stress can compound your risk of heart disease, cancer, and digestive problems, and it can even burn out your memory. Learning to manage it can actually help you live longer. In fact, people who have lived to 100 seem to have had better-than-average ways of dealing with stress. Several techniques can help you cope.

11 Don't fall victim to accidents and spills. First, drive safely and wear a seatbelt. If you're a man age 55 to 64, you're twice as likely to die in an auto accident as a woman your age. Driving risks are bound to increase if you develop vision or hearing problems or have slower reflexes. Around the house, you're at higher risk for falls as you get older. Remove clutter and other hazards underfoot, and exercise to improve your balance.

12 Think young. To remain vital, you need to stay actively engaged in life and break out of old routines. So find a passion or purpose and pursue it. Get involved in volunteer work. Try a new type of ethnic food, start a garden, adopt a pet. It's also important to challenge your faculties. Learning new things can actually stimulate new connections in your brain. Play bridge, do challenging crossword puzzles, join a book discussion group. Take up pottery or learn to play an instrument.

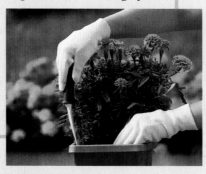

13 Preserve your pearly whites. Once upon a time, as people got older, they got dentures. If you'd rather keep your teeth, dental checkups and cleaning should be on your calendar at least once or twice a year. Daily flossing and brushing are also an important part of your preventive health care. Gum disease can actually spread infection to your heart and take years off your life.

A Little Effort Goes a Long Way

You don't have to become a health fanatic or overhaul your lifestyle to live longer and stay healthier. By gradually making some easy changes like the ones below, you'll be on your way to better health in no time.

SIMPLE STEP	TIME INVESTMENT	MAJOR BENEFIT
Add strawberries to your morning waffle	Minutes	■ Vitamin C helps prevent cataracts. It may also slow the progression of joint damage from osteoarthritis.
Switch to a cereal that contains 5 grams of fiber per serving	None	■ Cuts your risk of type 2 diabetes and heart disease and may help you lose weight.
Take a multivitamin that contains 400 micrograms of folic acid	Seconds	■ May cut the risk of colon cancer by up to 75 percent.
Do the crossword puzzle	20 minutes	■ Challenging your brain forces it to grow new dendrites, hairlike fibers that connect neurons. The more connections, the more agile your brain becomes.
Walk vigorously for 30 minutes six times a month	Three hours a month	■ Helps prevent osteoporosis and may cut the risk of premature death in half.
Get enough sleep	About 7 ½ to 8 hours	■ Strengthens your immune system and may lower your risk of premature death by as much as 30 percent.
Eat fish at least once a week	About 30 minutes	■ May cut your risk of heart attack by 40 percent. May also reduce the risk of several cancers and ease symptoms of rheumatoid arthritis.
Have an annual mammogram	About an hour	■ Cuts the risk of dying from breast cancer by up to 30 percent.

14 **Get enough sleep.** Restful, deep sleep can be more elusive than ever as you age. Yet adequate shuteye is crucial to aging well. Sleep has been strongly linked to proper immune system functioning and also to cardiovascular health. Learning more about your changing sleep patterns and how to preserve this precious restorative can add to the quality—and the quantity—of your life. See Chapter 11 for specific advice. Beyond sleep, you can repair both mind and body by learning how to relax and doing it more often.

15 **Stay connected socially.** Maintaining the ties that bind—with family and friends both old and new—is much more important than we realized, according to the most recent medical research. In fact, having a social network has been clinically proven to contribute to a longer life and reduce the need for doctor visits and trips to the hospital. If you have a support system, you're more likely to weather physical ailments, stress, and emotional problems—and derive more enjoyment from life. The more people you talk to daily or weekly, the better.

Solving the Mysteries of Aging

Hope springs eternal, but the human life span has built-in limits. Here are possible reasons why we won't live forever—yet.

What causes the body to age? Do our cells deteriorate from simple wear and tear? Or are they programmed to die off at a certain time? These are two major theories about what happens to us on the cellular level.

Free Radicals at Work

Dr. Denham Harman's theory on the effects of free radicals in the body has been called "the biggest discovery since germs." Free radicals are unstable oxygen molecules that have only one electron instead of the usual pair, so they try to latch on to other molecules. As they do this, they inflict damage on proteins, lipids, and DNA in the body's cells in a process known as oxidation. Think of an apple that's been cut open and left on the counter for a while. What happens to it? It turns brown.

That's what oxidation does, and it's happening inside your body.

Where do free radicals come from? Ironically, though free radicals are caused by all sorts of pollutants such as smog and tobacco smoke and even by fried foods, they are also a by-product of natural metabolic processes in the body. That's the paradox of oxygen: It gives us life and energy, but it also produces free radicals that repeatedly attack our cells every day. Over time, our damaged cells lose their ability to withstand infection and disease, and eventually they die. The good news is that antioxidants—vitamins, minerals, enzymes, and other compounds found in foods or produced in our bodies—may help neutralize free radicals. Since free radical dam-

What Free Radicals Do To Your Cells

Before and after free radical damage: On the left, a healthy cell has smooth protein strands and a flexible cell membrane. On the right, free radicals have damaged DNA in the nucleus, broken protein strands, and distorted lipids, making the cell membrane prone to destruction.

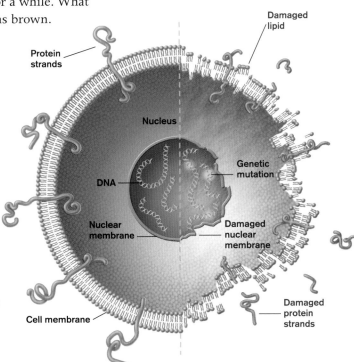

Protein strands

Damaged lipid

Nucleus

Genetic mutation

DNA

Nuclear membrane

Damaged nuclear membrane

Cell membrane

Damaged protein strands

age seems to increase as we age, we'd be wise to consume more antioxidant-rich fruits and vegetables.

The Ticking Clock

Another theory suggests that cells have an internal clock. Dr. Leonard Hayflick, a professor at the University of California, San Francisco, discovered that cells can divide only so many times (the "Hayflick limit"). The limit is different for each species. For example, a chicken's cells divide only 15 to 35 times. Human cells normally divide about 50 or 60 times before dying.

Why can't cells divide infinitely? Our chromosomes have tiny end segments called telomeres, which prevent our DNA from unraveling (picture the plastic piece on the end of a shoelace) and allow it to divide. Each time the cell divides, the telomere shortens. When the telomere is whittled down to nothing, the cell can no longer divide. You might say it then becomes an "old junker" cell. When these cells pile up, they start to interfere with other cells, causing tissues and organs to deteriorate.

The Hayflick limit might be foiled by an enzyme called telomerase, which can rejuvenate telomeres. The enzyme is normally manufactured in sperm and egg cells, but it is "turned off" in other body cells. Cancer cells also produce it. The challenge for scientists is to figure out how to harness the power of telomerase without unleashing cancerous growth. Such knowledge could help us learn how to replace burned or damaged skin, cure diseases such as macular degeneration, and even extend life.

In the meantime, avoid the things that cause telomeres to shrink faster:

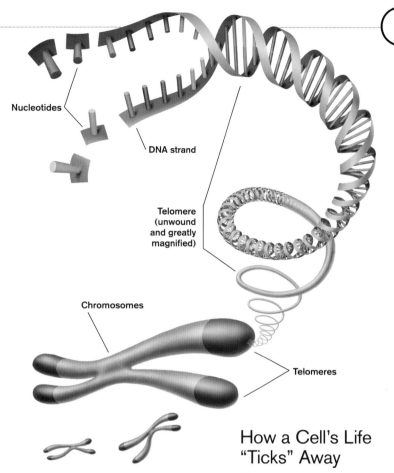

How a Cell's Life "Ticks" Away

Chromosomes are made up of DNA strands that replicate to create the genetic information for a new cell. Each time a DNA strand splits, its endcap, or telomere, shortens. When the telomere gets too short, the cell can no longer divide.

tobacco, sun and radiation exposure, stress, injuries, and infections. Also slow the pace of cell division by getting plenty of antioxidants (from broccoli, tomatoes, and green tea, for example) and perhaps taking supplements of vitamins C and E.

Can You Live Longer by Eating Less?

Pass up the pie if you want to help fight free radical damage and slow cell division. That's the theory of Dr. Roy Walford at the UCLA School of Medicine. In his experiments, mice given 40 percent fewer calories but all the nutrients they needed lived about 44 percent longer than those on higher-calorie diets. Rhesus monkeys on a reduced diet not only lived longer but had a lower incidence of diabetes and spinal arthritis. Though his theory hasn't been demonstrated in humans yet, Dr. Walford practices what he preaches. He's cut his own calorie intake back by 30 percent to 1,700 calories a day.

Rethinking Your Life Span

Did you ever think you'd live for a century? Don't dismiss the idea. It's much more likely today than ever before.

If you take charge of your health, how long can you expect to live? Very successful agers tend to push the boundaries of average life expectancy, which is now up to 79 in Canada (81.5 for women, 75.7 for men). In 1920, it was only 59.

Jeanne Calment, the longest-living person on record, certainly pushed the boundary. She lived to 122—now considered the maximum human life span. In most species, the life span is about six times the age of maturity.

The idea of living past 100 is hardly far-fetched. There are 3,130 centenarians in Canada now. In the U.S there are 70,000, and the number could be in the millions by 2050. What's more, scientists are expecting breakthroughs in the next 50 years that will snare what they call "The Big Enchilada," the key to extending human life. In the meantime the question is, how can you live longer and stay healthy enough to really enjoy all those extra years?

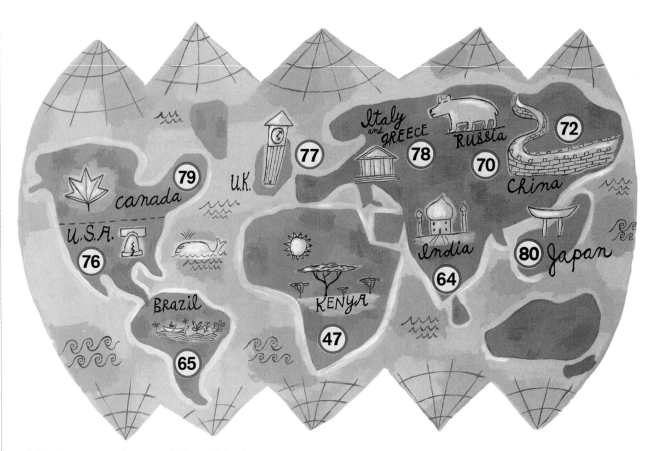

Life Spans Around the World Diet, lifestyle, standard of living, and health care are key factors influencing life expectancy. For example, the anti-aging secrets in the Asian and Mediterranean diets may help put Japan, Greece, and Italy ahead of the rest of us.

What the Centenarians Can Tell Us

Let's look to the people who made it to 100 or more for insight. Around the world, many of the oldest old are more vibrant than people who are decades younger. The Harvard Medical School New England Centenarian Study recently scrutinized the habits of centenarians. They learned that:

- most of them ate wisely and moderately (only 1 percent were obese)
- most of them lived most of their lives on the second or third floor, so they had to get their exercise and didn't become frail
- they didn't tend to smoke or abuse alcohol
- 25 percent had no cognitive disorder whatsoever
- about 15 percent were still living independently and about 35 percent lived with friends or family
- they tended to have a calm, optimistic, and positive attitude.

Centenarians share other habits as well. When scientists at the University of Georgia studied 157 centenarians for 10 years, they found that adaptability to life's challenges was critical to their longevity. What made them so adaptable? Such traits as optimism, compassion, a sense of humor, belief in God, indifference toward death, and satisfaction with life. Almost all of the centenarians also enjoyed close connections with family and friends.

Optimism may be especially important. Mayo Clinic researchers compared mortality rates for people who'd taken a personality test over 30 years ago and found that pessimists had a 19 percent greater risk of dying prematurely than optimists.

Why Do Women Live Longer Than Men?

Most centenarians are women—in fact, they outnumber men nine to one. To explain why, researchers have pointed to behavioral, biological, social, and psychological differences between the sexes. Consider these facts:

MEN

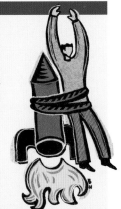

■ **Men take more chances.** Men are more likely to die from reckless or unhealthy behavior or violence, particularly when they're young (15 to 24) or middle-aged (55 to 64). Sex hormones may be involved too. Testosterone—often linked to aggression—is produced in higher amounts during that first mortality peak through ages 15 to 24. And by middle age, testosterone is thought to increase "bad" cholesterol and decrease "good" cholesterol, making men more vulnerable to heart disease and stroke.

■ **Men have faster clocks.** Men's faster metabolic rate may make their "ticking clocks" run faster, become more vulnerable to breakdown, and stop sooner.

WOMEN

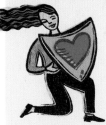

■ **Women have built-in protection.** Women have the heart-protecting advantage of estrogen, at least until menopause. It acts as an antioxidant, neutralizing the free radicals that damage cells and accelerate aging. The monthly menstrual cycle may also help women shed excess iron stores in their bodies, which contribute to the formation of free radicals.

■ **Women linger longer.** Women tend to have more chronic disorders (such as arthritis, osteoporosis, and autoimmune problems) and men have more fatal conditions, such as heart disease and stroke. That's not to say that more women aren't dying of heart disease than ever before, just that the proportion of fatal diseases is higher among men overall. More women end up living with their diseases than dying from them.

■ **Women have 'Xtra' help.** Stanford University researchers recently discovered a gene on the X chromosome that's critical to DNA repair. A man, with only one X chromosome, has only limited use of this capacity for repair. A woman's second X chromosome may compensate when genes on her first X chromosome have become damaged with age.

What Happens As We Age

Like death and taxes, aging is inevitable.
But most of the physical changes that accompany it are smaller than you think.

You're bound to experience some perfectly normal changes as you get older. The trick is to come to terms with the things you can't control and take charge of the things you can. Here's a quick summary of what's ahead.

Not So Bright Eyes The first indication that you're getting older may be how far away you have to hold the newspaper. If you hold it at arm's length and your eyes tire easily, you probably have presbyopia ("old eye"). The lenses in your eyes are less flexible now and can't shift as easily from distant to near sight. After age 40 you're also at higher risk for glaucoma, a buildup of pressure in the front of the eyes that can cause damage to the optic nerve and may produce blind spots or loss of peripheral vision. You may also develop cataracts that cloud your lenses and restrict your vision. Early detection is important in both problems.

What Was That? Hearing losses actually begin in your twenties. High-frequency sounds start to fade first, then by around age 65, you may start to miss low-frequency sounds before hearing loss becomes noticeable. Not everyone becomes hard of hearing, but more than a third of people over the age of 65 have significant problems. Changes in the inner ear can affect your balance too, so you have to be more careful to prevent falls.

Thin Skin As you age, you literally become thin-skinned. You gradually lose that youth-giving cushion of fat beneath the skin, along with the protein substances collagen and elastin and natural skin oils. As your skin gets thinner and more transparent, you may spot tiny little veins through it. You might also see some hyperpigmented areas, or liver spots, but these aren't harmful. What is harmful is the sun, which will worsen your wrinkles and overall skin condition, even if it doesn't lead to skin cancer.

Minimize these problems by drinking plenty of water, wearing sunscreen, eating a balanced diet rich in fruits and vegetables, and cleansing your skin gently. Although it won't give you back the skin you were born with, tretinoin (brand names Retin-A and Renova) can improve the texture and appearance of your skin. Available only by prescription, it peels away dead skin cells and boosts the production of collagen, ropelike protein strands that support the skin.

Ouchless You may find that your sense of touch isn't as fine-tuned as it used to be. Dietary deficiencies, circulation problems, and the normal effects of aging on your nervous system may all be involved in the decline. You may be unable to sense pain or extreme temperatures as quickly as when you were younger. That makes you more vulnerable to heatstroke,

Avoiding the Ups and Downs of Aging

Here's a quick look at what can happen to people as they age. Remember that many of these changes can be avoided by taking a proactive approach to your health.

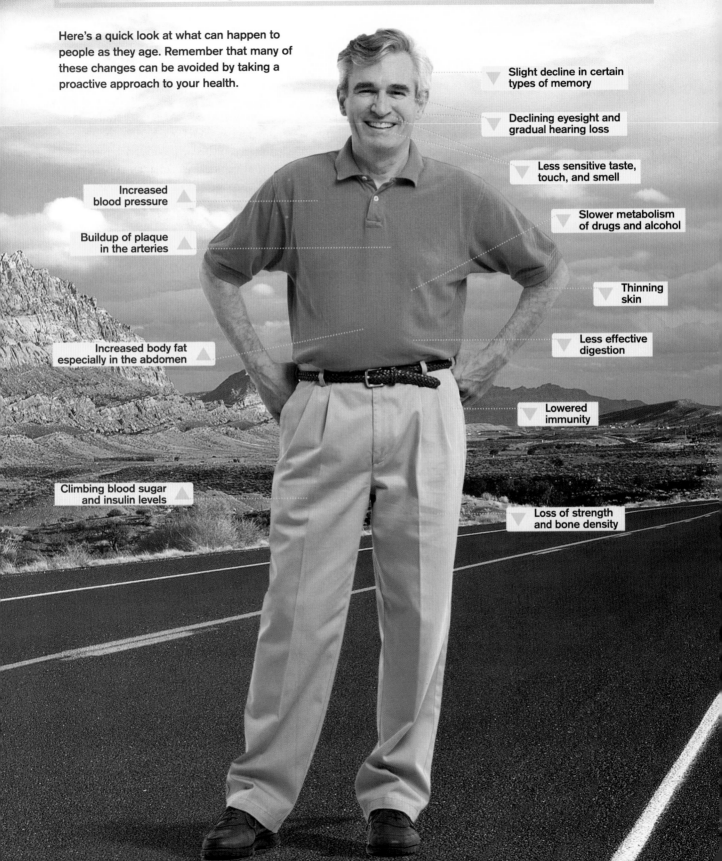

- Slight decline in certain types of memory
- Declining eyesight and gradual hearing loss
- Less sensitive taste, touch, and smell
- Slower metabolism of drugs and alcohol
- Thinning skin
- Less effective digestion
- Lowered immunity
- Loss of strength and bone density
- Increased blood pressure
- Buildup of plaque in the arteries
- Increased body fat especially in the abdomen
- Climbing blood sugar and insulin levels

Recharging Your Brain

At birth, your brain has about 100 billion neurons. Every neuron has branches, or dendrites, that reach out toward other neurons, moving messages and thoughts along. Even though your brain starts to lose neurons well before middle age, the loss is a tiny percentage of your total cells. Plus, your remaining neurons can be stimulated to grow new dendrites simply by working your mind more.

It's been proven: The more you think, the more new connections your brain will grow. Autopsy studies at UCLA showed that university graduates who had remained mentally active had up to 40 percent more brain connections than high-school dropouts. Learning a new language, persevering with that crossword puzzle, or just doing some new activity may be all the stimulation you need. Playing a musical instrument is an especially good challenge because it requires coordination between different areas of your brain. You have to do several things at once—read, listen, and play. No wonder lots of centenarians have musical skills.

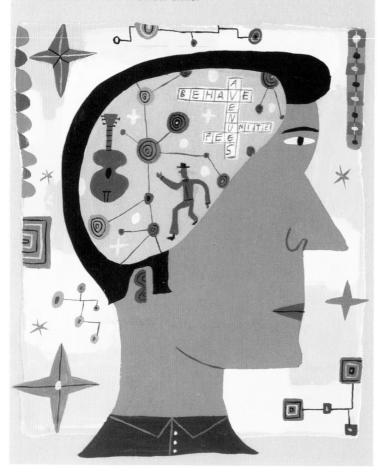

frostbite, and burns. So take extra care in extreme weather, and lower your hot-water thermostat.

 Was That Garlic or Onion? You may or may not have a problem with your ability to taste and smell, although the number of your taste-buds will definitely decrease and nerve endings in your nose may become less sensitive. Your sense of taste is related to your sense of smell, since your brain interprets signals from both to determine flavors. If either sense is impaired, it may dull your appetite and prevent you from getting all the nutrients you need. You may also find yourself over-salting your food.

 Clogging Up As you age, you might have some thick-ening and stiffening of your heart valves, heart walls, and arteries, as well as a slowing of your heart rate and perhaps some enlargement of the heart. The most common risk: Fatty deposits may accumulate on the inside of your coronary arteries, gradually harden-ing and narrowing the arteries so that your heart has to work harder to pump blood. This condition, called arteriosclerosis, can result in insuffi-cient blood flow to the heart, leading to temporary chest pain called angina. Bits of plaque may break off and block an artery, causing a heart attack or stroke. High cholesterol levels, high blood pressure, and smoking exacerbate the condition.

The good news? Unless you suffer from heart disease, your ticker can serve you nearly as well in your sev-enties, eighties, or nineties as it did in your twenties.

Give Me Air Like your heart, your lungs can function normally until you are quite old. However, the lungs, chest wall, and diaphragm become less elastic, so you may not be able to take in as much oxygen as when you were younger. But you might not even notice this except when you exercise or travel to high altitudes.

 Slower Motion Digestion takes slightly longer as you get older, but otherwise it too remains largely unchanged. You will probably have a slight decrease in digestive enzymes, meaning that a few nutrients, especially vitamin B_{12} and vitamin C, won't be fully absorbed from food. Your liver will take longer to metabolize drugs and alcohol. That means you'll feel the effects of both sooner.

 Brain Drain After about the age of 30, your brain begins to lose neurons. And by the time you're 80, your brain weighs about 7 percent less than it did when you were 25. But there are only a few cognitive losses that can be attributed to aging. First, as the brain ages, the speed at which it processes information slows. Second, certain types of memory do decline—for instance, the ability to recall a name or word. None of this has to make any difference in your thinking and mental functioning or your ability to remain independent.

No Bones About It Until about age 30, we manufacture more bone than we lose. After age 40, we may lose about 1 percent of our bone mass per year. Women may lose as much as 20

The good news: Unless you have cardiovascular disease, your heart can serve you nearly as well in your eighties and nineties as it did in your twenties.

percent of their bone density in the five to seven years following the onset of menopause, dramatically increasing the risk of fractures. Though your bone mass decreases, you can stave off much of this loss with calcium, weight-bearing exercise, and, for women, hormone replacement therapy.

 Reproductive Realities The reproductive changes you'll experience with age are gradual and need not hamper your ability to enjoy sex. Sexually active older men continue to produce sexual hormones and sperm at about the same levels as they did when they were younger. They may experience problems with the prostate, which enlarges and presses against the urethra. Women have a pronounced drop in hormone levels resulting in menopause, which has significant health implications.

Are You Immune? Your thymus gland, which governs the production of T-cells—your body's main line of defense against infection and disease—shrinks as you age. The result? You're less able to fight off illness. Fortunately, modern medicine has eliminated or reduced the impact of many infectious diseases. And simple measures, such as taking certain vitamins and herbs and getting enough sleep, can actually *increase* your immunity.

Fast Fact

By age 55, your metabolism starts to downshift. You need, on average, 145 fewer calories per day than you did in your mid-thirties.

SELF **TEST**

Assessing Your Health Risks

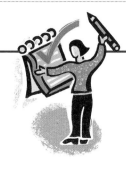

Ready to make your midlife and older years as vital as possible? Start by taking a good look at your health risks. See the box at right for instructions on how to calculate your overall health score.

◀**1.** What's your blood pressure?
  A 120-139/80 or under
  B 140-159/85
  C 160-170/90
  D 180/90 or over

◀**2.** What's your total cholesterol?
  A 4.2 to 5.2 mmol/L
  B 5.2 to 5.7 mmol/L
  C 5.7 to 6.2 mmol/L
  D 6.3 mmol/L or over

◀**3.** What's your HDL (good cholesterol)?
  A 1.2 mmol/L or over
  C 0.9 to 1.1 mmol/L
  D under 0.9 mmol/L

◀**4.** Have you had any of the following diseases?
  B Gingivitis or periodontitis
  C Diabetes
  C Heart disease
  C Osteoporosis
  D Diabetes with poor control
  D Heart disease with heart attack
  D Cancer
  D Stroke

◀**5.** Do you have a family history of diabetes, heart disease, stroke, hypertension, cancer, or osteoporosis?
  A None of the above
  B One of the above
  C Two or three of the above
  D Four or more of the above

◀**6.** How much weight have you gained since you were 18?
  A Less than 15 pounds
  B 16 to 25 pounds
  C 26 to 40 pounds
  D Over 40 pounds

◀**7.** Do you smoke?
  A No, or ex-smoker for 5 or more years
  C Exposed to passive smoke for an hour or more a day
  D Yes

◀**8.** Do you drink alcohol?
  A No, or up to 1 drink (women) or 2 drinks (men) a day
  D Yes, over 2 drinks a day

◀**9.** Do you use drugs?
  B Marijuana, occasionally
  C Marijuana, frequently
  D Cocaine or other hard drugs

◀**10.** What are your driving habits?
  A Always drive at or under speed limit
  B Often drive up to 15 miles above speed limit
  C Don't wear a seatbelt
  C Use a cell phone while driving
  D Often drive over 15 miles above the speed limit
  D Drive after drinking alcohol

◀**11.** How often do you exercise?
  A 5 or more times a week (for 30 minutes or more)
  B 3 to 4 times a week
  C 1 to 2 times a week
  D Never

◀**12.** How many of these food groups do you include in your daily diet?
  ● Whole grains (cereal, bread, pasta, rice)
  ● Fruits
  ● Meats/poultry/fish/beans and peas/nuts
  ● Vegetables
  ● Dairy products
  A 4 or more groups a day
  B 3 groups a day
  C 2 groups a day
  D Fewer than 2 groups a day

◀**13.** How often do you eat a healthy breakfast?
  A 5 or more days a week
  C 3 or 4 days a week
  D 2 or fewer days a week

◀**14.** How many fruits and vegetables do you eat?
  A 5 or more servings a day
  C 3 to 4 servings a day
  D 2 or fewer servings a day

◀**15.** How often do you eat red meat?
  A Once a week or less
  B 2 to 5 times a week
  C 6 to 7 times a week
  D Over 7 times a week

16. How often do you eat fish?

    A 2 or more times a week
    B Once a week
    D Once every two weeks or less

17. Do you regularly take vitamin and mineral supplements?

    Multivitamin
    A 1 a day
    B None

    Vitamin C
    A 160 mg or more a day
    D Under 160 mg a day

    Vitamin D
    A 600 to 800 IU a day
    B 400 IU a day
    D None

    Calcium
    A 1000 mg a day
    B 500 to 600 mg a day
    C 250 mg a day
    D None

18. Do you have a healthy emotional and social life?

    A You see friends or social groups 3 or more times a month.
    A You have a good sense of humor.
    B You see friends or social groups 1 or 2 times a month.
    C You tend to take things too seriously and worry a lot.
    D You're frequently depressed.
    D You see friends or social groups less than once a month.

19. What's your stress level?

    A You're not under any significant stress.
    C You have financial worries or other similar chronic stress.
    D You've had a major stressful event in your life (loss of job, death in the family, divorce, relocation, or major illness) in the past year.

20. What's your marital status?

    A Married
    C Single, divorced, or widowed

How to Read Your Report Card

Circle the appropriate answers, then determine your score by tallying the letters to the left of the boxes.

Mostly As: Congratulations! You're at lower risk for health problems than most people, so you have a head start on a healthier and longer life. Discover new ways to stay ahead of the aging process throughout this book.

Mostly Bs: Pat yourself on the back for doing better than a lot of people, but you could fall back into the pack if you're not proactive about your health.

Mostly Cs: You're probably aging the way most people do, which means you could easily develop problems if you don't take steps to become healthier. Don't worry, though: We'll give you plenty of help, and you may be surprised how easy it is.

Mostly Ds: You've got a long way to catch up with most of us. You're at high risk for health problems, so you'd better get moving. Be sure to take the advice in this book—it can make a big difference in your health.

Improve Your Grade!

Give yourself an extra A for each of the habits below that you practice. Does your overall score look a bit more optimistic now? That shows you what happens when you start taking even the smallest steps toward good health.

Do you...
- take an aspirin every day
- floss and brush your teeth daily
- eat several tomato products a week
- get a yearly flu shot
- have a fulfilling sex life
- get 7 to 8 hours of restful sleep a night
- practice yoga or meditation
- own a pet?

Have you...
- gotten your pneumococcal vaccine if you're 65 or older?

PART 1

YOUR GAME PLAN FOR GOOD HEALTH

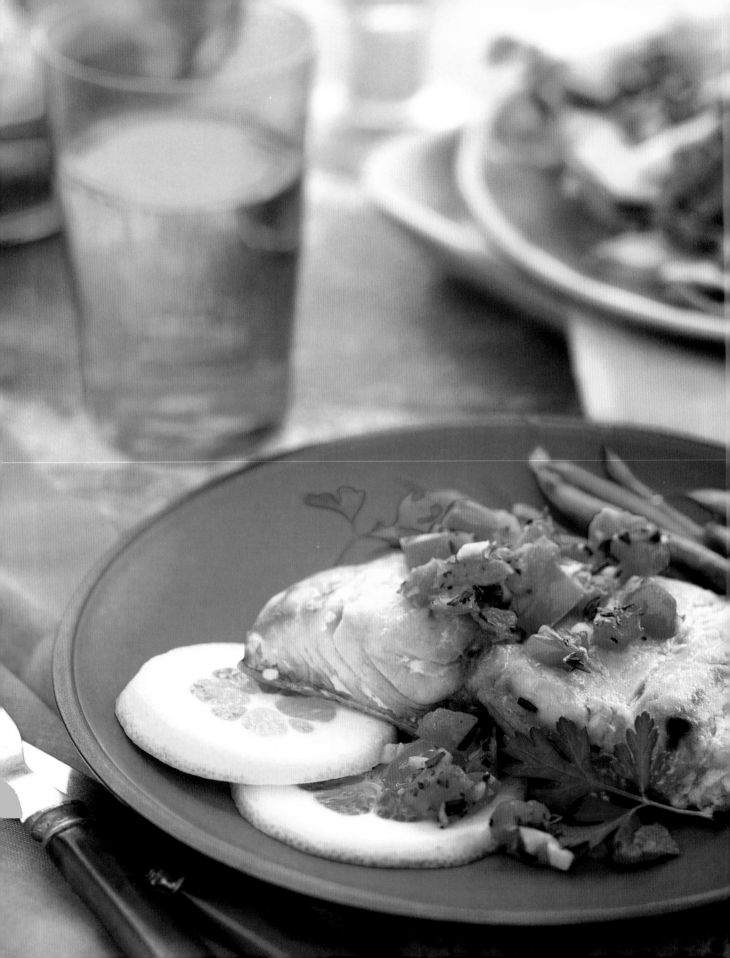

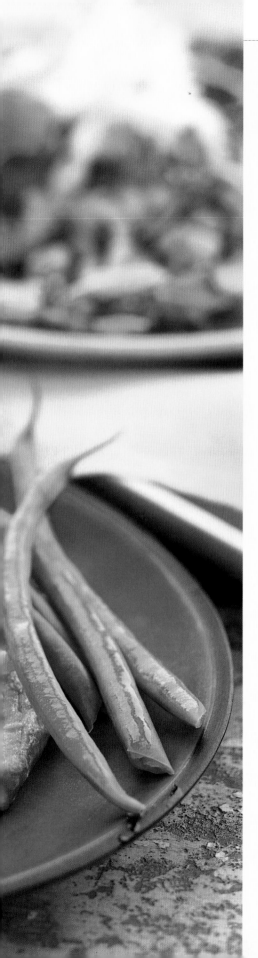

CHAPTER 1

EATING TO AGE WELL

What's a Healthy Diet?

Whoever said "eating well is the best revenge" was right in more ways than one. A healthy diet can help stave off aging and prevent the chronic illnesses to which humans are heir.

Eating is one of life's greatest pleasures. It's also a powerful way to enhance—or impair—your health. Over time, the food you eat affects your weight, cholesterol levels, blood pressure, insulin regulation, brain function, emotional health, and immune system. What you put on your plate, day after day, will play a major role, along with your genes, in determining whether you will live a long healthy life or succumb to a heart attack, a stroke, diabetes, or cancer.

Researchers at Georgia State University in Atlanta estimate that between one-third and one-half of the health problems experienced by older people are directly or indirectly related to nutrition. So use your fork to your advantage. Simply by making small changes such as eating fish at least once a week, adding an extra serving or two of vegetables to your daily diet, and changing your breakfast cereal, you'll go a long way toward giving your body what it needs to stay well.

Edible Medicine

Long before Ponce de Leon pounded the Florida Everglades in search of a fountain of youth, people have sought a diet that prevents disease and prolongs life. Today top scientific researchers are in on the act. Even Health Canada is involved. Here's what they've discovered so far about a healthy diet:

- It's rich in whole grains, fruits, and vegetables.
- It's low in saturated fat, which is found in fatty meats and full-fat dairy foods.
- It provides adequate but not excessive calories.

Canada's Food Guide to Healthy Eating is a graphic attempt to illustrate the proper balance of foods in a healthy diet. Grain products should form the cornerstone of your diet, along with fruits and vegetables, lower-fat dairy products and lean meat and alternatives round out the 4 food groups, with only the occasional serving of sugar and fat.

What's so wonderful about this approach to eating? It's associated with a lower risk for major illnesses, from heart disease to diabetes. Around the world, wherever researchers find people with low levels of chronic

---

A Pyramid for People over Age 70

Canada's Food Guide recommendations are based on, among other considerations, a person's age, sex, body size, and activity level. In Boston, USDA researchers have proposed a special Food Guide Pyramid for people over age 70, taking into account changes in nutritional needs. Here are the changes:

- **Water.** The bottom "tier" of the pyramid is 8 glasses of water. Why? Water is important for health at all ages. But as we age, thirst becomes a less reliable indicator of our body's need for liquid, so we need to remind ourselves to drink up.
- **Supplements.** At the top of the pyramid is a red flag, signaling supplements of calcium, vitamin D, and vitamin B_{12}. Does everyone need these supplements? Not necessarily, but there are good reasons to consider supplements or fortified foods at this stage of life. As we age, many of us lose the ability to absorb B_{12} from food, consume insufficient dietary calcium, and require more vitamin D.

disease, they discover the same eating pattern, often referred to as a "plant-based" diet.

There are variations on the theme, to be sure. The Mediterranean diet, with its emphasis on olive oil, is a richer diet than the Asian diet, in which the total fat level is quite low. But both patterns are replete with whole grains, fruits, and vegetables and very low in saturated fats. Dip-ping your ladle into these culinary traditions may not bring you eternal youth, but it's the best way to tip the odds in favor of a long, healthy life.

The Mediterranean Diet

For centuries, the people of the Mediterranean have been eating a joyful, flavorful diet—one that happens to protect them against the

Different People Need Different Amounts of Food

The amount of food you need every day from the 4 food groups and other foods depends on your age, body size, activity level, whether you are male or female and if you are pregnant or breast-feeding. That's why the Food Guide gives a lower and higher number of servings for each food group. For example, young children can choose the lower number of servings, while male teenagers can go to the higher number. Most other people can choose servings somewhere in between.

Grain Products
5–12 SERVINGS PER DAY

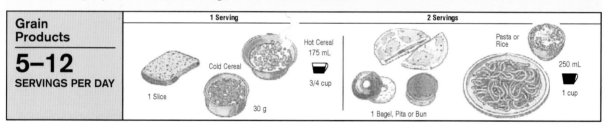

1 Serving — 1 Slice — Cold Cereal — 30 g — Hot Cereal 175 mL — 3/4 cup
2 Servings — 1 Bagel, Pita or Bun — Pasta or Rice — 250 mL — 1 cup

Vegetables and Fruit
5–10 SERVINGS PER DAY

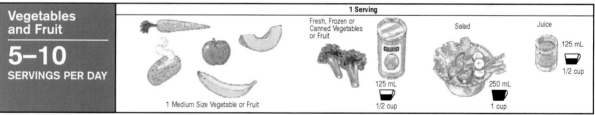

1 Serving — 1 Medium Size Vegetable or Fruit — Fresh, Frozen or Canned Vegetables or Fruit 125 mL 1/2 cup — Salad 250 mL 1 cup — Juice 125 mL 1/2 cup

Milk Products
SERVINGS PER DAY
Children 4–9 years: 2–3
Youth 10–16 years: 3–4
Adults: 2–4
Pregnant and Breast-feeding Women: 3–4

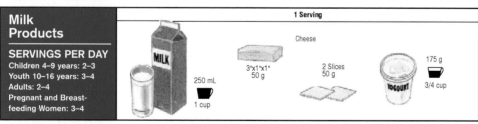

1 Serving — MILK 250 mL 1 cup — Cheese 3"x1"x1" 50 g — 2 Slices 50 g — 175 g YOGOURT 3/4 cup

Other Foods

Taste and enjoyment can also come from other foods and beverages that are not part of the 4 food groups. Some of these foods are higher in fat or calories, so use these foods in moderation.

Meat and Alternatives
2–3 SERVINGS PER DAY

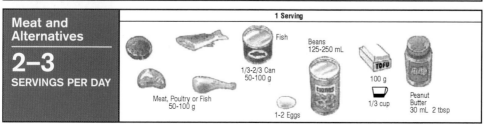

1 Serving — Meat, Poultry or Fish 50–100 g — Fish 1/3-2/3 Can 50–100 g — 1-2 Eggs — Beans 125–250 mL — TOFU 100 g 1/3 cup — Peanut Butter 30 mL 2 tbsp

© Minister of Public works and Government Services Canada,1997

In their own words

"There's a competition in scientific research between the Asian diet and the Mediterranean diet," says Harvard School of Public Health professor Frank Sacks, MD. "It's interesting to speculate about which one might come out a little ahead in terms of health. But that shouldn't distract us—both of these models are infinitely better than what we are eating now."

chronic diseases of modern times: heart disease, adult-onset diabetes, stroke, and colon and other cancers. In a recent Spanish study, men and women between 65 and 80 who followed the Mediterranean diet were 31 percent less likely to die over the next nine years, compared to those who did not.

The traditional diets of Greece, southern Italy, southern France, Spain, Portugal, and even Turkey and Israel are rich in bread, grains, beans, fish, vegetables, fruits, and olive oil, but they contain very little red meat, ice cream, or highly processed snack foods. The Mediterranean diet is not low in total fat. In fact, it's often as high in total fat as the usual North American diet. But the fat is mostly monounsaturated and comes mostly from olive oil, nuts, and fish—all "good" fats that don't promote heart disease, as saturated fats, like those in red meat, do.

New research finds that this dietary pattern is particularly

healthful for people who are at risk not only for heart disease, but also for type 2 diabetes. For them, a little more "good" fat is not only tasty but healthful.

As long as you don't overdo it and let the calories pile up, the Mediterranean diet—with grains, vegetables, beans, and fruits at the center of the plate and olive oil the primary source of fat—is healthy for everyone. Especially if you embrace another central feature of traditional Mediterranean life: plenty of physical activity!

The Asian Diet

Compared to rural China, death from heart disease in the United States, for example, is nearly 17 times more common in men and nearly 6 times more common in women. Researchers credit the traditional Asian diet, along with a more active lifestyle.

The traditional diets of China, Japan, and much of the rest of Asia are models of plant-based eating: rice or noodles at the center of the plate, a wide variety of fruits, greens, and other vegetables, and protein often in the cholesterol-lowering form of soy foods and heart-healthy fish. There is very little red meat or dairy, so saturated fats are generally low. (Calcium comes from calcium-rich vegetables and calcium-enriched soy foods).

Unlike the Mediterranean diet, the Asian diet is usually quite low in total fat. Because fat is high in calories, it's an eating pattern that's helpful if you're trying to keep your weight in check. As anyone who has delved into Asian cuisine knows, it's also a delicious way to eat. One caveat: Chinese restaurants in Canada often cater to our high-fat, meat-loving ways, so make it a point to order

Water, Water, Everywhere

Do you drink enough water? Everyone should strive to get 8 cups of liquid a day, and water is the best quencher. Drinking enough water greatly reduces your risk of developing kidney stones, even if you've already passed one or more. It may also reduce the risk of developing bladder cancer. Water helps regulate body temperature, too.

Is water itself the only source? Certainly not. Most fruits and vegetables are 80 to 95 percent water, so eat up. Fruit drinks also count, but steer clear of regular sodas, which have too much sugar. Even coffee and tea add to your total water intake, although they also act as diuretics, partially canceling out the benefits. Decaf tea and coffee are preferred over caffeinated.

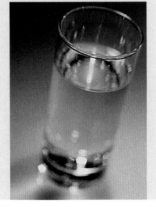

Changing Nutritional Needs

As our bodies change with age, so do our nutritional needs. Below are some of the nutrients we need more of. There are also some we need less of. For instance, we should limit sodium intake to 2,500 to 3,000 mg a day because our kidneys don't excrete the excess as efficiently. And we require less vitamin A because the body absorbs and stores this vitamin more readily, so limit supplement doses to 5,000 IU. We also need fewer calories due to a more sedentary lifestyle and a slower metabolism.

NUTRIENTS YOU NEED MORE OF	WHY	GOOD FOOD SOURCES
Calcium (For postmeno-pausal women and men over 65: 1,200 to 1,500 mg a day)	▪ Just as bone loss starts to speed up, our absorption of calcium from food starts to slow down.	▪ Dairy products, calcium-fortified juices and cereals, calcium-set tofu, dark-green leafy vegetables, sardines
Vitamin D (Ages 51-79: 400 IU a day; after age 80: 600 IU a day)	▪ As we get older, we're less able to produce vitamin D from sunlight. Also, lactose intolerance may cause us to decrease our intake of milk.	▪ Fortified milk and cereals, liver, eggs 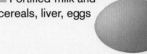
Vitamin E (15 mg or 22 IU a day)	▪ Cell damage from free radicals seems to escalate in later years. Vitamin E and other antioxidants may slow the process.	▪ Sunflower seeds, nuts (almonds, peanuts), vegetable oils, wheat germ, fortified cereals, avocados, mangoes
Vitamin C (Men: 90 mg a day; women: 75 mg a day. Add 35 mg if you smoke)	▪ See vitamin E, above. Vitamin C also helps maintain healthy connec-tive tissue.	▪ Citrus fruits and juices, potatoes, tomatoes, broccoli, dark-green leafy vegetables
Vitamin B_{12} (2.4 mcg a day)	▪ Our stomachs produce less acid, which helps digest B_{12}, important to mood, memory, immunity, and lower-ing high levels of the amino acid homocysteine, a risk factor for heart attack and stroke.	▪ Beef, pork, fish, milk, cheese, eggs. The synthetic form of vitamin B_{12} (found in fortified foods and in supplements) is better absorbed than that from food sources.
Folic acid (400 mcg a day)	▪ The vitamin helps counteract elevated homocysteine levels, which increase the risk of heart attack and stroke.	▪ Liver, beans, broccoli, dark-green leafy vegetables, cauliflower, oranges, orange juice. The form found in fortified foods and supple-ments is better absorbed than that from food sources.
Vitamin B_6 (Age 19-50: 1.3 mg a day; age 51+: 1.1 to 2 mg for women, 1.8 to 2 mg for men)	▪ See Folic acid, above. 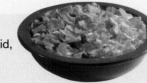	▪ Fortified cereals, liver, bananas, pork, chicken, fatty fish (salmon, tuna, mackerel), baked potatoes, canned chickpeas
Carotenoids such as beta-carotene, lutein, zeaxan-thin, lycopene (No RNI)	▪ Carotenoids are antioxidants with various anti-aging and disease-fighting properties.	▪ Cooked or canned tomatoes, dark-green leafy vegetables

SELF TEST

How Does Your Diet Rate?

This quiz will help you zero in on what you're doing right—and wrong—when it comes to eating for optimum health.

◀ **1.** How many servings of high-calcium foods do you eat per day? One serving consists of 8 oz of milk or calcium-fortified juice, ½ cup cooked greens (turnip, mustard, Swiss chard), ¾ cup yogurt, 2 oz cheese, 3 oz sardines, ½ cup tofu processed with calcium (check the label).
  A 3 to 4 servings or more
  B 1 to 2 servings
  C 0 to 1 serving

◀ **2.** When making sandwiches, the bread I most often use is:
  A 100 percent whole-wheat
  B Pumpernickel or rye
  C A hamburger or Kaiser roll

◀ **3.** What is the meat you eat most days of the week for dinner?
  A None, or skinless chicken or turkey breast
  B Top loin beef or pork
  C Ground beef

◀ **4.** How many servings of vegetables do you eat daily? One serving equals ½ cup cooked vegetables or 1 cup raw vegetables.
  A 4 or more servings
  B About 2 servings
  C 0 to 1 serving

◀ **5.** How many fruits do you eat daily? One serving equals one medium fresh fruit, ½ cup canned fruit, or 6 oz 100 percent fruit juice.
  A 4 or more servings
  B About 2 servings
  C 0 to 1 serving

◀ **6.** How many servings of alcohol do you drink daily? One serving equals 12 oz beer, 1 glass wine, 1 shot hard liquor.
  A 0 to 2 servings (men); 0 to 1 serving (women)
  C 3 or more servings (men); 2 or more servings (women)

◀ **7.** I eat beans or bean soups as my main meal for lunch or dinner:
  A 3 to 4 times a week
  B 1 to 2 times a week
  C Rarely or never

What's Your Score?

◀ **If you answered 7 to 10 questions "A":** Congratulations! You are eating a nutrition-savvy diet that will add years to your life.

◀ **If you answered 5 to 7 questions "A" and the rest mostly "B"s:** Not bad! Just a few additions here and a few subtractions there in your diet will bring you up to par.

◀ **If you answered 0 to 4 questions "A" and the rest "B"s and "C"s:** Your diet could use a makeover, but the fact that you are taking this quiz proves your interest in improving your eating habits. Keep reading to learn about foods that defy the aging process.

Answer Key

1. Each of these foods contains about 300 to 400 mg of calcium per serving. You need 3 to 4 servings daily to meet the new government recommendations of 1,200 mg of calcium for adults 51 years and older (under age 50, the daily requirement is 1,000 mg).

2. Only whole-wheat bread and other whole-grain breads are rich in fiber and whole grains. Most rye and pumpernickel breads are, like white breads, low in fiber.

3. Even lean red meat has three times more saturated fat than lean poultry.

4-5. Canada's Food Guide recommends 5 to 10 servings of fruits and vegetables a day. And this is supported by research and recommendations of the Canadian Cancer Society and the Heart and Stroke Foundation of Canada.

6. Moderate amounts of alcohol, particularly red wine, can have beneficial effects on the heart, especially for older people. A 5-oz glass of wine provides about a half ounce of pure alcohol, which raises levels of HDL ("good") cholesterol in the blood and reduces the likelihood of developing artery-clogging blood clots, which can lead to heart attack. Men who drink up to 2 alcoholic drinks a day have less heart disease than those who drink more or none at all. However, women at high risk for breast cancer should limit their intake to no more than

8. I eat fish for lunch or dinner:
   A 2 or more times a week
   B 2 to 3 times a month
   C Rarely or never

9. Check the following that apply to you:
   A I eat cookies, pastries, or other sweets no more than a few times a week, and I often have fruit for dessert instead.
   B I eat cookies, pastries, or other sweets in modest portions on many days of the week.
   C I often eat cookies, pastries, or other sweets.

10. I usually drink _____ with my meals and between meals.
   A water, skim milk, or fruit juice
   B tea, coffee, or diet soda
   C regular soda or sugary fruit drinks

three drinks per week. People who cannot control their alcohol consumption should not drink.

7. Beans and other legumes are low in fat, cholesterol free, rich in nutrients, and great sources of fiber and phytochemicals. Include beans in a main entree as an alternative to animal protein at least twice a week.

8. People who eat fish at least once a week are at substantially lower risk of developing heart disease.

9. Most Canadians eat too much sugar, adults included. It can crowd out more nutritious foods and add extra calories that go straight to your waist. And many sugary desserts and snacks are also rich in fat.

10. Water is so vital that it's considered an essential nutrient, even though it's calorie free and contains only trace amounts of minerals.

steamed dishes and extra vegetables, skip the deep-fried entrees, and put rice at the center of your plate. Better yet, cook in this style at home.

The New Dietary Guidelines

Canada's Food Guide is revised when scientific research shows that changes are needed. That is happening now. Canadian and American scientists have met to determine Dietary Reference Intakes (DRIs) which will ultimately replace our Canadian Recommended Nutrient Intakes (RNIs). In the meantime, it makes sense to consider these recent guidelines (in bold) recommended by experts:

● **Aim for a healthy weight.** As we age, we need fewer calories, and weight can creep up, increasing the risk of heart disease, diabetes, and other conditions. For weight-management tips, see Chapter 2.

● **Become physically active each day.** You can't separate eating (calories in) from activities (calories out).

● **Eat a variety of grains daily, especially whole grains.** People who eat at least three servings of whole grains daily are at lower risk of heart disease and diabetes.

● **Eat a variety of fruits and vegetables daily.** New research finds that eating a variety of high-fat or highly processed foods can lead to overeating. But eating a variety of fruits and vegetables actually helps people consume fewer calories.

● **Keep food safe to eat.** To avoid food-borne illness, discard old food, and keep hot foods hot and cold foods cold.

SimpleSolution

Does eating 5 to 10 servings of fruit and vegetables a day seem daunting? Just double or triple up. A "serving" of broccoli is a half cup, canned, fresh or frozen. Eat a cup and a half, you've already taken in three "servings." You can drink your fruits and vegetables, too. A ½ cup of fruit or vegetable juice counts as one "serving."

● **Choose a diet that is low in saturated fat and cholesterol and moderate in total fat.** Extremely low-fat diets are out; what matters most is cutting the amount of saturated fat you eat.

● **Choose beverages and foods that moderate your intake of sugars.** More and more of our calories are coming from sugar, especially in soft drinks. These provide no nutrition, just calories.

Pasta with Broccoli Rabe and Sun-Dried Tomatoes

Like regular broccoli, broccoli rabe is rich in antioxidant vitamins (beta-carotene and vitamin C) and a good source of fiber. You can substitute broccoli for the rabe. Cut the broccoli tops into small florets, peel the stems, and cut them into 1-inch pieces.

Makes 4 servings.

- ½ cup sun-dried tomatoes
- 1 large bunch of broccoli rabe (1¼ pounds), cut into 1-inch pieces
- 8 ounces fusilli pasta
- 1 tablespoon olive oil
- 4 cloves garlic, minced

- 1 to 1½ teaspoons crushed red pepper flakes
- 2 tablespoons no-salt-added tomato paste
- ¾ teaspoon salt
- ¼ teaspoon black pepper
- ⅓ cup golden raisins (optional)
- ⅓ cup grated Parmesan cheese

1. In a large pot of boiling water, cook the dried tomatoes for 5 minutes or until softened. Remove with a slotted spoon and set aside. When cool enough to handle, coarsely chop.

2. Add the broccoli rabe to the boiling water and cook for 4 minutes or until tender-crisp. With a slotted spoon, transfer to a colander.

3. Add the pasta to the boiling water and cook according to package directions. Reserving 1½ cups of the cooking water, drain the pasta and transfer to a large serving bowl.

4. Meanwhile, in a large skillet, heat the oil over low heat. Add the garlic and pepper flakes and sauté for 3 minutes. Add the tomatoes, rabe, tomato paste, salt, black pepper, and reserved cooking water. Cook, stirring, for 4 minutes or until the rabe is tender. Add to the hot pasta along with the raisins and Parmesan cheese, tossing well.

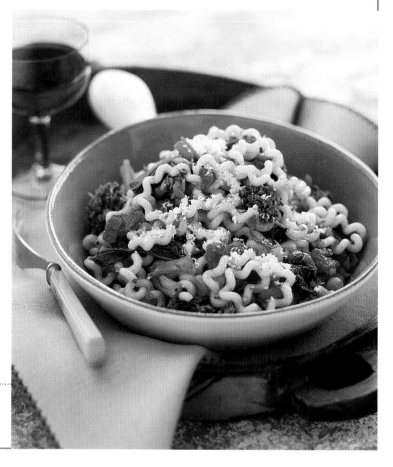

NUTRITION INFORMATION *Per Serving:* 339 calories, 16 g protein, 56 g carbohydrate, 9 g fiber, 6 g fat, 2 g saturated fat, 5 mg cholesterol, 580 mg sodium

Sweet and Sour Tofu with Vegetables

Soy protein can help lower elevated cholesterol levels. Serve this dish over brown rice or noodles, with a cool cucumber salad on the side.

Makes 4 servings.

2   tablespoons soy sauce
2   tablespoons fresh lime juice (1 large lime)
1/4   cup hot water
2   teaspoons sugar
4   green onions, thinly sliced (1/2 cup)
1/2   pound Napa cabbage, coarsely chopped
      (half a head, 4 cups chopped)
1   medium-size zucchini, trimmed, halved
      lengthwise, and sliced crosswise 1/4 inch thick
      (1 1/2 cups)
1   sweet red pepper, cored, seeded, and diced
      (1 cup)
1   can (16 ounces) pineapple cubes in juice,
      drained
12   ounces firm tofu, cut into 3/4-inch squares
1   tablespoon finely chopped fresh ginger
1/4   teaspoon salt
1/8   teaspoon ground red pepper (cayenne)

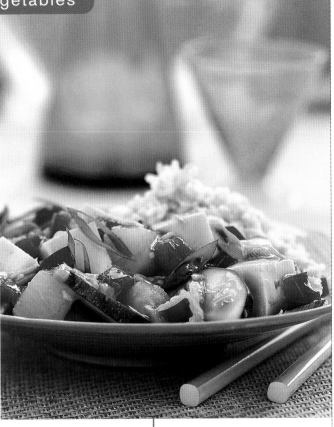

1. In a large saucepan, combine the soy sauce, lime juice, hot water, and sugar. Bring to a boil. Add green onions, cabbage, zucchini, and red pepper. Simmer, covered, for 4 minutes or until the vegetables are almost tender.

2. Add the pineapple, tofu, ginger, salt, and cayenne pepper. Cover and simmer, gently stirring from time to time, until heated through, about 3 minutes. Serve warm or at room temperature.

NUTRITION INFORMATION *Per Serving:* 164 calories, 11 g protein, 23 g carbohydrate, 5 g fiber, 4 g fat, 1 g saturated fat, 0 mg cholesterol, 681 mg sodium

● **Choose and prepare foods with less salt.** Reducing sodium, along with eating more fruits and vegetables and low-fat dairy foods, is a good way to control blood pressure. Losing weight is another.

● **If you drink alcoholic beverages, do so in moderation.** "Moderation" means up to one drink a day for a woman, two for a man.

Alcohol raises levels of beneficial HDL cholesterol, which carries LDL, or "bad" cholesterol, out of the body. It also inhibits the formation of blood clots that can cause heart attack and stroke. Red wine may have extra benefits. Its dark-red pigments are rich in antioxidants that prevent the oxidation of LDL, making it less likely to stick to artery walls.

The Skinny on Fat

Contrary to popular belief, not all fat is bad for you. In fact, certain types of fat even help your heart.

Should you eat a low-fat diet, one moderate in fat, or even one high in fat? Here's an emerging truth from the cutting edge of nutrition: It doesn't really matter, as long as you choose the right kinds of fats and control calories.

The "Bad" Fats

The fats to avoid are saturated fats, found in red meat, butter, cream, full-fat dairy products, lard, and tropical oils (palm, palm kernel, and coconut). Saturated fat raises artery-clogging LDL cholesterol, which increases your risk of heart disease. It has also been associated with lung, colon, and prostate cancer.

There is another kind of bad-guy fat, one that lurks in an overwhelming number of processed foods. It's called a trans fat, an artificially hardened vegetable oil also known as partially hydrogenated oil, and it's just as bad for your heart as saturated fat. Trans fats are found in stick margarine, vegetable shortening, fried fast foods, and virtually all crackers, cookies, chips, and baked goods as well as other processed foods.

The "Good" Fats

While saturated fats and trans fats increase heart disease risk, unsaturated fats actually lower it by reducing LDL ("bad") cholesterol. The best type, called monounsaturated fat, is plentiful in olive oil, canola oil, nuts, seeds, and avocados. Highly polyunsaturated fats, such as those in corn and safflower oil, also lower cholesterol, but excessive amounts may increase cancer risk, so use them in moderation. Another "good" fat is found in fatty ocean fish. Called omega-3 fatty acids, these protect against heart disease and may also offer some protection against certain cancers. Researchers estimate that switching just 5 percent of your calories from saturated to unsaturated fats may decrease the risk of a fatal heart attack by as much as 42 percent.

Olive oil: 14%, 9%, 77%
Canola oil: 6%, 36%, 58%
Corn oil: 13%, 62%, 25%
Sunflower oil: 11%, 69%, 20%
Safflower oil: 9%, 78%, 13%

Saturated fat   Polyunsaturated fat   Monounsaturated fat

Choosing a Cooking Oil All vegetable oils aren't created equal. Olive and canola oil have a high percentage of heart-healthy monounsaturated fat and should be your first choice in cooking and baking. Corn, sunflower, and safflower oils are higher in polyunsaturated fats, which are less stable and more likely to produce harmful free radicals.

Quick Chocolate Cake with Raspberries

Who says dessert has to be sinful to taste terrific? This mouth-watering treat has only 2 grams of fat per serving.

Makes 9 servings.

1½ cups all-purpose flour
½ cup unsweetened cocoa powder
1 teaspoon baking powder
½ teaspoon baking soda
½ teaspoon salt
1¼ cups sugar
½ cup unsweetened applesauce
1 egg or 2 egg whites
1 cup skim milk or water
2 teaspoons vanilla extract
¼ cup seedless raspberry jam
  Confectioners' sugar
1 pint fresh raspberries

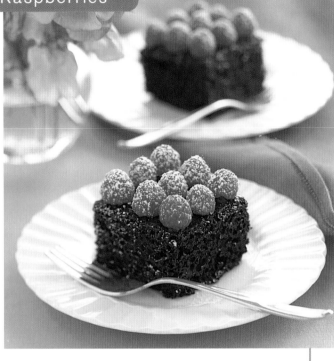

1. Preheat the oven to 350° F. Lightly spray an 8 x 8 x 2-inch baking pan with nonstick cooking spray. Dust with cocoa powder.

2. In a medium-size bowl, whisk together the flour, cocoa powder, baking powder, baking soda, and salt.

3. In a large bowl, using an electric mixer on low speed, beat together the sugar, applesauce, and egg until smooth. Beat in the milk and vanilla until blended. Add the flour mixture and beat until blended. Turn the batter into the prepared pan.

4. Bake for 40 to 45 minutes, or until a pick inserted in the center comes out clean. Cool in the pan on a wire rack for 10 minutes. Turn the cake out onto the rack or a serving plate to cool completely.

5. To serve, melt the jam in a saucepan over low heat. Brush over the top of the cooled cake. Top with raspberries and dust with confectioners' sugar.

NUTRITION INFORMATION *Per Serving:* 256 calories, 5 g protein, 58 g carbohydrate, 4 g fiber, 2 g fat, 1 g saturated fat, 24 mg cholesterol, 268 mg sodium

Easy Ways to Trim the Fat

In Cooking
- Remove poultry skin.
- Roast, bake, broil, or stew meats instead of frying them.
- Use nonstick pans to eliminate the need for cooking oil.
- Buy a defatting cup to skim the fat from stocks and gravies, or refrigerate them and skim the fat after it rises to the surface and hardens.
- Use pureed potatoes instead of cream to add body and richness to "cream" soups.

In Baking
- Instead of one whole egg, use two egg whites.
- Reduce the oil in recipes by one third, or replace up to half of it with yogurt or applesauce.
- Try reduced-fat cream cheese or ricotta cheese instead of the full-fat varieties.
- In place of cream, use evaporated skim milk.

Your Energy Foods

Carbohydrates have gotten a bad rap in recent years, but in fact, they form the cornerstone of a healthy diet.

Carbohydrates are the building blocks of a healthy diet. They fuel the body, which turns them into the basic currency of energy: glucose, or blood sugar. If you restrict your intake of carbohydrates, your body will turn part of the protein and a little of the fat you eat into blood sugar—in effect converting them into carbohydrates through a complicated, wasteful process. It's much more efficient and healthful to give your body the right amount of carbohydrates in the first place. Not too much, of course—too many calories from carbohydrates, like too many calories from fat or protein, can lead to weight gain. It's especially easy to overeat carbohydrate-based snacks like cookies and crackers.

So choose quality food sources. Whole-grain breads, brown rice, and cereals still have the nutritious germ and fiber-rich outer layers intact.

Whole starchy vegetables like potatoes, corn, and beans are rich in nutrients and fiber and low in sugar. Shoot for three servings of whole grain foods each day to lower the risk of heart disease and diabetes. Harvard University researchers report that a woman age 55 to 69 who eats whole grains three times a day is 30 percent less likely to have a heart attack over the next 10 years.

No one is yet sure how whole grains protect us, but we do know they're better for us than refined grains, such as white bread, which are stripped of most of their beneficial fiber as well as vitamin E, folate, B_6 and other essential vitamins that become especially important as we age. A diet low in complex carbohydrates and high in refined grains (such as white bread, white rice, pasta, and sugar) increases your risk of developing diabetes.

A few tips for adding more fiber-rich whole-grain carbohydrates to your diet:

- Read labels carefully. Make sure "whole-wheat" or "whole-grain" flours are the first or second ingredient. (Even in some wheat breads, it isn't.)
- Try replacing one-third of the white flour with whole-wheat flour in homemade pancakes and baked goods.
- Give wheat germ a whirl. It's crunchy and nutty and has all the nutritional advantages (vitamin E and other vitamins, minerals, and fiber) missing in refined bread. Add a tablespoon to breakfast

Fiber-rich whole-grain breads and cereals offer protection against heart disease and diabetes.

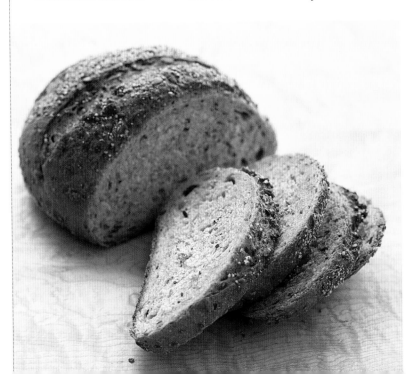

Fruity Tabbouleh

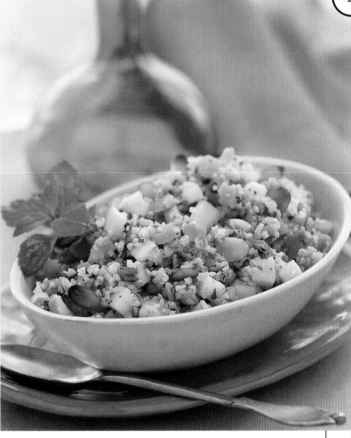

One serving provides 10 grams of fiber and a healthy dose of vitamin C (supplied by the apricots) and vitamin E (from the almonds).

Makes 4 servings.

- 1 cup coarse bulgur (cracked wheat)
- 1/2 teaspoon salt
- 2 1/2 cups boiling water
- 1 apple, cut into small dice
- 1 tablespoon fresh lemon juice
- 1/2 cup sliced almonds, lightly toasted
- 1/2 cup dried apricot halves, cut into fine bits
- 2 green onions, very finely chopped (1/4 cup)
- 1 tablespoon chopped fresh parsley
- 1 tablespoon chopped fresh mint
- 1 tablespoon canola oil or light olive oil

1. Place the bulgur in a medium bowl. Stir in the salt. Cover with boiling water and set aside for 1 hour.

2. Meanwhile, in a large bowl, toss the apples in the lemon juice until well coated. Add the almonds, apricots, and onions. Mix the parsley and mint, and stir in, along with the oil.

3. Drain the soaked wheat if necessary. Toss and gently stir into the fruit mixture. Refrigerate for at least 1 hour or overnight. Serve chilled.

NUTRITION INFORMATION *Per Serving:* 283 calories, 8 g protein, 45 g carbohydrate, 10 g fiber, 10 g fat, 1 g saturated fat, 0 mg cholesterol, 302 mg sodium

cereals, quick breads, muffins, pancakes, and yogurt.
- Opt for brown rice now and then, and enjoy its rich nutty flavor.
- A baked potato, topped with low-fat cheese, yogurt, or sour cream, or even a teaspoon of butter or margarine, is nutritious and fiber-rich. So are sweet potatoes, which are loaded with beta-carotene.
- Beans, lentils, and peas are rich in protein, making them excellent meat substitutes, and high in fiber. Rinse canned beans thoroughly (soak dried beans) to reduce the gas factor and the salt;

dry lentils don't need presoaking.
- No need to thaw frozen peas (good sources of fiber). Just separate them under cold running water and toss into simmering soups and stews a few minutes before serving.

Focus on Fiber

Fiber is the part of carbohydrates that our bodies don't readily digest, yet it's essential to health. Fiber is in all whole-plant-based foods: whole grains, vegetables, fruits, beans, nuts, and seeds. Animal products (meat, poultry, fish, dairy) have none.

SELF TEST

How Much Fiber Do You Eat?

◄ **1.** What fruits do you eat most days of the week?
   A Apples, oranges, bananas, or berries
   B Grapes or watermelon
   C Orange juice or other juice

◄ **2.** What are you most likely to eat for breakfast?
   A Whole-grain cereal or oatmeal with milk
   B A bagel with cream cheese
   C A doughnut or muffin

◄ **3.** Which category of vegetables do you eat from most often each week?
   A Peas, carrots, broccoli, dark leafy greens

   B Lettuce and tomatoes
   C French fries

◄ **4.** I eat at least one ½ cup serving of beans (black, kidney, garbanzo) in a main dish, soup, or salad:
   A Once a day
   B 2 to 3 times a week
   C 1 to 2 times a month

◄ **5.** The type of bread I eat most days of the week is:
   A 100 percent whole-wheat or 7-grain bread
   B Pumpernickel or rye
   C White, Italian, or French

What's Your Score?

◄ If you answered 4 or 5 questions "A": Great job! You're reducing your risk of heart disease, diabetes, and bowel problems by eating plenty of fiber.

   ◄ If you answered 3 questions "A" and the rest mostly "B": Good, but you can do better—and gain valuable health protection.

   ◄ If you answered 1 or 2 questions "A" and the rest "B" and "C": Time to get on track. Begin by changing just one habit. Switch to a whole-grain cereal, or make your sandwich on whole-wheat bread instead of white.

Answer Key

1. Berries are rich in fiber per 1 cup serving (raspberries, 8 grams; blueberries, 4 grams). Apples, bananas, and oranges contain about 3 grams of fiber each; grapes and watermelon have only 1 gram of fiber per cup; and fruit juice (even with pulp) has virtually none.

2. Whole-grain cereal, whether hot or cold, is the best way to start your morning, with anywhere from 3 to 10 grams of fiber per serving. A 3½-inch bagel contains 2 to 3 grams, while a doughnut contains less than 1 gram (and of course, plenty of sugar and fat).

3. Peas, broccoli, and greens are among the highest-fiber vegetables, with about 3 to 4 grams per serving. Lettuce and tomatoes have less. Eat a wide variety of both high- and lower-fiber vegetables, since all are stocked with vitamins, minerals, and phytochemicals. French fries, however, are mostly fat, with plenty of calories.

4. Beans are loaded with fiber, containing about 7 grams per ½ cup serving.

5. Look for breads labeled "100 percent whole wheat" or "whole grain," both fiber-rich. Color is not a reliable indicator since some dark breads contain added coloring. Reading the food label is your best bet.

There are two types of fiber. Soluble fiber—found in beans, lentils, apples, pears, and oats—helps stabilize blood sugar and lower cholesterol levels. Insoluble fiber—found in many grains, cereals, seeds, and vegetables—improves bowel health by speeding food through the colon.

Until recently, it was believed that a high-fiber diet helped prevent colon cancer, but recent studies have not confirmed the effect. However, other benefits are proven: prevention of constipation, prevention and treatment of diverticulitis (a painful inflammation of small pouches along the colon wall), reduction of blood cholesterol, improved control of blood sugar, and reduced risk of heart disease and diabetes. A few words of advice:

- Increase fiber intake gradually, over several weeks, working up to 25 to 35 grams a day. Drink plenty of water, or the extra bulk provided by the fiber may slow or block bowel function.
- Skip the fiber supplements. If you increase your intake of high-fiber fruits and vegetables, you won't need to take supplements.
- If you must take a supplement for regularity, consider psyllium, available in drugstores. A heaping tablespoon daily (about 10 grams) lowers high blood cholesterol by about 5 percent as it helps you become more regular.

The Sweets Story

Canadians love sugar, a simple carbohydrate. We consume about 10 to 15 percent of total calories from added sugars. However, many experts recommend a limit of only 6 to 10 percent.

Is sugar bad for you? While there's nothing toxic about it, it adds calories without vitamins or minerals. Sugary foods also may elevate triglyceride levels, blood fats that increase the risk of heart disease. While sugar itself doesn't cause diabetes, a diet high in sugar and refined grains and low in fiber-rich whole grains may increase your risk of adult-onset diabetes. And of course, sugar, especially the sugar in sticky foods, promotes cavities. Worst of all, sugary foods add extra calories, making weight control much harder. They also crowd out more nutritious foods from your diet.

Sugar is everywhere. It's in many processed foods—even in ketchup, soups, and salad dressings. So moderating your intake requires a conscious effort. Here are some ways to begin.

- Limit nondiet soft drinks (they account for one-third of the added sugar in our diets), sweetened fruit punch and iced tea, and lemonade.
- On packaged food labels, look for hidden sugars: brown sugar, corn sweetener, corn syrup, fructose, fruit juice concentrate, glucose (dextrose), high-fructose corn syrup, honey, invert sugar, lactose, maltose, molasses, raw sugar, table sugar (sucrose), and syrup. If one is listed as the first or second ingredient, or if several are listed, that food is high in added sugar.
- Cut sugary fruit juices with water or seltzer. Unlike fruit juice, whole fruit has fiber in addition to natural sugars, so it doesn't raise your blood sugar as much.
- Watch out for "low-fat" foods that are high in sugar and calories.
- Use less sugar in coffee or tea.

Is Protein a Priority?

Everyone needs protein, but not much. Requirements for protein vary according to age, weight, and health. In an ideal balanced diet, only 10 to 12 percent of daily calories should come from protein.

So choose the most nutritious protein sources, including beans, lentils, peas, soy foods, fish, shellfish, lean poultry, and very lean cuts of beef or pork. You'll get fiber from the plant protein in the legumes and soy, heart-healthy omega-3 fats from the fish and seafood, and good quality protein from lean poultry and red meat without much artery-clogging saturated fat. Low-fat and fat-free dairy foods and egg whites are also excellent protein sources.

Produce Power

Mom was right when she told you to eat your vegetables. Filling your plate with produce is one of the best ways to prevent cancer and other diseases.

Even a Martian dropped on Earth for one day would probably hear that it's a good idea to eat more fruits and vegetables. The reasons mount as you get older. Produce is not only nutritious—a rich source of vitamin C, beta-carotene, folate, potassium, magnesium, and fiber, with little or no fat or sodium and few calories—but also a unique source of some powerful phytochemicals that protect you from disease. Here are some of its benefits.

- **Weight.** Eating more produce is a key weight-management strategy. Fruits and vegetables are low in calories and high in fiber and water, both of which are filling. Researchers at Tufts University found that the greater the variety of vegetables that people eat, the thinner they are.

- **Heart Disease.** Fruits and vegetables are rich in fiber, potassium, folic acid, and antioxidants—all of which protect against heart disease. In population studies around the world, people who eat the most fruits and vegetables are between 15 and 40 percent less likely to develop heart disease, compared with people who eat the least produce.

- **Blood Pressure.** One effective way to lower high blood pressure is to eat 8 to 10 small servings of fruits and vegetables a day, along with at least 3 low-fat dairy servings. The effect is as pronounced as that achieved by many blood-pressure-lowering drugs. And eating this way often leads to weight loss, which may also help reduce blood pressure.

- **Cancer Protection.** People who eat five or more servings a day of fruits and vegetables are only half as likely to die from cancer as those who eat one serving or none. Certain types of produce may provide even greater protection. In population surveys, the vegetables most associated with a lower risk of cancer include onions, garlic, carrots, green vegetables, tomatoes (especially cooked tomatoes), and cruciferous vegetables (vegetables in the cabbage family) including

Antioxidant Superstars

Deeply colored fruits and vegetables are rich in antioxidants, which help protect against chronic illness and may even slow down the aging process. Antioxidants are positively charged molecules that combine with negatively charged free radicals, making them harmless. The USDA Human Nutrition Research Center on Aging at Tufts University recently measured the antioxidant potential of fresh fruits and vegetables, scoring each for its "oxygen radical absorbance capacity," or ORAC. The higher the number, the greater its ability to neutralize free radicals. The ORAC scores are based on a serving size of 3.5 ounces. Here are the top 14 scorers.

FRUITS		VEGETABLES	
Blueberries	2400	Kale	1770
Strawberries	1540	Spinach	1260
Raspberries	1220	Brussels sprouts	980
Plums	949	Broccoli florets	890
Oranges	750	Beets	840
Red grapes	739	Red bell peppers	710
Cherries	670	Yellow corn	400

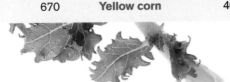

Cherry-Berry Yogurt Muffins

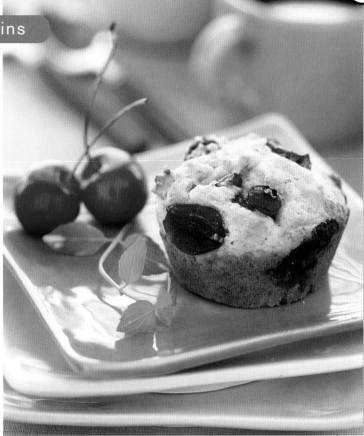

Fight those free radicals with these delicious muffins, chock-full of antioxidant-rich cherries and blueberries and wheat germ for a dose of fiber and vitamin E.

Makes 1 dozen muffins.

$1\frac{1}{2}$ cups all-purpose flour
$\frac{1}{2}$ cup toasted wheat germ
1 tablespoon baking powder
$\frac{3}{4}$ teaspoon salt
$\frac{1}{2}$ teaspoon baking soda
1 cup low-fat plain yogurt
1 egg or 2 egg whites
3 tablespoons canola oil or light olive oil
$\frac{1}{2}$ cup sugar
1 cup fresh or frozen cherries, coarsely chopped and drained
$\frac{1}{2}$ cup fresh or frozen blueberries

1. Preheat the oven to 400° F. Lightly coat 12 muffin cups with nonstick cooking spray or line with paper liners.

2. In a large bowl, whisk together the dry ingredients. Set aside.

3. In a small bowl, whisk together the yogurt, egg, oil, and sugar. Stir into the flour mixture just until blended. Gently stir in the cherries and blueberries. Divide the batter evenly among the muffin cups.

4. Bake for 20 minutes or until golden brown and a pick inserted in the center of a muffin comes out clean. Cool the muffins in the pan for 5 minutes, then turn muffins out onto a wire rack for 15 minutes. Serve warm.

NUTRITION INFORMATION *Per Muffin:* 168 calories, 5 g protein, 27 g carbohydrate, 1 g fiber, 5 g fat, 1 g saturated fat, 19 mg cholesterol, 313 mg sodium

---

broccoli, cabbage, kale, Brussels sprouts, bok choy, and cauliflower. One study found that men who ate three or more servings of cruciferous vegetables a week had a 41 percent lower risk of prostate cancer than men who ate less than one serving per week.

● **Longevity.** Fruit lovers have an added advantage: A recent Swedish study of men age 54 to 80 found that those who ate the most servings of fruit lived longest.

Filling Your Plate

It's not hard to add more fruits and vegetables to your diet. Just stock up on fresh or frozen produce (there's a greater variety of frozen produce available now than ever before) on your next trip to the supermarket, then try these suggestions.

Ways to eat more vegetables
● In the winter, soup up your soup with extra frozen vegetables straight from the freezer.

WARNING

Fresh fruits and vegetables can carry microorganisms that cause illness. Wash produce thoroughly in cold running water—especially fruits and vegetables like lettuce and berries that will be eaten raw. When buying fruit juice, make sure it's pasteurized.

Nutrition Note

Fruits rich in vitamin C include apricots, cantaloupe, grapefruit, honeydew melon, kiwis, mangos, oranges, pineapple, plums, strawberries, tangerines, and watermelon.

- In the summer, toss your salad with snow peas and sugar snap peas for crunch and color. Cook them briefly first, then refresh them under cold running water.
- Salsa, anyone? It's a great dance— and an easy, nutritious topping for broiled chicken or fish.
- No time to wash salad greens? Supermarkets stock a variety of pre-cleaned, ready-to-eat salads. Studies have found that these pre-washed greens are cleaner than you'd probably get them if you washed them yourself.

- Make pasta with vegetables, using one part pasta to two parts veggies.

Ways to Eat More Fruits

- Put fruit in a big, attractive bowl on your kitchen counter or on the top shelf of your fridge. Research shows that when fruit is most visible, it's more likely to be eaten.
- Cereal and yogurt are lonely without fruit: Slice in half an apple or banana, or add some fresh berries or dried cranberries.
- Skip that candy bar and snack on mixed dried fruit (raisins, apri-

Crab, Corn, and Avocado Salad

Avocado provides heart-healthy monounsaturated fat, crab is a good source of protein, and watercress may help fight cancer.

Makes 4 servings.

- 1   **can (15.25 ounces) corn kernels, drained**
- 2   **tablespoons salsa**
- 1   **green onion, finely chopped (2 tablespoons)**
- 1   **bunch watercress, trimmed**
- 1   **avocado, halved, peeled, pitted, and sliced**
- 1   **tablespoon fresh lemon juice**
- 8   **ounces (about 2 cups) cooked lump crabmeat**
- 2   **tablespoons finely chopped cilantro (coriander)**
- 40 **baked tortilla chips**

1. In a small bowl, combine the corn, salsa, and green onion; set aside. On four salad plates arrange the watercress. Top with avocado slices. Sprinkle with lemon juice.

2. Add the corn mixture and crabmeat to the plates. Sprinkle evenly with cilantro. Place the chips to the side of the plates and serve.

NUTRITION INFORMATION *Per Serving:* 298 calories, 17 g protein, 39 g carbohydrate, 6 g fiber, 10 g fat, 1 g saturated fat, 57 mg cholesterol, 493 mg sodium

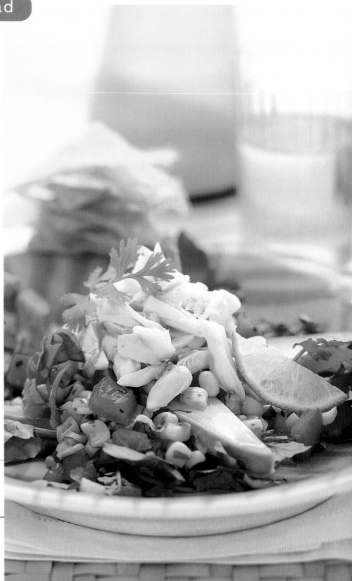

SELF TEST

What Color Is Your Diet?

◀ **1.** You're sitting down to your usual morning meal. What natural hues can you find in your breakfast foods?
   A Red, yellow, or orange, and brown
   B Tan and white

◀ **2.** You just stopped by the salad bar for lunch. If you described your salad plate like an artist's palette, what would it most look like?
   A Green on the edges, with dapples of red, orange, and more green speckled throughout the plate
   B Varying shades of green
   C Green around the edges with white blotches in the middle

◀ **3.** How often do you eat snacks containing bright neon colors (orange, red, blue) that leave a stain on your mouth or fingers?
   A Rarely
   B Once a week
   C Once a day

◀ **4.** Look into the produce drawer in your refrigerator. How many different colors do you count?
   A 4 or more
   B 3
   C 1 or 2

◀ **5.** Take a close look at your next dinner plate. How many different colors do you see?
   A 4 or more
   B 3
   C 1 or 2

What's Your Score?

◀ Mostly "A"s: Excellent! Your diet is chock-full of health-protective plant chemicals.

◀ Mostly "B"s: Pretty good. You're probably eating the same two or three fruits and vegetables every week. Be more adventurous. Try one new fruit or vegetable each week.

◀ Mostly "C"s: Don't feel bad. Most people fit into this category. Linger in the produce aisle and discover what you've been missing!

Answer Key

1. Typical breakfast fare—toast, English muffins, pancakes, waffles—is starchy and white or tan in color. Fruits add naturally vibrant colors to your breakfast meal. Add strawberries, blueberries, or kiwi to your cereal or yogurt instead of the usual banana and get an extra boost of fiber and nutrients.

2. A salad bar can be a nutrition gold mine—or a land mine. There's nothing wrong with selecting just salad greens (B), but you miss out on many different flavors, textures, and nutrients. If you lean toward the white stuff loaded with mayonnaise (C)—macaroni, potato, and egg salad—you end up with loads of fat and calories. Yet salad bars offer an extensive variety of veggies that you probably wouldn't keep in your fridge. So take advantage and load your plate with at least five different vegetables.

3. Snack foods doused in bright added coloring (e.g., cheese puffs, "fruit" drinks, many candies) are usually highly processed and high in sugar and/or fat. Try deeply colored fruit like fresh blueberries instead.

4. It's a natural wonder that fruits and vegetables are imbued with beautiful colors. They need all the help they can get because although they are among the most nutritious foods around, they take a backseat in the typical Canadian diet. Make up your mind to eat at least four different fruits and vegetables each week.

5. A typical dinner of chicken, mashed potatoes, corn, and bread can get pretty monotonous—in color and in nutrients. The more color in your meal, the greater the variety of nutrients you are eating. Aim for at least four different colors in your next dinner.

cots, cherries, prunes) instead. Don't overdo it, though, since dried fruit is high in calories.

● Start a blender habit: Fruit smoothies are quick and delicious.

● Bring back the melon appetizer before dinner. It's a lovely first course.

● Opt for fruit-based desserts, such as cobblers or baked apples.

Nine Superstar Foods

Want to fight disease with your fork? Make sure your diet includes these nine foods, all of which have been found to have special health-enhancing power.

Eating to age well means more than eating nutrient-rich foods without excess calories. Certain foods contain specific compounds that just might convince Father Time to slow down a bit. Scientists call these unique compounds phyto-chemicals, a technical word for plant chemicals. They are a big reason why fruits and vegetables are so good for your health.

1 **Soy.** If you haven't yet discovered soy, now's the time. Like all beans, soybeans are rich in minerals (including iron) and trace elements. Many soy foods, including most tofu and soy milk, are processed with or enhanced with calcium, which is vital to both men and women as they age. Soy is also an excellent source of protein, important if you're cutting back on meat.

But what really sets soy apart is that it contains plant estrogens called isoflavones, which seem to offer unique health-protective properties. For instance, they may guard against osteoporosis by building bone, and some studies suggest they may help reduce hot flashes. They also are being investigated for their potential to protect against certain cancers.

Soy effectively lowers high cholesterol levels. According to a health claim approved by the United States FDA, 25 grams of soy protein can usually lower your total cholesterol by 5 to 10 percent. You can get that much in 12 ounces of tofu, 1 quart of soy milk, 4 ounces of edamame (baby soybeans, pronounced eh da MOM

ay), or four heaping tablespoons of soy protein isolate powder.

Here's how to get started:

- Pour soy milk (made from crushed, cooked soybeans) on your favorite cereal. (Look for a calcium-fortified brand.) You can also use soy milk instead of dairy milk in recipes for custards and baked desserts.
- Use firm tofu in stir-fries and soft or silken tofu in dips and spreads.
- Try a melted soy cheese sandwich.
- Edamame are very rich in isoflavones. Buy shelled, blanched edamame in bags and add to salads, grain dishes, soups, and stir-fries.
- Many "veggie" burgers are soy-based. If you don't like one brand, try another—the taste does differ.
- Soy "meats" such as bologna may not contain high levels of isoflavones (check the label), but they are good alternatives to meat. Select brands with lower sodium and fat content.
- Tempeh (pronounced TEM peh), a fermented soy food, is firm and chewy—great for stir-fries. Or just braise in soy sauce and eat. Try smoked tempeh as a pork alternative in bean soups like split pea.
- Miso (pronounced MEE soh), fermented soybean paste, can be used as a soup base or added to chicken broth for the start of a great soup. Miso can be high in sodium; look for a brand that isn't.

2 **Fish.** You probably know that fatty fish is good for your heart. Ocean fish fat, rich in omega-3 fatty

WARNING

Tofu sold loose in open tubs of water is often contaminated with bacteria. Opt instead for containers of packaged tofu in the produce section of your supermarket.

Disease-Fighting Plant Chemicals

Scientists have isolated some powerful chemicals found in plant foods that, based on animal studies or preliminary studies in humans, are thought to help fight disease. Fortunately, you don't need to learn to pronounce their names to benefit from them. Just eat a wide variety of fresh fruits, vegetables, whole grains, beans, and soy foods, along with some seafood and an occasional egg or two.

FOODS	PHYTOCHEMICAL	BENEFIT
Soy foods, beans, tea	Isoflavones	Estrogen-like compounds that may help protect against heart disease, osteoporosis, and certain cancers.
Flaxseeds, wheat germ, soy	Lignans	Similar to isoflavones, above.
Tea (green, oolong, and black)	Catechins and theaflavins	Powerful antioxidants that may help prevent the oxidation of LDL ("bad") cholesterol, therefore helping to prevent heart disease.
Berries, red grapes, apples, nuts	Ellagic acid	A powerful antioxidant.
Citrus fruits	Tangeretin and nobiletin	Antioxidants. They may also inhibit blood clotting, possibly helping to prevent heart disease.
Citrus fruits	Limonene	Inhibit the activity of proteins that trigger cell growth, possibly helping to prevent cancer.
Blueberries, strawberries, raspberries, blackberries, cherries, red grapes	Anthocyanins	Antioxidants. They may also inhibit cholesterol synthesis.
Yellow onions, broccoli, kale, berries, tea, apples	Quercetin	A very powerful antioxidant that may offer protection against heart disease and cancer.
Broccoli, cabbage, Brussels sprouts, kale	Isothiocyanates, such as sulforaphane and indoles	Perhaps the strongest cancer-protective food compounds yet discovered.
Garlic and onions	Allicin and other allylic sulfides	May reduce the tendency of blood to clot, possibly offering protection against heart attack and stroke.
Legumes, soy, seeds, whole grains	Protease inhibitors	May help repair DNA and curb out-of-control cell growth, possibly helping to guard against cancer.
Tomatoes, red peppers, pink grapefruits, guavas, watermelons	Lycopene	Antioxidants being studied for their ability protect against cancer, especially prostate cancer.
Kale, broccoli, Brussels sprouts, spinach, collard greens, peaches, corn, egg yolks	Zeaxanthin and lutein	May help prevent macular degeneration (an age-related eye disorder).
Soy foods, nuts, seeds, wheat germ	Sterols	Lower blood cholesterol levels.
Nuts, soy foods, legumes	Saponins	Help lower blood cholesterol levels.

Good Fats in Fish

Oily fish are better sources of heart-healthy omega-3 fatty acids than white fish. Here's a short rundown.

GREAT SOURCES	MODERATE SOURCES	POOR SOURCES
Mackerel	Bass	Cod
Salmon	Bluefish	Flounder
Sardines	Halibut	Haddock
Sturgeon	Striped sea bass	Snapper
Trout (lake or rainbow)	Swordfish	Sole
Tuna (albacore or bluefin)	Tuna (yellowfin)	Trout (brook, sea)

acids, protects against heart disease by lowering high triglyceride levels (a risk factor for diabetes, too) and reducing the tendency of blood to form artery-clogging clots. Eating as little as one fish meal a week was linked to a whopping 40 percent reduction in heart disease in one study, and it may even help prevent sudden death from heart attacks. It also seems to help people who have had one heart attack avoid a second. In a two-year

Mackerel with Tomatoes, Garlic, and Herbs

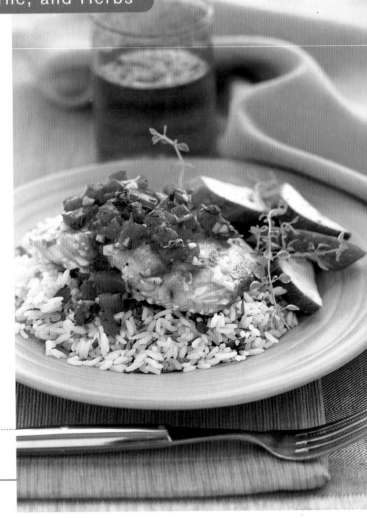

You can substitute any fatty fish—swordfish, tuna, shark, bluefish, halibut, catfish, or trout—for the mackerel. You can also use milder fish such as cod or snapper if you prefer.

Makes 4 servings.

- 1¼ pounds mackerel fillets
- ¼ teaspoon salt
- 3 ripe plum tomatoes, seeded and coarsely chopped
- 2 teaspoons finely chopped garlic
- 1 tablespoon fresh lemon juice
- 1 tablespoon chopped fresh rosemary leaves or 1 teaspoon dried
- 1 tablespoon chopped fresh thyme leaves or 1 teaspoon dried

1. Preheat the oven to 425° F. Place fish in a glass or ceramic baking dish and sprinkle with salt. Top with the tomatoes and garlic. Sprinkle with the lemon juice, rosemary, and thyme.

2. Bake for 8 to 12 minutes, depending on the thickness of the fillets, or until the fish is opaque in the center and flakes easily.

NUTRITION INFORMATION *Per Serving:* 252 calories, 30 g protein, 6 g carbohydrate, 1 g fiber, 12 g fat, 3 g saturated fat, 68 mg cholesterol, 267 mg sodium

Tropical Soy Smoothie

Here's a delicious way to add some soy to your diet. The fruit supplies a good amount of vitamin C and beta-carotene.

Makes 1 (12-ounce) serving.

¼ **cup pineapple cubes**

¼ **cup mango cubes**

2 **strawberries, hulled**

1 **cup plain low-fat soy milk**

Juice of ½ lime (1 tablespoon)

1. Combine the pineapple, mango, strawberries, soy milk, and lime in the container of a blender or food processor. Whirl until smooth, stopping to scrape down the sides of the container if necessary. Pour into a tall glass.

NUTRITION INFORMATION *Per Serving:* 193 calories, 5 g protein, 42 g carbohydrate, 3 g fiber, 3 g fat, 0 g saturated fat, 0 mg cholesterol, 98 mg sodium

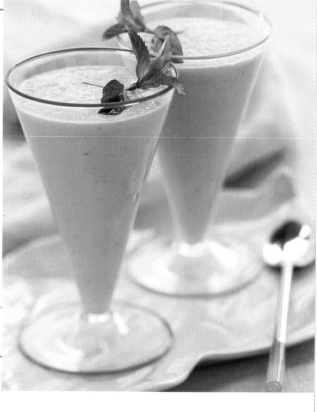

study of heart attack survivors, those who ate fish at least twice weekly were 29 percent less likely to have a second heart attack.

And that's not all. A diet that includes seafood has also been linked with a lower risk of cancer, especially cancer of the esophagus, stomach, and colon. And new research finds that it may even help ward off depression by boosting the body's production of serotonin, a key mood-affecting brain chemical. A recent large-scale Finnish study found that people who ate fish less than once a week were 31 percent more likely to suffer from mild to severe depression than people who ate fish more frequently. Some fish tips:

- Strive for at least one seafood meal a week. (Fish Fridays, anyone?)
- Don't let fear of fat drive you away from fatty fish. It's often lower in fat and calories than the leanest meats.

- Good choices: bass, trout, herring, bluefish, tuna, mackerel, salmon, and swordfish.
- Shellfish is fine. Even shrimp, relatively high in cholesterol, is low in saturated fat and contains some omega-3 fats, so it belongs in a cholesterol-lowering diet.
- Lean fish such as cod and flounder is okay—it's an excellent source of protein with almost no saturated fat.
- To keep calories low, choose fish that's baked, broiled, poached, steamed, or grilled instead of fried.

3 Garlic. Like to cook with garlic? Good for you! It's a great way to add flavor without increasing fat, calories, or sodium. And you may be getting additional health benefits. Several (though not all) studies find that a clove a day can lower high

SimpleSolution

To get the most omega-3 fatty acids in tuna fish, choose water-packed tuna. If you choose oil-packed tuna, those heart-healthy oils will dissolve in the packing oil— and go down the drain. Also choose higher-fat versions of water-packed tuna—different species vary greatly.

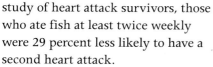

YOUR GAME PLAN FOR GOOD HEALTH

cholesterol, and there is evidence that garlic also reduces the tendency of the blood to clot, another potential heart benefit. People who eat a lot of garlic (and onions) also seem to be at lower risk of stomach cancer and possibly breast cancer. Eat garlic raw, or, to maximize the active ingredient in garlic in cooked dishes, try this: Cut or chop or smash the clove and let it sit for about 10 minutes before adding it to your dish to allow time for allicin, the sulfur compound from which all of garlic's unique potential benefits derive, to form.

4 **Broccoli and Its Cabbage Cousins.** All green vegetables promote health, but broccoli and its cabbage-family cousins are special. They are not only loaded with vitamins and fiber, they also contain a class of phytochemicals called isothiocyanates. Some studies suggest that these compounds protect against a wide range of cancers by stimulating the liver to boost production of cancer-fighting enzymes. The cabbage family of cruciferous vegetables is a big one, including arugula, Brussels sprouts, cabbage, cauliflower, collard

Crustless Broccoli Quiche

You can cut this quiche into smaller squares to serve as an appetizer or hors d'oeuvre. You can also substitute chopped cooked kale, collards, or other greens for the broccoli.

Makes 4 servings.

- 8 ounces liquid egg substitute or 4 whole eggs
- 1 cup reduced-fat ricotta cheese
- 1 teaspoon mustard
- 1/2 teaspoon salt
- 1/8 teaspoon pepper
- 2 cups chopped cooked broccoli
- 1 cup shredded low-fat Swiss cheese

1. Preheat the oven to 350° F. Lightly coat a 9-inch square baking dish with nonstick cooking spray. In a large bowl, beat together the egg substitute, ricotta cheese, mustard, salt, and pepper.

2. Scatter the broccoli and Swiss cheese over the bottom of the pan. Pour the egg mixture over them.

3. Bake for 40 to 50 minutes or until a knife inserted in the center of the quiche comes out clean. Let the quiche stand for 10 minutes before slicing and serving.

NUTRITION INFORMATION *Per Serving:*
204 calories, 27 g protein, 10 g carbohydrate, 3 g fiber, 7 g fat, 4 g saturated fat, 23 mg cholesterol, 986 mg sodium

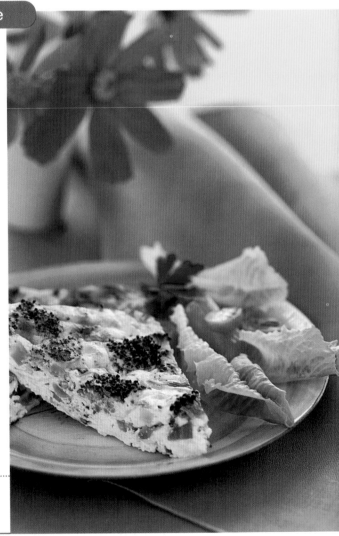

Spinach Salad with Pears and Walnuts

Spinach is rich in folic acid, beta-carotene, and vitamin C, and along with the pear provides a significant amount of fiber. The yogurt provides a calcium boost, and garlic and walnuts are both good for your heart.

Makes 4 servings.

- 3/4 **cup plain low-fat yogurt**
- 1 **clove garlic, crushed**
- 1 **tablespoon olive oil**
- 1/4 **teaspoon Dijon mustard**
- 1 **pound spinach, rinsed, trimmed, and torn in bite-size pieces**
- 1 **ripe pear, cored and thinly sliced (1 1/3 cups)**
- 1/4 **cup coarsely chopped walnuts (1 ounce)**

1. In a food processor or blender, whirl the yogurt, garlic, oil, and mustard for 30 to 60 seconds or until smooth. In a large bowl, combine the spinach, pear, and walnuts. Pour the dressing over the salad and toss until coated.

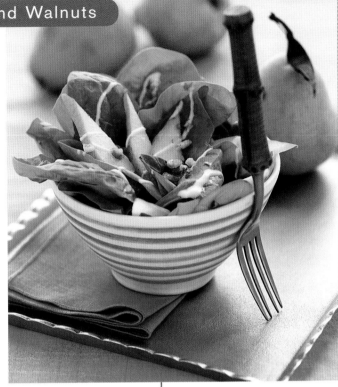

NUTRITION INFORMATION *Per Serving:* 153 calories, 7 g protein, 15 g carbohydrate, 4 g fiber, 9 g fat, 1 g saturated fat, 1 mg cholesterol, 131 mg sodium

---

greens, kale, kohlrabi, mustard greens, radishes, rutabaga, Swiss chard, turnips, and watercress.

Broccoli is rich in an isothiocyanate called sulforaphane, one of the most powerful of these protective compounds yet discovered. So dig in! Since sulforaphane will survive the heat of cooking, serve your broccoli any way from tender-crisp to well cooked; just don't boil it for hours. To get even more sulforaphane, add some broccoli sprouts (steam them lightly first to kill any bacteria) to your salad or sandwich; they have 20 to 50 times the sulforaphane per ounce as broccoli, and they are now widely available in supermarkets.

Watercress contains a particular isothiocyanate that is easily destroyed by heat. Cooked watercress is still very nutritious, but eat some raw or just lightly steamed, too.

5 Tomatoes. The substance that turns a tomato red may help keep your body healthy. It's a plant pigment called lycopene, a potent antioxidant. Some studies suggest that lycopene may reduce the risk of prostate cancer. A recent review concluded that on average, men who ate 10 weekly servings of tomato products were 35 percent less likely to develop the disease. There is also some evidence that lycopene may help ward off cancers of the lung, pancreas, and digestive tract. And population studies suggest that people who eat more tomatoes are also less likely to develop heart disease. Some tomato tactics:

Nutrition Note

One cup of cooked broccoli has more vitamin C than a medium navel orange (100 mg versus 80 mg).

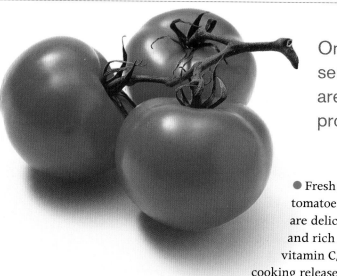

On average, men who eat 10 servings weekly of tomato products are 35 percent less likely to get prostate cancer.

Want to live to a ripe old age? Eat tomatoes. They contain a compound called lycopene that may help fight cancer and boost the immune system.

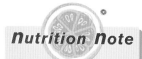

Nutrition note

If your peanut butter doesn't separate at room temperature, it's made with hydrogenated oils, which contain cholesterol-raising trans fats. Opt instead for "natural" brands.

- Fresh tomatoes are delicious and rich in vitamin C, but cooking releases the lycopene from tomato cell walls so our bodies can best absorb it.
- Commercial tomato sauces contain lycopene in a highly absorbable form, so go ahead and fill the pantry with your favorite brand.
- To spiff up canned tomato sauce, sauté a chopped onion in a little olive oil until soft, add the sauce, and toss in a large chopped fresh tomato with a little freshly chopped garlic and some dried oregano. Toss with fresh pasta.
- For a super-healthy pizza, make it or order it with extra tomato sauce and vegetables, and skip the cheese.

6 Spinach. Popeye had it wrong. Spinach won't make you strong. But preliminary research suggests it may help you keep your eyesight. It guards against macular degeneration, the most common cause of blindness in people over age 65. In one study, people who ate spinach (and other dark greens like kale, collard, mustard, and turnip greens) two or four times a week were 46 percent less likely to develop macular degeneration than people who eat these foods less than once a month. The sight savers? Scientists suspect lutein and zeaxanthin, two phytochemicals in the carotenoid family; they may help the macula (a tiny spot in the center of the retina) screen out potentially damaging ultraviolet light. That's not the only reason to love spinach. It's a good source of fiber, folic acid, and vitamins A, C, and E.

- Always wash spinach carefully to remove any grit. Place the leaves in a large bowl filled with water, then lift them out; repeat with fresh water until no sand appears.
- Try sizzled spinach. Place a bit of olive oil in a large nonstick skillet and heat it until it is hot but not smoking. Toss washed, drained fresh spinach into the skillet and stir until the spinach wilts, about two minutes.
- Don't forget spinach salad.

7 Tea. Who would have guessed that tea is so healthful? It's rich in antioxidant compounds called catechins, which may protect you against heart disease, stroke, and cancer. Green tea is the richest in catechins (27 percent dry weight), with oolong a close second (23 percent). But black tea (4 percent) still has enough of these compounds to have an effect. So reach for a cup of tea when the desire for a hot beverage hits.

Don't worry too much about tea's caffeine content. A cup of black tea has just 35 mg of caffeine, less than even weak coffee. Green tea has only

25 mg. (The longer you steep tea, the more caffeine it will contain.) Some ideas for tea time:

- Try a high-quality green tea. It's a mild, refreshing beverage. No need for sugar or milk.
- To make good tea, black or green, bring fresh cold water to a boil and pour over tea leaves; let black tea steep 4 to 5 minutes, green tea 3 to 4 minutes.

8 Blueberries. All berries— blueberries, strawberries, raspberries—are rich in vitamin C, fiber, and antioxidants, which protect against heart disease and cancer. But blueberries are extra special. Like cranberries, blueberries may guard against urinary tract infections by preventing the bacteria that cause them from attaching to cell walls. One animal study even suggests that berries may help prevent age-related cognitive decline, and that blueberries help improve balance.
A bit of berry advice:

- Wash all berries gently in cold water before eating them to remove any bacteria.
- Add blueberries to your cereal or yogurt for a burst of sweetness.
- Stock up on frozen blueberries. In many supermarkets they are now sold "individually quick frozen," in bags, not solid blocks. Toss a half cup over low-fat ice cream or add to muffin batter or quick-bread dough.

9 Nuts. Nuts are nutty. High in fat and calories, they seem like nutritional no-no's. In fact, they're not. Population studies find that men and women who eat nuts several times a week, compared to people who rarely eat nuts, are much less likely to die of heart disease. In fact, eating a handful of nuts such as walnuts four to five times a week could lower your risk of heart attack by up to 40 percent according to some research. That's most likely because the fat contained in nuts is the heart-healthy kind—unsaturated, with some omega-3 fatty acids (almonds and walnuts contain the most). Nuts are also packed with vitamin E and magnesium, unique health-protective phytochemicals, and compounds, such as saponins, that may protect against cancer.

So toss some into your salad (see Spinach Salad with Pears and Walnuts, page 55). You can toast nuts for extra flavor. Toasting is easy: Just add sliced or chopped nuts to a dry skillet over medium heat for two or three minutes. Shake the pan often to prevent scorching. Then add the toasted nuts to your favorite salad or mix them into home-baked breads and desserts.

A tablespoon or two of nuts is plenty. No need to munch a bunch: A half cup of nuts may top 400 calories. So don't just *add* them to your diet; use them *instead* of other high-fat foods, like bacon or cheese.

Berry, berry good: Of all the fruits and vegetables that have been studied, blueberries have the most potent antioxidant power.

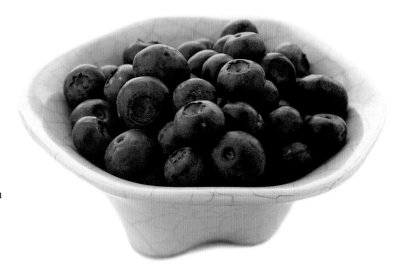

Functional Foods

Supermarkets are beginning to stock their shelves with foods enriched with various health-protective compounds (so-called functional foods). But buyer beware: some are a waste of money.

et your medicine be your food, wrote Hippocrates, the Greek "father of medicine," two thousand years ago. But he probably never envisioned that we would actually add medicine to our food. Yet that's just what you'll find on grocery shelves in North America.

First developed by the Japanese, so-called "functional foods" contain nutrients that have a special health benefit. They range from bone-building orange juice to eggs enriched with the heart-healthy fats found in fish. But you may also find some clunkers that won't add to your health—but will subtract from your wallet.

Medicine or Marketing?

Depressed? Try snack chips made with St. John's wort. Or maybe you'd like to boost your brain power with fruit juice spiked with ginkgo. Sound far-fetched? Not anymore. These products are now readily available in U.S. stores. In Canada, however, they do not fit the much narrower definition for functional foods. Still, you may find them in some health food stores in this country.

Are they a good idea? No. Herbal supplements are best used for specific purposes in controlled doses for limited periods of time. The amount

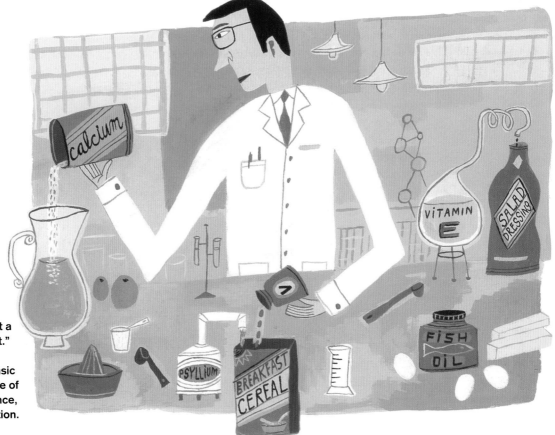

Functional foods are not a "magic bullet." Continue to follow the basic dietary advice of variety, balance, and moderation.

of St. John's wort in those corn chips is probably so low that it won't do you any harm, but it won't do you any good either, and the chips will add calories to your diet.

In Canada, functional foods are foods that have health benefits in addition to providing basic nutrients and nutritional benefits. For example, foods made with oat bran not only provide carbohydrates and certain vitamins, but because they contain beta glucan, they also lower blood cholesterol.

Certain functional foods may enhance an anti-aging diet. Here's what to look for:

- It should be a healthful food that you would include in a well-balanced diet anyway. Example: calcium-fortified orange juice. Orange juice is already a nutritious food, so if you need extra calcium, it's a great way to get it.
- The added ingredient should be scientifically established to have benefit. Research shows that calcium fits the bill. So do omega-3 fatty acids to lower high cholesterol. There is good evidence that psyllium and soy protein to protect against heart disease, and margarines with stanols or sterols to lower high cholesterol, offer a health benefit.

Good Bets

1 Heart Foods. If you have high cholesterol, diet can lower it, and adding certain functional foods to your diet can lower it an extra 5 to 10 percent or more. For example:

- Two cholesterol-lowering margarines, Benecol and Take Control (not yet available in Canada), have been approved in the U.S. by the Food and Drug Administration to carry a claim that they may lower elevated cholesterol levels. They contain plant compounds (sterols, stanols) that interfere with the absorption of cholesterol.
- Psyllium-enhanced cereals, rich in soluble fiber, lower high cholesterol, as does oat bran. Certain "heart-healthy" cereals now contain psyllium.
- Foods enriched with soy protein can be beneficial. In the U.S., the FDA has approved a claim that eating 25 grams of soy protein a day can lower cholesterol. Soy-enriched foods are not currently available in Canada. Watch for them in the future.

2 Vitamin-Enhanced Foods. Some hens are now fed on a flax-seed diet which results in eggs with a high level of vitamin E.

3 Bone Builders. Calcium was once found in our diet mainly in dairy foods. But today you can find it added to orange juice as well.

In general it's a good thing: Most Canadians get too little calcium, important for preventing osteoporosis and keeping blood pressure in check. So go ahead and drink calcium-fortified juice. But remember: Calcium needs vitamin D to be truly effective, so if you don't drink much milk (fortified with D) and don't get out in the sun for 15 minutes a day (without sunblock), consider a vitamin D supplement. And don't overdo calcium; a safe limit is 2,500 mg a day.

4 A Better Egg. Some eggs now contain omega-3 fatty acids, the "good" fats found in fish.

Fast Fact

Functional foods do not include foods fortified or enriched with nutrients to meet dietary needs. For example, meal replacements, sports nutritional foods, and nutrient-dense ready-made dinners for seniors are not classed as functional foods in Canada.

Food, Friends, and Joy

Healthy eating isn't just about disease-fighting nutrients. Sharing a meal with family and friends provides benefits beyond those of the foods on your fork.

Eating to age well? You'll want to focus on more than just nutrients. The act of eating can be a shared bond between family and friends. In fact, the word *companion* stems from the Latin words meaning with ("con") and bread ("pane"). Breaking bread with others is an occasion for conversation, a social experience, a source of simple pleasure, an opportunity for relaxation. For many people, though, the frenzied pace of life makes it difficult to plan meals together. For others, isolation means they often eat alone.

Loneliness is a risk factor for poor nutrition. Studies show that older people who live by themselves are more likely to skip meals and eat poor-quality diets. In Tennessee, when researchers created a "loneliness index" for 61 people age 60 and older, those who scored highest were most likely to consume too few calories and too little calcium.

On the other hand, marriage seems to confer an extra health advantage: better nutrition. In a study of more than 4,000 Americans age 55 or older, both men and women living with their spouses consumed a better diet than those cooking for one. If you are recently widowed, this is a particularly vulnerable time. Studies show that even up to two years after the loss of a spouse, widowed older adults eat significantly poorer diets.

Whatever your social circumstances, make the most of mealtime. Make lunch plans with a new acquaintance. Try forming a dining club with friends, and invite a friend or two over for an informal potluck dinner every now and then. You'll nourish your friendships and your body at the same time.

Although it's a great idea to watch what you eat, there's no need to obsess about food and health. Eating well should not feel like deprivation. The pleasure you get from food is important, especially if it leads you to sample a wide variety of foods. Recent research reveals that the more varied your

Any meal that brings together friends or family is, in one respect, a healthy one.

Roast Pork and Vegetable Fajitas

Want to invite a friend or two over to dinner at the last minute? Here's a fun, healthy meal to serve.

Makes 4 fajitas.
Recipe for marinade follows.

1   **pork tenderloin ($^3/_4$ pound)**

1   **clove garlic, halved**

2   **sweet red peppers, halved, seeded, and cut into $^1/_4$-inch-wide strips**

2   **small red onions, halved and cut into $^1/_4$-inch-wide slivers**

1   **large zucchini, sliced $^1/_4$ inch thick**

4   **fat-free 8-inch flour tortillas, warmed (see note)**

Fresh salsa, low-fat yogurt or sour cream, and chopped cilantro (coriander) for garnish (optional)

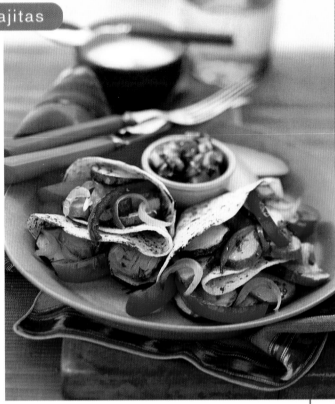

1. Preheat the oven to 450° F. Pour half of the marinade into a plastic food-storage bag. Rub the pork with the garlic, then place the meat in the bag of marinade. Seal the bag and set aside at room temperature while preparing the vegetables.

2. Mix the peppers, onions, and zucchini with the remaining marinade in a large bowl. Line a 15 x 10-inch jelly-roll pan with aluminum foil. Lightly coat the foil with nonstick cooking spray. Spread the vegetables evenly on the foil. Roast for 35 to 40 minutes, stirring occasionally.

3. Remove the pork from the marinade and place it in a small roasting pan. Roast for 20 to 25 minutes or until the internal temperature of the pork registers 160 degrees on an instant-read meat thermometer.

4. Remove the pork from the oven and let it stand for 5 minutes before slicing. Divide the sliced pork and vegetables evenly among the warm tortillas. Wrap and serve with garnishes, if you like.

Marinade In a measuring cup, combine $^1/_4$ cup lemon juice, 2 tablespoons red wine vinegar, 1 tablespoon olive oil, 2 tablespoons ground cumin, 1 teaspoon salt, $^1/_4$ to $^1/_2$ teaspoon coarse black pepper, and 2 cloves garlic, chopped.

Note: Stack the tortillas and wrap in aluminum foil. Place the foil packet in the oven along with the meat and vegetables during the last 5 minutes of roasting time.

NUTRITION INFORMATION *Per Serving:* 278 calories, 22 g protein, 34 g carbohydrate, 3 g fiber, 6 g fat, 1 g saturated fat, 50 mg cholesterol, 634 mg sodium

diet—especially if it includes a broad and changing assortment of fruits and vegetables—the more likely it is to keep you healthy. On the other hand, people who eat a very limited variety of foods are more likely to develop heart disease.

An unprecedented array of foods is available in supermarkets today, so go ahead and experiment. Take a tip from the Japanese: Their government suggests eating 30 different foods a day to get a wide variety of nutrients and avoid overdoing any one food.

Eight Weeks to Better Eating

Eating habits are just that—*habits*. Try to alter them all at once and you'll be back to your old ways in no time. But by making a few small changes every week over the course of eight weeks, you'll find yourself with a new way of eating you can embrace for life.

SUNDAY	MONDAY	TUESDAY

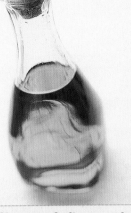

1

Your task this week: Buy a bottle of extra-virgin olive oil. Start using it in place of butter or margarine in sautés and stir-fries. Make your own low-fat vinaigrette using 4 tablespoons olive oil, 2 tablespoons vinegar, and salt, pepper, and dried herbs to taste.

2

Choose a fruit or vegetable that you don't normally eat, and try it this week. Pick something that's in season, whether it's mango (great in salads and an excellent source of beta-carotene) or kale (a superstar antioxidant that you can throw into soups at the last minute for maximum retention of nutrients).

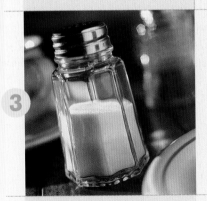

3

If you're like most Canadians, you consume far too much sodium. Most of it comes not from the salt shaker but from processed foods, like canned soups. Start reading food labels to realize just how much is sneaking into your diet. Your desire for salt will decrease as you cut back your intake.

4

Your next project: Start weeding trans fats from your diet. This will be tricky, since manufacturers add them to crackers, chips, and many other packaged foods. Check labels for "partially hydrogenated oil." When possible, use olive or canola oil in place of shortening or stick margarine.

Garlic may lower blood pressure and even inhibit certain cancers. Whisk a crushed clove into salad dressings. For garlic mashed potatoes, add peeled, halved cloves to potatoes while they boil, then mash.

WEDNESDAY	THURSDAY	FRIDAY	SATURDAY

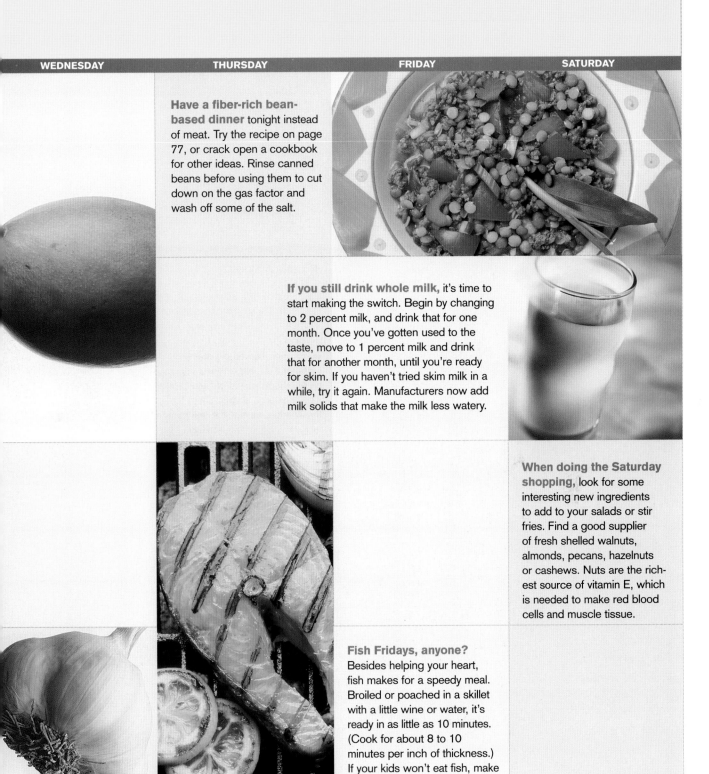

Have a fiber-rich bean-based dinner tonight instead of meat. Try the recipe on page 77, or crack open a cookbook for other ideas. Rinse canned beans before using them to cut down on the gas factor and wash off some of the salt.

If you still drink whole milk, it's time to start making the switch. Begin by changing to 2 percent milk, and drink that for one month. Once you've gotten used to the taste, move to 1 percent milk and drink that for another month, until you're ready for skim. If you haven't tried skim milk in a while, try it again. Manufacturers now add milk solids that make the milk less watery.

When doing the Saturday shopping, look for some interesting new ingredients to add to your salads or stir fries. Find a good supplier of fresh shelled walnuts, almonds, pecans, hazelnuts or cashews. Nuts are the richest source of vitamin E, which is needed to make red blood cells and muscle tissue.

Fish Fridays, anyone? Besides helping your heart, fish makes for a speedy meal. Broiled or poached in a skillet with a little wine or water, it's ready in as little as 10 minutes. (Cook for about 8 to 10 minutes per inch of thickness.) If your kids won't eat fish, make them a separate meal.

Eight Weeks to Better Eating

SUNDAY	MONDAY	TUESDAY

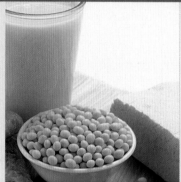

5   **Pick a soy food to try.** If you've avoided tofu because of its texture, try the firm or extra-firm variety. Freeze tofu and crumble it into chili. Try steamed whole green soybeans, available frozen. Add miso (soybean paste) to soups. Or have a soy burger. Experiment to find a brand you like.

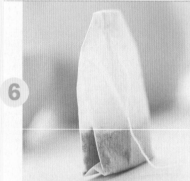

6   **Do you drink coffee?** If so, try substituting tea for one of your daily cups of java. Tea offers antioxidant benefits that coffee doesn't and may even protect against heart disease and cancer. Green tea offers the most health benefits, but black tea is also healthful. Experiment with different varieties of tea, sold loose or in tea bags.

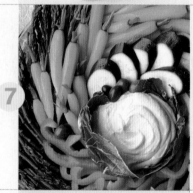

7   **Attack your snack habit.** Keep baby carrots in the fridge; a handful will meet your vitamin A needs for the day. Try low-fat vanilla or lemon yogurt sprinkled with wheat germ. Or enjoy toasted almonds. Place a handful of unsalted almonds on a cookie sheet and toast in a 350° F oven for 3 to 5 minutes. Remove and salt lightly.

8   **Make this Sunday dinner** an excuse to gather with family or friends. It doesn't matter what you serve (try lasagna made with roasted vegetables such as eggplant, zucchini, and sweet peppers). Just enjoy this time together.

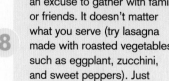
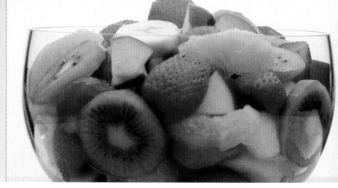

| WEDNESDAY | THURSDAY | FRIDAY | SATURDAY |

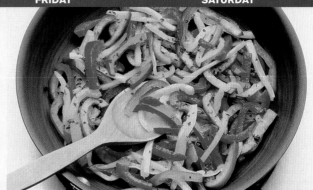

Fill your freezer with frozen vegetables. They make an instant addition to meals (add them to stir-fries) and will help you reach your goal of 5 or more servings of fruits and vegetables a day. Since freezing is the best way to preserve the nutrients in fresh foods, they're often just as nutritious as—or even more nutritious than—produce that's been sitting in the grocery store.

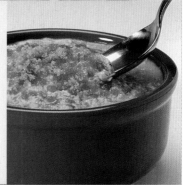

Give your breakfast a makeover. Opt for heart-healthy oatmeal, or buy a new breakfast cereal. (Look for one that contains 3 or more grams of fiber per serving and less than 3 grams of fat.) Add fresh berries or dried cranberries for extra appeal. Avoid granola unless you buy the low-fat variety. Or make your own: Mix 2 cups rolled oats with 1 cup dried fruits and seeds and a little brown sugar. Toast for 3 to 5 minutes in a warm oven.

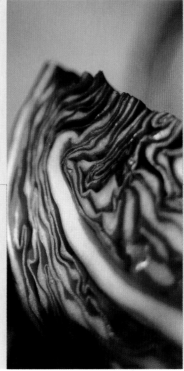

Add a cancer-fighting cruciferous vegetable to one meal this week. Choose from broccoli, cabbage, Brussels sprouts, kale, Swiss chard, mustard greens, and water-cress (great in salads and sand-wiches). To spice up broccoli, add toasted sesame seeds (toast on the stove in a pan, shaking, for 1 to 2 minutes) and red pepper flakes.

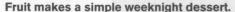

Fruit makes a simple weeknight dessert.
Try fresh fruit salad or a fruit crisp or cobbler. Baked apples make a delicious fall dessert. (Cortlands or Granny Smiths work well.) Core the apples and peel off a ½-inch strip at the top of each. Into each apple, place 1 teaspoon of sugar or honey, 1 teaspoon cinnamon, and a few raisins or currants (optional). Place in a shallow baking dish with ½ inch of water. Bake at 350° F until very tender, about 45 minutes.

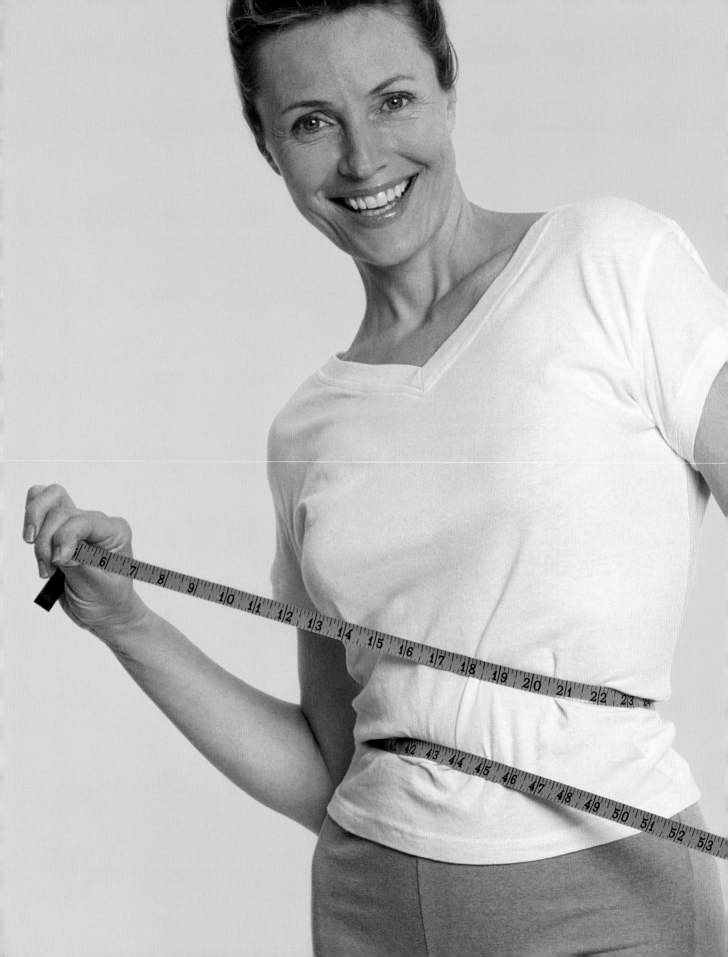

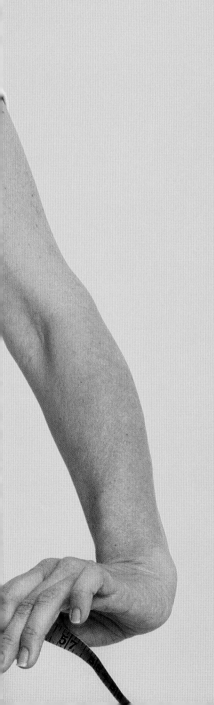

CHAPTER 2

WATCHING YOUR WEIGHT

Fighting the Battle of the Bulge

Battling the infamous middle-age spread? If your belt no longer goes the distance, your problem isn't just cosmetic—it's putting your health at risk.

Oh, that widening waistline! Those sagging saddlebags! Do you wince at the mirror and wonder how that extra weight got there? It didn't happen overnight. Pounds begin to pile on in our mid-thirties, when we start to become less active. As we lose muscle, our body's metabolic furnace cools and we burn fewer calories, even at rest. Every 10 years after age 50, we need about 100 fewer calories a day to maintain the same weight. But most of us continue to eat just as we always have, so week after week those extra ounces of fat settle in. The result? Most North Americans gain about 10 pounds per decade after their twenties.

As much as we may resent our gray hair and wrinkles, the flab, sag, and spread of aging is a more fear-some enemy because it threatens our health. In addition to sapping your energy, lugging around excess poundage boosts your risk of just about every major disease, including high blood pressure, heart disease, ischemic stroke, type 2 diabetes, breast and uterine cancer, colon cancer, and gallstones. Even low-back pain and arthritis can be exacerbated by extra weight.

Are You Overweight?

Neither the fit of your waistband nor your mirror's frank gaze can really tell you whether or not you need to worry. Even the bathroom scale won't give you a dependable answer. Nor will traditional weight charts. That's because what's most important isn't how much you weigh, it's how

WARNING

A five-pound weight gain can increase your risk of type 2 diabetes by 10 percent.

Do you have high blood pressure? By losing just 10 pounds, you may lower your reading—possibly by enough to decrease your blood-pressure medication or even stop taking it.

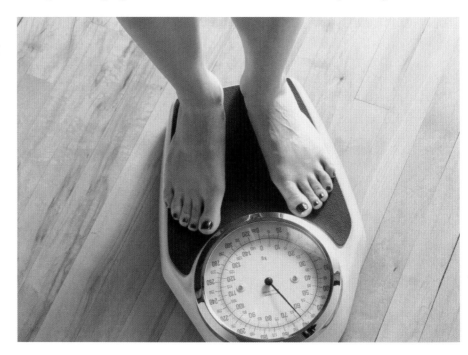

Every 10 years after age 50, we need about 100 fewer calories a day to maintain the same weight.

much body fat you have. Since muscle weighs more than fat, you may tip the scales and still be healthy if you have a very muscular build.

Unfortunately, there's no easy, reliable way to measure your percentage of body fat. Instead, the best tool for grading your girth is the body mass index (BMI), a mathematical formula based on height and weight. To learn how to calculate your BMI, see How Lean Are You? (right).

Apples vs. Pears

Where you carry your fat may be just as important as how much you carry. If your fat is concentrated around the abdomen, where it creates an apple-shaped silhouette, it is more dangerous to your health. Apples are at higher risk for high cholesterol, hypertension, cardiovascular disease, type 2 diabetes, and possibly breast and endometrial cancer. Pear-shaped people, who wear more of their excess fat on the buttocks, hips, and thighs, seem to be less vulnerable to these health problems.

Though many men tend to be apples and many women, pears, either sex can have either shape. To find out which fruit category you fit into, calculate your waist-to-hip ratio (WHR). Divide your waist measurement at the narrowest point in inches by your hip measurement at the widest point in inches for your WHR. If your WHR is over 0.80 (for men) or 0.90 (for women), you're an apple.

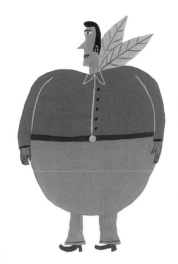
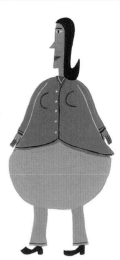

How is your fat distributed? If your body shape looks more like an apple than a pear, you're at greater risk for heart disease and other serious health problems.

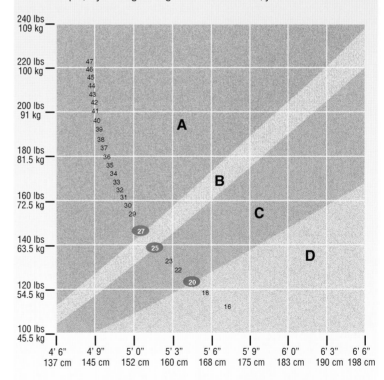

How Lean Are You?

Use the formula weight (kg) ÷ height (m²) to calculate your BMI. Alternatively, locate the point on the chart where your weight and height intersect. Draw a line to the number closest to that point for your approximate BMI. For example, if you weigh 69 kg and are 173 cm tall, your BMI is around 23.

Zone	BMI	Health Effects
A	>27	Increased risk of developing health problems
B	25-27	May lead to health problems in some people
C	20-25	Good weight for most people
D	<20	May be associated with health problems for some people

YOUR GAME PLAN FOR GOOD HEALTH

The Way to Lose Weight

If you want to lose weight, crash dieting isn't the answer. Instead, gradually change the way you think about eating—and exercise.

The only "trick" to losing weight is to take in fewer calories than you burn. Sounds simple enough, right? So why the scores of books, pills, and programs each year touting new ways to lose weight?

The truth is, there are no quick fixes. In order to budge your pudge—and keep the pounds from creeping back—you have to permanently change your approach to eating and add physical activity and exercise to your daily routine. Don't try to change your lifestyle all at once or you're less likely to succeed.

A Two-Pronged Approach

Counting calories isn't the answer, but it's a start. To figure out roughly how many calories you need to maintain your current weight, multiply your weight in pounds by 10 if you're sedentary, 15 if you're fairly active, or 20 if you're exerting yourself energetically all day long. (To convert kilos to pounds, multiply your weight in kilos by 2.2, then proceed with the multiplying factor of 10, 15, or 20.) To shed a pound a week, subtract 3,500 calories a week, or 500 a day, from your current total.

The best way to do this is not just by eating less, but by eating less and burning more calories. Instead of trying to cut 500 calories a day from your diet, it's smarter to cut 250 calories and then burn off the other 250 calories through exercise. Why is exercise so important? Most dieters who fail to exercise eventually gain back their excess weight. When researchers at Baylor College of Medicine in Houston studied overweight people who dieted, exercised, or did both, those who exercised without dieting kept off the most weight for the longest time.

⚠️
WARNING

See your doctor if you have an unexplained weight gain. It could be linked to an underlying disorder, such as an underactive thyroid. Signs and symptoms include dry skin, always feeling run-down or cold, constipation, and numbness and tingling in your fingers or toes. Another tip-off: Your basal body temperature is below 97.6° F three days in a row. (Take your temperature in the morning, before getting out of bed.) Other conditions that can cause weight gain include heart, kidney, or other endocrine disorders.

How Fast Is Your Metabolism?

Most of the calories you consume—about 60 to 65 percent—go toward keeping your heart beating, maintaining your body temperature, and performing other essential bodily functions. To find out how many calories your body needs to fuel these tasks, calculate your basal metabolic rate (BMR).

STEP 1	STEP 2	STEP 3
■ Convert your weight from pounds to kilograms by dividing it by 2.2.	■ Multiply the result by 0.9 (men should skip this step).	■ Multiply the result by 24.

That's how many calories you need a day without allowing for physical activity and exercise. If you add these in, you'll need 30 to 50 percent more calories. But if you're not active and are taking in more calories than your BMR, you're probably putting on weight. Boosting your lean muscle mass through strength training can increase your BMR so that you burn calories faster, even at rest.

Health Canada recommends 60 minutes a day of physical activity. But you can break up your activity into several shorter segments of 10 or 15 minutes and still get results. If you do more strenuous activities, such as aerobics, jogging, or hockey, 20 to 30 minutes four times a week is adequate. If the activity is light walking, easy gardening, or stretching, aim for 60 minutes a day.

Why Muscle Matters

Exercise also helps preserve muscle, and the more muscular you are, the more calories your body will use up, even at rest. If you "diet off" about 8 percent of your body weight over the course of several months without exercising, as much as 40 percent of the weight you lose comes from lean muscle tissue. But if you cut calories and add exercise, only 23 percent of your weight loss will be lean body mass. That means you'll trim more inches from your figure (since fat is less compact than muscle) while also boosting your metabolism (so you'll be able to enjoy an occasional snack).

Researchers at the University of Alabama found that middle-aged adults who worked out with weights three times a week for six months built enough muscle to raise their resting metabolism by 80 to 150 calories a day—about the equivalent of a 20- to 40-minute workout.

You don't have to pump a lot of iron to reach your goal. Using elastic resistance bands, working out in a pool, or climbing hills can provide the resistance you need to build muscle strength. But for the most benefit, do one or two sets of 8 to 12 repetitions for each major muscle group at least twice a week, and try to lift

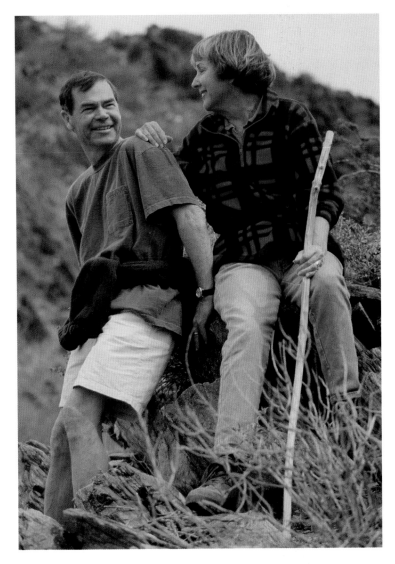

progressively heavier weights. Turn to pages 128 to 133 for a strength-training routine you can do at home.

Secrets to Success

Knowing how to take off pounds is one thing; doing it is another. In order to change your weight, you need to change your ways, which means changing the habits that put on the weight in the first place. Though breaking habits is never easy, psychologist James Prochaska, head of the Health Promotion Part-

Exercise doesn't have to be a chore. Make it a fun part of your lifestyle and you're much more likely to stick with it.

Fast Fact

A pound of muscle burns about 45 calories a day. A pound of fat burns fewer than 2 calories a day.

Fast Fact

If you've gained 10 pounds over a decade and you don't exercise, the problem may be worse than you think. Chances are you've also lost 5 pounds of muscle, which means you've really gained 15 pounds of fat—not 10. And since muscle burns far more calories than fat does, the loss of muscle means you're likely to amass even more weight in the years to come.

DRUG CAPSULE

If your BMI is 27 or more and you have high blood pressure, high cholesterol, or diabetes, your doctor may prescribe a drug to help you kick off your weight-loss plan. Two drugs are available. Sibutramine (Meridia) affects two brain chemicals that regulate appetite. It helps you feel full sooner. Orlistat (Xenical) interferes with a digestive enzyme that breaks down dietary fat so that 30 percent of the fat you eat is never absorbed.

nership at the University of Rhode Island, has identified six stages of successful habit-changing.

1. Precontemplation: In this stage, you're not yet convinced you need to change. Bone up on the pros and cons of your current flab factor and decide if it's really time to shape up.

2. Contemplation: Okay, you've decided that you should trim some inches, but you're not yet committed to taking action. Visualize exactly how your life will improve once you lose weight. Add up the benefits of slimming down—all the gains to your health, vitality, and looks—and get pumped up about the possibilities.

3. Preparation: Readiness is everything. Make a plan for changing your diet and exercise habits that you can stick to. Pick a start date. Set realistic goals for each day and each week, another for the first month and for three months from now. Keep the goals small and specific (for example, buy a food scale, change from 2 percent to 1 percent low-fat milk). Write down a detailed plan, including how you'll deal with each obstacle to your goals. Now add a six-month and a

one-year goal. Announce your intentions to co-workers, friends, and family, and enlist their support.

4. Action: Plan your weekly menus, and write detailed shopping lists. Pack a gym bag. Arrange your home exercise equipment to make it easy to use. Enlist a workout buddy or a lunch partner who shares your goals. Plan satisfying treats, like a piece of your favorite chocolate or a leisurely bubble bath, so you won't feel deprived. Reward yourself for sticking to your plans each day and each week. And be patient: New behaviors can take six months to "groove."

5. Maintenance: Here's where you turn your changes into habits. Mentally shift into a new gear. Research shows that identifying yourself as an exerciser or a healthful eater is important to making your new habits a permanent lifestyle change.

6. Termination: This stage puts the past behind you. You've gained reassurance that a lapse is not a relapse. By now you are truly a healthier person with a different look—and a different outlook—than the one you started with.

Beating the Odds

Your chances of losing weight and keeping it off are probably better than you think. The most widely quoted statistic on weight loss states that more than 90 percent of all dieters gain back the weight they lost. But that figure came from a 1959 survey conducted at a hospital nutrition clinic, as well as from university studies. People who enlist in such research programs tend to have more chronic, hard-core weight problems than the general population. Those who successfully lose weight on their own usually don't get counted in such studies.

That's changing, though. The Weight Control Registry, based at the University of Pittsburgh Medical School in the U.S., has been studying thousands of people who have kept off at least 30 pounds for a year or more. You can do it, too.

The Skinny on Popular Diets

You can hardly turn around today without bumping into a new diet book offering the "answer" to weight loss. Before you hitch your hopes to one of them, ask yourself, "Is this an eating plan I can live with permanently?" If the answer is no, chances are you'll put the weight back on when the diet is done. The best diet is a health-promoting way of eating that you can follow forever. Whatever choices you make, be sure they're balanced and varied. Here's the lowdown on some popular weight-loss approaches.

WEIGHT-LOSS TACTIC	PROS	CONS	COMMENTS
Low-fat, high-fiber *Eat More, Weigh Less* *The 20/30 Fat & Fiber Diet* *Volumetrics*	■ Most widely endorsed by experts.	■ Diets that advocate very low fat content (less than 10 percent) may lead to deficiencies of healthful fats and can be impractical because they are overly restrictive.	■ Some people have had great success with these diets. The less extreme versions of this approach (like Volumetrics) reflect the most current scientific findings.
High-protein, low-carbohydrate *The 5-Day Miracle Diet* *Sugar Busters* *Dr. Atkins' New Diet Revolution* *The Zone*	■ You are likely to lose weight fairly quickly on these diets.	■ Rigid and restrictive. Most people soon tire of eating burgers without buns and hardly any fruits or vegetables. ■ Nutritionally unbalanced. High-protein diets are often low in vegetables and whole grains—important sources of essential vitamins, minerals, and glucose (the primary source of energy for the brain and nervous system). ■ Potentially dangerous. When the body is forced to burn fats instead of glucose for fuel, it produces ketones, fat-burning compounds that tax the kidneys and leach calcium from bones. Eventually this can lead to bad breath, nausea, vomiting, confusion, unconsciousness, even death. Some of the diets emphasize foods high in cholesterol and saturated fats—the fats that clog your arteries—and skimp on calcium and disease-fighting plant nutrients.	■ Although some people have success with these diets, use them with caution. Initial weight loss is due to water loss when carbohydrates are drastically reduced, then as a result of calorie restriction, not from eating fewer carbohydrates. But there is some evidence that your protein needs do increase when you restrict calories.
Base your diet on your blood type *Eat Right for Your Type*	■ None.	■ Nutritionally unbalanced. Depending on your blood type, you're advised to shun certain food groups and compensate for nutritional losses with supplements. For example, people with type O blood are told to eat animal protein (except dairy) and to avoid grains.	■ This approach is not based on sound science. There is no substantiation of the supposed link between blood type and digestion.

Eating for Losers

It's not just about eating less—it's about eating differently. More fiber, less fat, and, yes, smaller servings should make up your new notion of nourishment.

Trimming your meals doesn't just mean cutting calories from them. Although calorie counting works for some people, it's tedious, and there are other ways to streamline your diet without making yourself crazy. If you stop to apply the following tactics to every meal you plan, you'll automatically cut down on calories—without any superhuman sacrifices.

1 Add More Fiber

In one study reported in the *Journal of the American Medical Association*, people who ate a high-fiber diet over a 10-year period gained the least weight, regardless of how much fat they consumed. By slowing the absorption of nutrients into the bloodstream, fiber helps curb insulin production after a meal. The higher insulin levels associated with low-fiber diets seem to help promote weight gain by stimulating fat storage and increasing appetite.

Health Canada recommends eating 25 to 35 grams of fiber a day. According to Dietitians of Canada, the average Canadian intake is 13 to 15 grams a day. By contrast, studies conducted in rural Africa, where obesity is rare, found that the Africans consume about 80 grams of fiber daily. Boosting your intake by even a few grams a day may make a difference: An English study found that lean adults averaged 19 grams of fiber daily, while obese adults averaged only 13.

Another benefit of fiber is that it may help you feel fuller longer. To test this hypothesis, researchers fed overweight subjects 350 calories of oatmeal or cornflakes, then three hours later allowed them to drink as much as they wanted of a nutritional shake. The people who ate oatmeal, which is higher in fiber, sipped 40 percent less of the shake than the cornflake eaters.

So stock up on high-fiber foods, and try to turn your thinking upside down: Make fresh and cooked vegetables and fruits, as well as whole grains and beans, the stars of your meals. Relegate meat and poultry to a supporting role as often as possible.

2 Fool Your Eye— And Your Stomach

Some experts believe that people tend to eat the same amount of food in weight every day, regardless of the food's fat or calorie content. So concentrate on eating bulky foods that

7 Easy Ways to Eat More Fiber

INSTEAD OF EATING:	FIBER (IN GRAMS)	EAT THIS:	FIBER (IN GRAMS)
Total Corn Flakes	0	Fiber One	13
Farina	0	Quaker Oat Bran	6
Plain bagel	0	Low-fat bran muffin	4
Medium cantaloupe	1	Medium orange	7
Progresso Hearty Tomato soup	1	Progresso Hearty Black Bean soup	10
1 white pita bread	.3	1 whole wheat pita bread	4.4
1 slice white bread	0	1 slice whole-wheat bread	2

100-Calorie Chinese Chicken Soup

You can make a delicious vegetarian version of this soup by substituting tofu for the chicken and vegetable broth for the chicken broth.

Makes 4 servings.

- **8 ounces boneless, skinned chicken breast halves, cut into bite-size pieces**
- **2 teaspoons soy sauce**
- **½ teaspoon Oriental sesame oil**
- **2 cans (14½ ounces each) fat-free, reduced-sodium chicken broth**
- **2 large cloves garlic, finely chopped**
- **¼ teaspoon Chinese five-spice powder**
- **1 small carrot, pared and thinly sliced**
- **2 cups shredded spinach leaves (thick stems removed)**
- **2 green onions, thinly sliced**

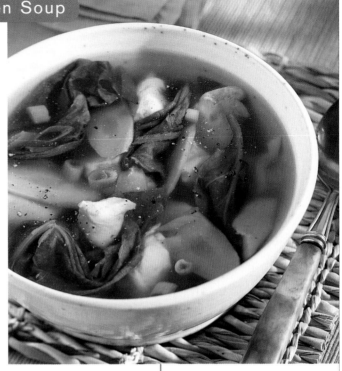

1. In a small bowl, toss the chicken with the soy sauce and sesame oil. Set aside for 5 minutes.

2. In a large saucepan, heat the broth, garlic, and five-spice powder to a boil over medium heat.

3. Add the chicken with its juices and the carrot. Reduce the heat to medium-low and simmer for 5 minutes. Stir in the spinach and green onions. Simmer 1 minute longer. Serve hot.

NUTRITION INFORMATION *Per Serving:* 90 calories, 13 g protein, 4 g carbohydrate, 1 g fiber, 2 g fat, 0 g saturated fat, 31 mg cholesterol, 766 mg sodium

---

are high in nutrition (not calories) relative to their weight. That means foods that contain plenty of fiber, water, and/or air.

For example, instead of eating a handful of calorie-dense raisins, choose water-dense grapes. Instead of a compact slab of meat or cheese, opt for a plateful of beans and vegetables. If you make pasta salad, pile it high with vegetables to lower its energy density. Instead of french fries, try whipping up some winter squash with skim milk. Make chili with an emphasis on fiber-rich beans and vegetables instead of ground beef. Snack on light, unbuttered, air-popped popcorn (sprinkled with garlic salt) rather than calorie-dense potato chips or nuts.

3 Downsize Your Portions

We live in the era of "super-sizing." Burgers are whoppers, and movie popcorn comes in jumbo-size tubs. Marketers realize that super-sizing sells more food. And studies show that people will eat more when presented with a bigger portion. So while economy-size packaging may seem to spare your wallet, it certainly won't spare your waistline.

SimpleSolution

Keep a food diary. Several studies show that recording what you eat is the best predictor of successful weight loss. It helps you become more aware of how much you eat and track the situations that trigger overeating.

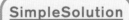

North Americans consistently underestimate the number of calories they consume by as much as 25 to 50 percent.

To combat the negative effects of this bigger-is-better sell, we have to retrain our brains. Studies show that we routinely underestimate our caloric intake by as much as 25 to 50 percent.

Even nutrition students can be fooled. Marion Nestle, chair of the Department of Nutrition and Food Studies at New York University, and her colleague Lisa Young conducted a study in which college students taking a nutrition course were told to bring in a bagel, baked potato, muffin, or cookie that they considered medium in size. The students then compared these foods to the U.S. Department of Agriculture (USDA) serving sizes. The results: A typical potato weighed 7 ounces, whereas one serving of potato according to the USDA is 4 ounces. A medium bagel was 4 ounces, or two servings. A typical muffin was almost 6 ounces, or three servings.

If you look at food labels to track what you eat, make sure you take into account how many servings the package contains. Often something that looks like one serving is actually labeled as two, so if you eat the whole thing, don't forget to double the calories listed.

Restaurants are perhaps the biggest offenders when it comes to oversize portions. One survey found that the average restaurant portion of spaghetti with tomato sauce measured $3\frac{1}{2}$ cups and contained 849 calories. Since Health Canada bases its Food Guide Rainbow guidelines for pasta on $\frac{1}{2}$ cup per "serving," this would equal seven of its servings—enough of that entire food group (bread, rice, cereal, and pasta) for a whole day. Solution? Ask the waiter to put half the meal into a doggie bag before you start eating.

4 Cook It Smart

Whether you're cooking at home, eating out, or ordering in, it's not just what and how much you eat but how the food is prepared that counts. Here are the leanest cooking methods—and the ones to avoid.

Smarter Snacking

North Americans love to nibble. In fact, we eat an average of three snacks a day. While there's nothing wrong with snacking per se, all too often we fill up on high-calorie, high-fat snack foods, then either skimp on meals and lose out on nutrition or eat regular-size meals and overdo our total calorie intake.

There is a way to snack smartly: Choose nutritious snacks and think of them as part of your daily food intake rather than as "extras." This will satisfy your cravings and also help you meet your nutrition needs. Instead of potato chips, try a piece of fruit, or give one of these ideas a whirl.

SNACK	CALORIES
8 ounces tomato juice	40
5 fat-free saltines	60
1 frozen fruit juice bar (no sugar added)	25
3 cups plain, air-popped popcorn	55
13 mini pretzels	100
6 baked tortilla chips	110
4 tablespoons salsa	20
4 ounces fat-free chocolate pudding	100
½ cup applesauce	80
1 cup plain, low-fat yogurt with ½ cup strawberries	170
8 medium-size baby carrots	30

Avoid these treats—they may seem light, but they pack a high-calorie wallop:

1 small croissant	230
3 cups buttered popcorn	210
1-ounce bag potato chips	150
1-ounce bag cheese puffs	155

Tex-Mex Black and White Bean Salad

Fool your eyes and stomach with this satisfying dish high in fiber and water.

Makes 4 servings (about 6 cups).

1   clove garlic, halved

1   can (15 ounces) black beans, drained and rinsed

1   can (15 ounces) white beans, drained and rinsed

1   can (8.25 ounces) no-salt-added whole kernel corn, drained and rinsed

1   small jalapeño chile, cored, seeded, and finely chopped

2   ripe tomatoes (about 8 ounces each), cored, halved horizontally, seeded, and diced (about 2 cups)

1   cucumber, peeled, seeded, and diced

2   scallions, trimmed and finely chopped (about ¼ cup)

1½ teaspoons ground cumin

1   teaspoon salt

¼   teaspoon black pepper

3-4 tablespoons lime juice (3 to 4 limes)

¼   cup chopped fresh cilantro (coriander)

4   packed cups shredded romaine lettuce, from 1 head

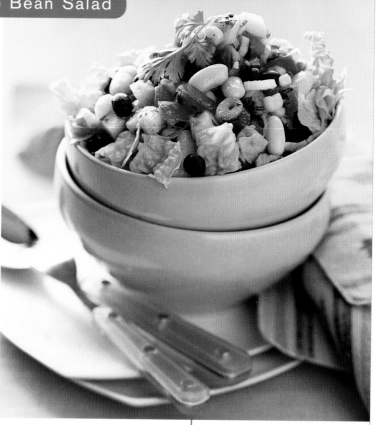

1. Rub a large bowl with the cut garlic. In the bowl, fold together the beans, corn, chile, tomatoes, cucumber, scallions, cumin, salt, and pepper. Fold in the lime juice, to taste.

2. Just before serving, fold in the cilantro. For each serving, spread 1 packed cup shredded romaine lettuce on a plate, and spoon about 1½ cups of the salad over the romaine.

NUTRITION INFORMATION *Per Serving:* 189 calories, 10 g protein, 37 g carbohydrate, 10 g fiber, 2 g fat, 0 g saturated fat, 0 mg cholesterol, 217 mg sodium

Best Ways

Baking: Keep fat to a minimum and boost flavor by pouring wine, fruit juice (such as orange or apple juice), or even tea over fish, squash, or potatoes before baking.

Broiling: Use soy sauce, fruit juice, water, or even melted fruit preserves to baste meat or fish instead of oil or butter when broiling.

Grilling: Let the fat drip off your meat. Avoid oil-based marinades. Try wrapping seasoned food in foil packets so it steams in its own juices and stays moist as it cooks.

Microwaving: This quick-cooking method preserves the flavors and essential nutrients contained in vegetables and fruits.

Poaching: Poach in broth, wine, or

SimpleSolution

Before you eat, ask yourself, "Am I hungry?" If the honest answer is no, then find another activity to satisfy your need. The calories you eat when you're not hungry are processed differently than the ones you eat when you are. They are more likely to be stored as fat than used as energy.

fruit juice and season the poaching liquid with herbs for even more flavor. This is the tastiest and leanest way to cook fish, fowl, or fruit desserts. It's great for eggs, too.

Pressure cooking: Ideal for beans, grains, soups, stews, and dried vegetables. Chill soups after cooking, then skim the fat away.

Roasting: Brings out a toasty or caramel flavor in vegetables and grains. Use a rack to let fat run off meat, fowl, or fish.

Sautéing: Prepare your food without adding fat by substituting a bit of water, wine, or broth for oil.

Steaming: Use a steamer basket to prevent nutrients from leaching into the water.

Stewing/braising: This slow-cooking method allows meat to give off fat. Chill the dish after cooking, then skim the fat away.

Good Ways

Boiling: You'll trim calories with this cooking method, but you'll also lose water-soluble nutrients, especially if the food is chopped. Try boiling whole potatoes in their skins. Use boil-in-bag vegetables (choose a brand without butter or cream sauce).

Cider-Baked Acorn Squash with Apple Stuffing

With its high water content, squash provides bulk without the calories, but with plenty of nutrients. You can make this sweet, satisfying side dish with butternut or dumpling squash instead of acorn, but you may have to adjust the cooking time.

Makes 4 servings.

2   **small acorn squash (about 1 pound each), halved lengthwise and seeded**

$1/2$ **cup apple cider or apple juice**

$1/2$ **teaspoon salt**

1   **apple pared, cored, and chopped**

1   **tablespoon light-brown sugar**

$1/4$ **teaspoon cinnamon**

$1/8$ **teaspoon nutmeg**

1. Preheat the oven to 350° F.

2. Place the squash halves cut-side down in a 13 x 9-inch baking dish. Add the cider to the pan.

3. Bake in the preheated oven for 30 minutes. Remove the pan from the oven and leave the oven on. Carefully turn the squash cut-side up and sprinkle with salt.

4. Combine the apple, sugar, cinnamon, and nutmeg in a small bowl. Spoon this mixture evenly into the squash halves. Drizzle the cider from the baking pan over the mixture, using a baster if you have one. Add a couple of spoonfuls of water to the pan.

5. Bake the squash, stuffed-side up, for 30 minutes longer or until tender.

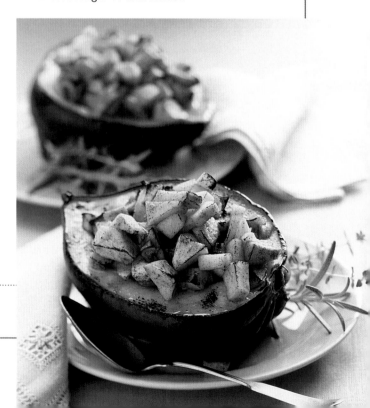

NUTRITION INFORMATION *Per Serving:* 123 calories, 2 g protein, 32 g carbohydrate, 7 g fiber, 0 g fat, 0 g saturated fat, 0 mg cholesterol, 298 mg sodium

Foil-Baked Salmon with Lemon and Dill

You can prepare the foil packets earlier in the day and refrigerate them until ready to bake. A 1-inch-thick fillet takes about 10 minutes to cook through. Thinner fillets cook in less time and thicker fillets take a couple of minutes longer. Add 2 or 3 minutes to baking time if the packets are baked cold from the refrigerator.

Makes 4 servings.

- 4   salmon fillets (6 ounces each)
- $1/2$ teaspoon salt
- $1/8$ teaspoon pepper
- $1/4$ cup finely chopped green onion
- $1/4$ cup finely chopped fresh dill or 2 tablespoons dried dill
- 8   thin slices lemon
- $1/4$ cup water, fish bouillon, or chicken broth

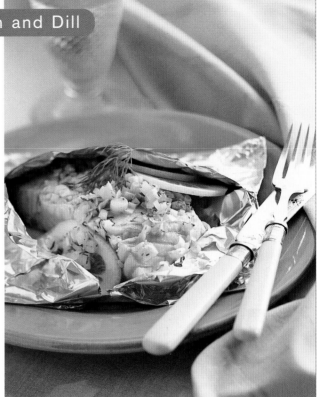

1. Place a baking sheet on the middle rack in the oven and preheat the oven to 400° F.

2. Tear off 8 sheets of aluminum foil, each 12 x 12 inches. Using double layers of foil, place a salmon fillet in the center of each foil square. Sprinkle evenly with salt and pepper. Combine the green onion and dill in a small cup. Sprinkle evenly over the fillets. Top with lemon slices. Drizzle each fillet with 1 tablespoon of the water, bouillon, or broth.

3. Seal each packet by bringing two opposite sides of the foil up and over the fish. Fold the edges over twice, then fold the side edges twice. Place the packets on the preheated baking sheet.

4. Bake for 10 to 15 minutes, depending on the thickness of the fillets. Before serving, partially open the packet to check that the center of the fish is cooked through.

5. To serve, place each packet on a dinner plate and allow diners to open their own packets. Or transfer the contents of the packets to the plates and serve at once.

NUTRITION INFORMATION *Per Serving:* 192 calories, 32 g protein, 2 g carbohydrate, 1 g fiber, 6 g fat, 1 g saturated fat, 83 mg cholesterol, 399 mg sodium

---

Stir-frying: Use this quick-cooking method to seal in the flavor of vegetables, tofu, meats, or fowl. Minimize fat by using a little bit of water or stock instead of oil.

Worst Ways

Deep frying: Avoid this high-fat disaster. If you must deep fry, drain the food well on paper towels.
Pan frying: Cut back on fat by using

nonstick pans, spraying pans with nonstick cooking spray, or wiping a small bit of oil onto the pan with a paper towel for an ultralight coating.
Overgrilling: Avoid barbecuing foods to a crisp. When you allow the fat from meats or marinades to drip onto hot coals, the resulting smoky, charred bits contain dangerous carcinogens. Trim fat from meats, and move food away from open flames.

Fast Fact

Just 50 excess calories a day will increase your weight by 50 pounds over a 10-year period. On the other hand, cut 100 calories a day (the amount in one tablespoon of mayonnaise) and you'll lose 7 pounds in a year.

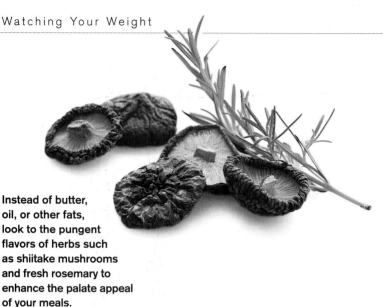

Instead of butter, oil, or other fats, look to the pungent flavors of herbs such as shiitake mushrooms and fresh rosemary to enhance the palate appeal of your meals.

Do Your Meals a Favor by Adding Flavor

The more flavorful a dish, the less fat it needs to taste good. Here are six surefire ways to please your palate.

1 Build your menu around fresh seasonal fruits and vegetables at their peak of ripeness, and their flavor will stand alone.

2 Choose recipes that highlight your favorite herbs and spices, either fresh or dried.

Chicken Stir-Fry with Broccoli and Tomatoes

You can substitute lean slices of beef or pork loin for the chicken, and sweet red or yellow peppers for the tomato, if you like. If you use sweet peppers, add them to the skillet at the same time as the broccoli. Serve this dish with brown rice or buckwheat noodles.

Makes 4 servings.

- 2 teaspoons canola oil or other vegetable oil
- 1/4 teaspoon salt
- 1 pound boneless chicken breast, cut into 1-inch cubes
- 1 tablespoon soy sauce
- 2 teaspoons finely chopped garlic
- 1 teaspoon finely chopped fresh gingerroot or 1/4 teaspoon ground ginger
- 3 cups broccoli flowerets
- 1 cup reduced-sodium chicken broth
- 1 tablespoon cornstarch
- 4 firm-ripe plum tomatoes, quartered lengthwise

1. Heat the oil and the salt in a 12-inch nonstick skillet or wok. When the oil is very hot, add the chicken breast and stir-fry for 3 minutes. Add the soy sauce, garlic, and ginger and stir well.

2. Add the broccoli, then slowly add 1/2 cup of the chicken broth. Cover and cook for 2 to 3 minutes or until the broccoli is just tender.

3. Meanwhile, mix the cornstarch into the remaining broth until dissolved. Stir the tomatoes and the cornstarch mixture into the skillet. Simmer for 2 minutes or until the sauce thickens and clears. Serve hot.

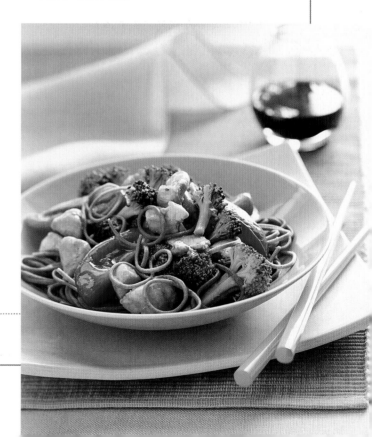

NUTRITION INFORMATION *Per Serving:* 190 calories, 26 g protein, 9 g carbohydrate, 2 g fiber, 6 g fat, 1 g saturated fat, 64 mg cholesterol, 504 mg sodium

Fruit Parfait with Ginger Tea Cream

More volume than calories, this milky gelatin dessert is fun to make with fruity herbal teas such as lemon, orange, or berry flavor, or with aromatic teas such as jasmine, black currant, or Earl Grey.

Makes 4 servings.

2   **cups skim milk**
1   **envelope unflavored gelatin**
2   **ginger herbal tea bags**
3   **tablespoons sugar**
$^1/_8$ **teaspoon salt**
4   **cups mixed fruit such as cantaloupe cubes, sliced strawberries, and blueberries**

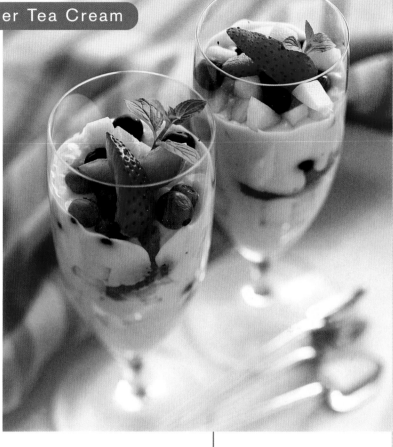

1. In a large saucepan, bring 1 cup of the milk to a boil. Meanwhile, place the remaining 1 cup of milk in a small bowl. Sprinkle the gelatin over the cold milk. Set aside for 5 minutes or until the gelatin softens.

2. Add the tea bags, sugar, salt, and softened gelatin mixture to the boiling milk, stirring with each addition. Remove from heat and stir for 1 minute to dissolve the gelatin and sugar. Set aside for 3 minutes to allow the tea to steep.

3. Let the milk mixture cool to room temperature, then refrigerate for 1 to 1½ hours or until it begins to set. Spoon ¼ cup of the tea cream into each of four large wine goblets or dessert cups. Top with fruit and remaining tea cream. Refrigerate at least 1 to 2 hours longer, until the tea cream is set and chilled.

NUTRITION INFORMATION *Per Serving:* 144 calories, 7 g protein, 30 g carbohydrate, 3 g fiber, 1 g fat, 0 g saturated fat, 2 mg cholesterol, 146 mg sodium

3 Add chopped onion or garlic to your dish for an extra flavor note—and added health benefits. Roasting these vegetables is a good way to bring out their sweetness and soften their bite.

4 Add a splash of wine, sherry, or vinegar to sauces to add flavor without adding fat. Simmer sauces slowly until reduced to concentrate and intensify their taste.

5 Use soaked dried mushrooms to add texture and a distinctive accent to savory dishes. The soaking liquid makes a delicious addition to soup stock.

6 Stir miso (fermented soybean paste) into soups, stews, and dressings, or use it in sauces for stir-fried vegetables or noodles. You can find miso in the refrigerated section of your grocery store.

SimpleSolution

Want to eat less junk? Keep it out of sight. In one study, when the lid stayed on the ice cream cooler in a large hospital cafeteria, only 3 percent of obese subjects and 5 percent of normal-weight subjects chose ice cream. When the lid came off, the numbers rose to 17 and 16 percent. The same principle works in reverse, so keep a bowl of fresh fruit out on the counter for snacking.

YOUR GAME PLAN FOR GOOD HEALTH

20 Easy Weight-Loss Tips

Weight loss is not a simple matter, but there are many simple things you can do to help make it happen. Here are 20 of them.

1 Drink water. People often mistake thirst for hunger, so next time you feel like noshing, reach for water first. Drinking also helps you feel full. Some experts suggest sipping water (or iced tea) just before you sit down to a meal. Continue drinking as you eat to add volume and weight to your meal.

2 Set realistic goals. One or two pounds a week maximum is doable. Top weight-loss programs advocate stopping after the first 10 pounds and maintaining that loss for about six months before trying to lose any more.

3 Build in splurges. If you allow yourself to eat whatever you want for 2 meals out of every 21, you won't inflict enough damage to subvert your weight loss. And you'll feel less deprived.

4 Count to 10. Studies suggest that the average craving lasts only about 10 minutes. So before caving in to your urge, set your mental timer for a 10-minute time-out. Use the time to tackle an item on your to-do list; choose one that will give you a sense of accomplishment—and get you out of the kitchen.

5 Eat more often. People who have kept their weight off for more than a few years tend to eat an average of five times a day. Light, frequent meals curb your appetite, boost your energy, improve your mood, and even speed your metabolism, since the process of digestion itself burns calories.

6 Make weekly resolutions. Don't try to overhaul your diet overnight. If you make too many changes at once, chances are you'll get frustrated and throw in the towel. Instead, make one change, such as eating at least one piece of fruit daily, every week.

7 Start with 10 percent. People who start by focusing on achieving just 10 percent of their long-range weight-loss goal may have the best chance of ultimate success. Losing those first pounds yields the biggest health gains, too, since belly fat is usually the first to come off and is the most dangerous.

At restaurants, order some light appetizers rather than a main course, or share an entree and add an extra salad (with low-fat dressing on the side).

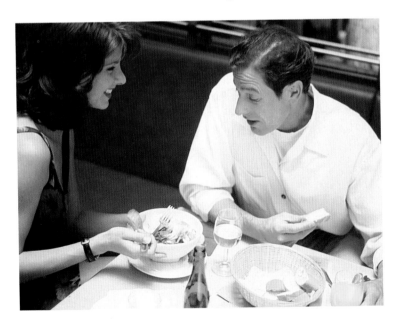

What's Your Dietary Downfall?

Most people have an Achilles' heel when it comes to weight control. What's yours? Here is some advice on how to overcome common problems.

PROBLEM	SOLUTION
You can't resist snacking. 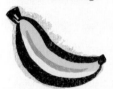	■ Don't worry—snacking isn't forbidden. Snacks can help control your appetite. Just don't add snacks to three full meals a day. Instead, break your meals into smaller portions and eat them over the day as snacks. For example, save half a banana from your breakfast cereal and eat it midday. When the snacking urge strikes, reach for cut veggies, low-fat yogurt, whole-grain crackers, air-popped popcorn, or pretzels. (See Smarter Snacking, page 76.)
You love your junk food.	■ Give in—a little! Thinking of foods as "good" or "bad" often creates more problems than it solves. Depriving yourself will simply trigger the urge to overeat something else. Any food is okay in moderation. When you treat yourself to a small portion occasionally, it can reward you for keeping up your healthier habits.
There's no time to cook.	■ Take advantage of pre-cut, frozen, or canned veggies. Add frozen vegetables or canned beans to your favorite canned soup to make an instant, filling meal. Buy pre-washed salad-in-a-bag. Cook ahead on the weekend, or just double the ingredients of your Sunday-night supper. Freeze serving-size portions so they'll be quicker to thaw and reheat. And don't forget the microwave. A baked potato topped with broccoli, for instance, takes only a few minutes to make.
You eat when you're stressed. 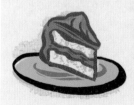	■ Boredom, fatigue, depression, and stress are common triggers for eating too much. To break the hand-to-mouth habit, look for other ways to address your needs. If you're tired, try a brisk walk (or a nap if possible). If you're having a tough day, call a friend or write in your journal. If you're feeling down, try renting a funny movie. Or, once in a while, save your favorite treat for just such a situation. Dietitians of Canada can help you find a dietitian who knows all about the emotional side of eating. Call 416-596-0857 or go to www.dietitians.ca.
Your family won't give up their french fries.	■ Start by letting your family know how important it is to you right now to maintain a healthy diet, and enlist their support. Then make sure there is at least one healthy food at every meal, and serve yourself a hearty portion of it while skimping on the rest. Also, doctor your menus in ways your family won't notice, such as using evaporated skim milk instead of cream in sauces and thickening "cream" soups with puréed potato. Finally, try baking thin potato slices coated with oil as an alternative to those french fries.

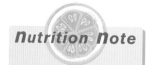

Nutrition Note

The worst diet tactics:
- Omitting entire food groups
- High-fat diets
- Any diet that lacks variety, balance, and moderation

YOUR GAME PLAN FOR GOOD HEALTH

8 Spike your meals with salsa. This spicy condiment can stand in for mayo to deliver plenty of flavor without the fat. Mix it with a bit of low-fat yogurt to make tuna salad. Spread it on a veggie burger, or serve it with chicken or fish.

9 Take one-third off. When you eat dinner out, reduce the temptation to clean your plate by setting aside one-third of your meal. Ask the server for a doggie bag, and take it home for lunch the next day. Try serving yourself one-third less at home, too. This simple tactic could subtract more than 500 calories a day.

10 Go easy on the alcohol. Remember that alcohol is a source of calories. A 12-ounce beer has about 150 calories; a 3.5-ounce glass of wine, around 85. A margarita packs a bigger caloric punch. Even worse offenders are creamy cocktails, such as Brandy Alexanders and Mudslides—equivalent to drinking a rich dessert. If you're trying to lose weight, stick with water.

11 Write notes to yourself. To help you stay on track, post notes to yourself on the fridge and the pantry. Put up a little stop sign or make tags with questions like, "Do you want this food enough to wear it?" and "Are the calories worth the consequences?"

12 Stay away from sodas. Soft drinks are a major source of empty calories in the North American diet. We drink twice as much soda as milk and nearly six times more soda than fruit juice. But fluids don't satisfy your appetite as well as solids. A study at Purdue University found that when people were fed 450 calories daily as jelly beans or as soda, the soda drinkers gained a significant amount of weight, but the jelly-bean eaters compensated for the extra calories by cutting back on other food. So if you crave something sweet, you're better off chewing it than gulping it. If you're truly thirsty, reach for water or unsweetened iced tea instead of soda.

13 Don't just eat—dine. Eating on the run or in front of the tube invites mindless munching. Instead, set the table every time you eat. Make a conscious choice to sit down and savor every bite. Placing a portion of chips on your best china helps focus your attention so you don't eat the whole bag.

14 Up your protein (a little). Research suggests that protein prolongs the feeling of fullness better than carbohydrates or fats do. Studies in Scotland, Denmark, Sweden, and England found that people who ate a high-protein breakfast or lunch were less hungry at their next meal. Protein also requires a few more calories to digest. Just don't go overboard. Stick to low-fat protein sources like low-fat yogurt or cottage cheese, low-fat soy drinks or snacks, or thinly sliced turkey breast.

15 Learn how to measure. It's easy to misjudge portion sizes. Pull out the measuring spoons and cups, especially for full-fat salad dressings, dairy foods, and mayo.

16 Make smart substitutions. Look for nutritious low-calorie alternatives to sugary, high-fat treats. Try frozen grapes instead of candy.

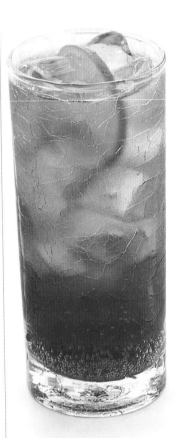

Are you hooked on soda? Try this fizzy substitute instead: Mix one part cranberry juice to three parts seltzer, and top it off with a squeeze of fresh lime.

Use air-popped popcorn instead of oil-popped. Dip fresh strawberries in fat-free fudge sauce for a sensuous chocolaty treat.

17 Have a "party plan." When attending a party, offer to bring a plate. Arriving armed with chopped fresh veggies and a low-fat dip—or any other low-calorie snack—ensures that you'll have something to snack on without feeling guilty.

18 Think positively. Experts note that low self-esteem is a major cause of overeating. Train yourself to focus on your best points rather than your weak spots. Buy clothes that fit and flatter you at your current weight. Update your hairstyle and get a makeup consultation so you feel attractive today.

19 Give yourself a break. No one says you have to reach your goal without making mistakes along the way. Tell yourself you can succeed in losing weight by taking things one step at a time and starting fresh whenever you slip up. If you overeat one night, just get back on track in the morning by focusing on what's worked for you in the past.

20 Relax! Some people binge when they're stressed. A Yale University study found that women who secreted the most cortisol (a hormone released during stress) ate the most high-fat food after stress. The combination of cortisol and insulin prompts the body to store fat in preparation for possible starvation—just what you don't need. If stress has a stronghold on your life, try learning yoga, meditation, or simple breathing exercises.

7 Light Meals to Make in 20 Minutes

- **Stuffed Baked Potato** Microwave a large potato, then split it and fill it with steamed vegetables mixed with low-fat sour cream and a pinch of garlic salt or chopped fresh herbs.
- **Nicoise Salad** Layer a bed of lettuce with sliced tomatoes and sliced boiled or microwaved potatoes. Arrange blanched green beans, canned tuna, halved hard-boiled eggs, and anchovies (optional) on top, and drizzle with low-fat vinaigrette.
- **Grilled Chicken Pita** Slit and fill a whole-wheat pita round with sliced, grilled, or broiled chicken breast, lettuce and tomato, and a sauce of spicy salsa mixed with low-fat mayonnaise.
- **Easy Vegetable Pasta** Sauté chopped peppers, zucchini, onions, and fresh tomatoes until soft. Add prepared tomato pasta sauce and a handful of torn basil leaves. When warm, serve over pasta and top with a sprinkle of Parmesan cheese.
- **Mediterranean Chicken Wrap** Prepare a mixture of chopped, cooked chicken breast, fresh alfalfa sprouts or spinach, tomato, chopped peppers, sun-dried tomatoes, and mozzarella cheese. Place it on a large tortilla. Drizzle with low-fat balsamic vinaigrette and wrap tortilla around filling, tucking in the sides to make a long package.
- **Spicy Turkey Quesadilla** Top a large flour tortilla with strips of sliced smoked turkey, finely diced tomato, chopped fresh cilantro (coriander), and reduced-fat cheddar or Monterey Jack cheese. Drizzle on your favorite hot sauce, then place another tortilla on top. Heat in an oven or toaster oven until cheese is melted, then cut into wedges and serve with low-fat sour cream and more hot sauce if desired.
- **Grilled Vegetable and Goat Cheese Sandwich** Brush sliced eggplant, peppers, and mushrooms with olive oil, and grill or broil until cooked through. Sprinkle the vegetables with balsamic vinegar and pile on a slice of toasted bread that has been spread with goat cheese.

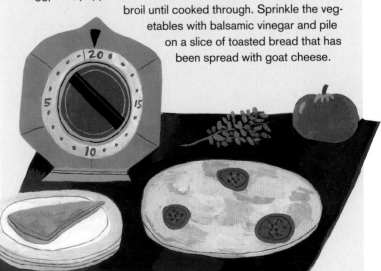

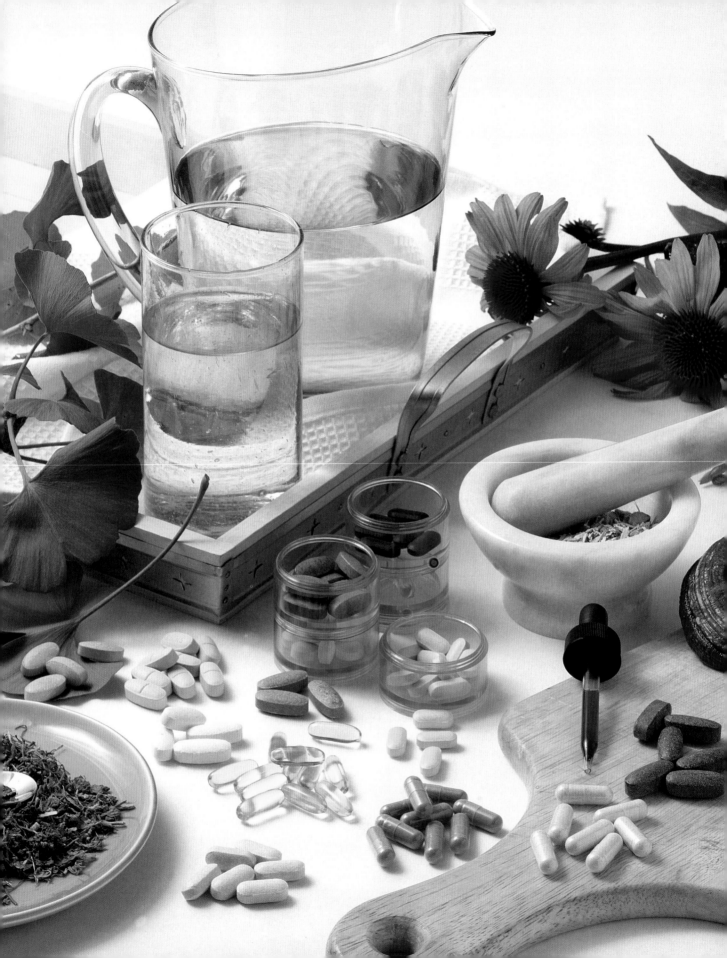

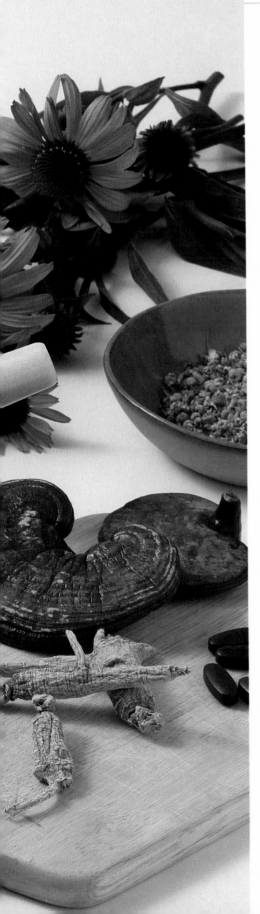

CHAPTER 3

THE ROLE OF SUPPLEMENTS

Using Vitamins and Minerals

Can nutritional supplements really help you live longer? Here's the true story on their benefits—and limitations.

sn't a healthy diet supposed to take care of all your nutritional needs? Theoretically, yes. No supplement can ever begin to replace a sound diet. But chances are, you could use a little help from supplements. According to one survey, people from Quebec average just 4 servings of fruits and vegetables a day. Nova Scotians fare even worse. Surveys show they consume about 140 grams of vegeta-bles and 164 grams of fruit a day. Even if you eat the recommended 5 to 10 servings of fruits and vegeta-bles a day, you still might benefit from supplements, perhaps because you're among the 20 percent or so of North Americans who are dieting, or because high stress levels or smoking is causing your body to consume antioxidants faster than normal.

Scientists are learning that even mild deficiencies of many vitamins and minerals may increase your risk for a variety of ailments—a strong argument for taking a daily multivit-amin, no matter what your eating habits. Preliminary findings show that a multivitamin and mineral tablet may, for example:

- boost immunity
- help counter depression
- lower high blood pressure
- provide protection against heart attacks and strokes.

You may also benefit from individual supplements, depending on your circum-stances. The people who fall into one of the following categories are good candi-dates for either a mul-tivitamin or additional sup-plements.

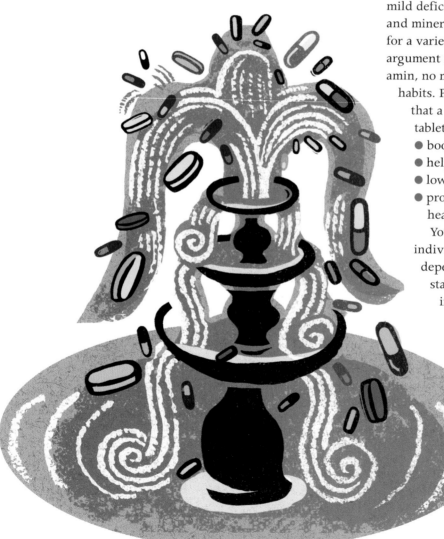

Are supplements the fountain of youth? Not exactly. But they can probably boost your health and maybe even help you live longer.

Do you skimp on fruits and vegetables? A supplement can never replace the hundreds of nutrients in fresh produce, but it may prevent a vitamin or mineral deficiency. Take a multivitamin, and start adding one serving of fruit or vegetables daily until you reach at least five a day.

Do you avoid dairy foods? Unless you really love collard greens, kale, canned sardines or salmon with bones, or calcium-fortified orange juice, you're probably not getting the recommended 1,000 to 1,500 mg of calcium you need. Take a 500 or 600 mg calcium tablet twice a day. (See page 94 for advice on choosing a calcium supplement.)

Are you a vegetarian? Depending on how strict a vegetarian you are, you may or may not need supplements. If you eat no animal products at all, you may fall short on vitamin B_{12} and zinc; if so, a multivitamin will cover you. If you don't eat dairy foods, follow the advice above.

Do you smoke? If you smoke, your body uses up more vitamin C, which is mobilized to fight the cancer-causing effects of tobacco. The government recommends getting 35 extra mg on top of the Dietary Reference Intakes (DRIs) of 75 mg for women and 90 mg for men, but many scientists suggest higher levels. Unless you eat a lot of foods rich in vitamin C, supplement with 250 to 500 mg of C daily.

Are you exposed to passive smoke? Studies show that inhaling second-hand smoke lowers your blood levels of vitamin C, although not as much as if you yourself smoked. No recommendations have been set for people who breathe in passive smoke, but, to be on the safe side, follow the recommendation for smokers.

Are you a woman who might become pregnant? If you are, you should take 400 IU of folic acid a day. This B vitamin helps prevent neural tube defects that affect between 2 and 4 of every 1,000 babies born in Canada. Folic acid supplements are better absorbed by the body than the vitamin (called folate) found in food.

Are you over 60? After age 60, your ability to absorb certain vitamins from food may decline because your stomach may start producing less acid. At the same time, your needs for certain nutrients, such as vitamin D and B_6, increase. Many people over age 60 have a particular problem absorbing vitamin B_{12} from food; your doctor can determine if you do and will prescribe supplements if that's the case. B_{12} is important for keeping your immune system functioning efficiently. Deficiencies of this vitamin may contribute to depression and may affect concentration and memory.

Vitamin D requirements shoot up after age 70 to 600 IU, more than some multivitamins provide. Canadian researchers recommend taking calcium and vitamin D supplements if you are over age 70 and your diet does not provide adequate amounts. As well, everyone over 70 should take a B_{12} supplement or eat foods fortified with B_{12}.

Are you a chronic medication user? The following medications affect the absorption or retention of certain nutrients. If you regularly take any

---

Fast Fact

Vitamin C may help lower blood pressure, according to a study at Oregon State University. People with high-normal blood pressure or stage 1 hypertension who took 500 mg of vitamin C experienced an average drop of 9 percent in systolic pressure (the first of the two blood pressure readings) and a smaller drop in diastolic pressure.

SimpleSolution

If you take any of the fat-soluble vitamins (A, D, E, or K), take them with the fattiest meal of the day (usually dinner) for better absorption.

Fast Fact

If you're a smoker, you may have heard that taking beta-carotene supplements can increase your risk for cancer. But don't worry about the amount of beta-carotene found in your multivitamin. The level is only a fraction of the amount (20 to 30 mg) taken by the smokers in the studies.

If you are over age 60, you may be a good candidate for supplements of vitamin B$_{12}$. To find out, ask your doctor to check your blood levels of this vitamin, important to mood, memory, and immunity.

of them, ask your doctor if you need a supplement beyond a multivitamin.

- **Antihypertensives** that contain hydralazine can diminish levels of vitamin B$_6$.
- **Anticonvulsants** that contain phenytoin, such as Dilantin, can diminish folate and vitamin D.
- **Antacids** that contain aluminum hydroxide can deplete phosphate, vitamin D, and folate. Chronic antacid use may decrease stomach acid to the point of interfering with the absorption of vitamin B$_{12}$, especially if you're over 60.
- **Cholesterol-lowering drugs** that contain cholestyramine bind with fat and deplete the fat-soluble vitamins A, E, D, and K, as well as B$_{12}$ and folate.
- **Diuretics** that contain thiazide or furosemide deplete potassium, zinc, and magnesium.
- **Glucocorticoids** decrease calcium absorption and increase the excretion of calcium into the urine.
- **Laxatives** Mineral oil depletes fat-soluble vitamins, calcium, and phosphorus. Stimulant laxatives such as bisacodyl and phenolphthalein deplete calcium and vitamin D. You're better off with a fiber-based bulk-forming laxative.

Do you drink heavily? Since alcohol depletes nearly every nutrient, especially the B vitamins, a multivitamin is in order. The tricky part is that alco-

holism alters the normal metabolism of certain vitamins, such as vitamin A, depleting it in some tissues and increasing it in others, so taking too much can be toxic to some organs. Your best move is to get help to stop drinking. Vitamins cannot overcome the damage, only slow it.

Are you anemic? Anemia is sometimes—but not always—caused by a lack of iron, vitamin B$_{12}$, or folic acid. After a blood test confirms which nutrient you're lacking, your doctor can prescribe a supplement.

Shopping for Supplements

Shopping for supplements makes bathing suit shopping (if you're a woman) look easy. Aisles of products with varying ingredients and price tags can be overwhelming. In Canada, vitamins, minerals, and some herbs are classified as drugs. They must meet government standards for safety, effectiveness, potency, purity and quality. If you're shopping in the U.S., the problem is that supplements aren't closely regulated by any federal agency. So there's no guarantee that what's in the container matches what's on the label in terms of quality and potency.

The product label should give you all the information you need to know before buying and using a supplement. This isn't always the case in Canada, but it is improving. According to Health Canada, labels should use plain, truthful language that the layperson can understand.

Here's some information to help you shop for supplements:
- In Canada, all vitamins and minerals must include on their label an

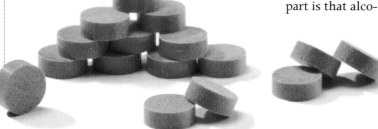

expiration date, the amount of active ingredient, and the Drug Identification Number or DIN. The DIN means that Health Canada has approved the product for sale based on extensive reviews of effectiveness and safety. If you're shopping in the U.S., look for "USP" on the product label. USP stands for U.S. Pharmacopeia, the organization that sets quality standards for drugs and supplements. In the case of supplements, it's up to the manufacturer to voluntarily comply with the standards. While "USP" on the label doesn't guarantee a better pill (since there is no independent verification that the supplement has in fact met the USP standards), it's the best assurance you have. Keep in mind that for some supplements, there are no USP standards. Also, the absence of USP on the label doesn't necessarily mean the product fails to meet USP standards.

- Don't be swayed by meaningless terms. The following marketing terms have no meaning agreed upon by experts or by regulations governing the sale and manufacture of supplements: "clinically proven," "guaranteed potency," "highly concentrated," "maximum absorption," "natural," "pure," "quality extract," "essential."
- An expiration date is required by law for all drugs. It is a pledge from the manufacturer that the products will remain "fresh" up to that point.
- Price alone isn't always a good guide; some inexpensive supplements may be as good as pricier versions. Most drugstore and generic brands are perfectly fine.

- Most supplements should be stored in a cool, dry, dark place. This means they shouldn't be stored in either the bathroom or the refrigerator. If a product requires refrigeration, it will say so on the label. Keep supplements out of the reach of children.

Choosing a Multivitamin

When purchasing a multivitamin, instead of sorting through 20-plus ingredients on the label, scan for these 10 nutrients and make sure the amounts are close to recommended levels (the DRIs). Many of these are the ones people tend to fall short on. (Remember, buying much more than these amounts can be a waste of money.) The nutrients not covered here are usually found in good supply in all multivitamins or are easily found in foods.

Iron Start here, because if this number is wrong, there's no need to read further. Iron is critical for healthy blood and preventing anemia. Premenopausal women who lose iron through menstruation need the most. Other people don't need much, unless they have iron-deficiency

In their own words

"There are compelling reasons to take a supplement," says Jeffrey Blumberg, Ph.D., professor of nutrition at Tufts University in Boston. "I certainly don't mean 'Take a pill and forget about food.' Foods also contain other substances such as fiber and phytochemicals. You need the whole nutritional package. Dietary supplements are just what they say they are—supplements, not substitutes."

Terms to Know

- **Dietary Reference Intakes (DRIs)** are a set of scientifically based nutrient reference values established by scientists in Canada and the U.S. Their aim is to achieve a set of harmonized dietary reference values for both countries. The Dietary Reference Intakes are comprised of four reference numbers: Estimated Average Requirements (EAR), Recommended Daily Allowances, (RDA), Adequate Intakes (AI), and Tolerable Upper Intake Levels (UL). The DRIs will ultimately replace Canada's current Recommended Nutrient Intakes (RNIs), which have been in place since 1977.

WARNING

Don't take individual supplements of vitamin E if you take blood thinning medication such as aspirin or warfarin (Coumadin). The vitamin can cause a dangerous increase in the action of these drugs.

anemia. High levels may be associated with an increase in heart attacks and possibly an increase in colon cancer. If your breakfast cereal is heavily fortified with iron, you may not need iron in your supplement. **Recommended level:** no more than 18 mg if you're premenopausal; no more than 8 mg if you're a postmenopausal woman or a man of any age.

Vitamin A and beta-carotene

Vitamin A is actually a cluster of compounds called retinoids that have varying degrees of vitamin A "activity." One of the most active of the retinoids is beta-carotene, a plant pigment. It's also an antioxidant, meaning it fights those unstable oxygen molecules called free radicals that have been linked with chronic disease. Beta-carotene is converted in the body to vitamin A as needed, and since it's not toxic and does not convert to toxic levels, manufacturers often use it to make up a portion of

the vitamin A in supplements. Vitamin A can be toxic at doses of about 50,000 IU a day. **Recommended level:** 900 mcg (or 3,000 IU) for men, 700 mcg (or 2,333 IU) for women.

Folic acid

Folic acid Large-scale surveys show that men and women age 50 and older get only about half the folic acid they need. This B vitamin appears to protect us from heart disease by reducing blood levels of the amino acid homocysteine, which contributes to clogging of the arteries. Low blood levels of the vitamin have been linked with cervical and colon cancer. And 15 to 38 percent of people with depression are deficient in it. Folic acid seems to improve the efficacy of Prozac and similar antidepressants. **Recommended level:** 400 mcg (or 0.4 mg, which is equivalent).

Vitamin B₆

Vitamin B_6 This vitamin also helps lower blood levels of homocysteine. Deficiency may contribute to depression. **Recommended level:** 1.5 mg for women, 1.5 to 1.7 mg for men.

Vitamin D

Vitamin D We get this vitamin two ways: from sunlight, which allows our bodies to manufacture it, and from vitamin D, found in fortified milk or cereal. Sunblock, a dark winter, and aging skin all curtail the body's ability to manufacture vitamin D from sunlight, and it's hard to get enough from food. Vitamin D is essential for directing calcium into bones and may also help keep blood pressure and blood fats in check. Don't get more than the recommended dosage because excess can be toxic. **Recommended level:** 400 IU if you're 51 to 70; 600 IU if you're over 70.

Do You Need a Special Multivitamin?

Should you be taking a "men's," "women's," or "senior" multivitamin? The answer is no to the men's and women's formulas; they're often more expensive and don't reflect a scientifically based need for a different pill. Some women's multivitamins are particularly bad buys. They may offer more generous doses of iron—which you don't need if you're post-menopausal—and calcium, but leave out other important nutrients. The senior supplements, on the other hand, are the best choice for post-menopausal women and men past the age of 55. In these supplements, iron levels are reduced and levels of certain B vitamins are enhanced.

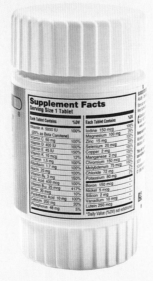

Don't Be Fooled by Bells and Whistles

Why does Brand X multivitamin cost $10, while Brand Y costs $20? Probably because Brand Y is ripping you off. More expensive is not necessarily better when it comes to supplements. Neither are high doses of nutrients, nor the addition of herbs and unproven substances. Here's a partial listing of ingredients taken straight from the label of an actual U.S. product, with comments.

A multivitamin should come in one tablet, not two or three. You just pay more for these "divided doses."

3 TABLETS PROVIDE

VITAMINS

Vitamin A (Beta-Carotene, Palmitate)	10,000 IU
Vitamin D (Calciferol)	100 IU
Vitamin E (natural)	100 IU
Vitamin C (Magnesium Ascorbate)	1000 mg
Pantothenic Acid	60 mg
Pyridoxine (Vitamin B_6)	40 mg
Riboflavin (Vitamin B_2)	34 mg
Thiamin (Vitamin B_1)	30 mg
Folic Acid	400 mcg
Cyanocobalamin (Vitamin B_{12})	200 mcg

MINERALS

Magnesium (Oxide, Ascorbate, Amino Acid Chelate)	300 mg
Calcium (Carbonate, Amino Acid Chelate, Gluconate)	150 mg
Potassium (Chloride)	40 mg
Iron (Amino Acid Chelate)	18 mg
Zinc (Gluconate, Amino Acid Chelate)	15 mg
Manganese (Amino Acid Chelate)	2.5 mg
Copper (Amino Acid Chelate)	200 mcg
Iodine (Kelp)	150 mcg
Selenium (L-Selenomethionine)	50 mcg

OTHER DIETARY INGREDIENTS

Bioflavonoids (mixed citrus)	100 mg
Choline Bitartrate	40 mg
PABA (Para-Aminobenzoic Acid)	30 mg
Lecithin	30 mg
L-Glutamine	24 mg
Hesperidin Complex	10 mg
DNA	1 mg

GREEN FOODS/SUPERFOODS

Spirulina	1000 mg
Bee Pollen	150 mg
Wheat Grass	100 mg
Kelp	24 mg
Chlorophyll	7.5 mg
Alfalfa Concentrate	6 mg
CUSTOM HERBAL BLEND	243 mg

A good multivitamin, should provide around 100% of the recommended level for most nutrients. Because B vitamins are inexpensive, manufacturers may pile them on to make their product seem more impressive. Nutritionally, there's no need for the high doses.

The Dietary Reference Intakes (DRIs), the new guidelines that are being developed by Canadian and U.S. experts, have tolerable maximum upper limits for vitamins and minerals. That is because health experts today are aware of the serious dangers of overdosing on supplements. Choose a brand with levels below the safe upper limits.

Spirulina, bee pollen, and other extraneous ingredients, mostly unproven or in amounts too small to make a difference, just crowd out the really important nutrients. No wonder you need three tablets.

Other Red Flags:

▪ "Unique form of chelated iron...": Chelated minerals are bound with another substance, supposedly for better absorption, but there's not much research proving they work better. If you have to pay more for it, forget it.

▪ "Free of corn, yeast, soy, and dairy products...": Many of these products don't appear in regular supplements, or appear in such minuscule amounts that they won't hurt you unless you're allergic. And starch is a good thing, helping the tablet disintegrate in your stomach.

▪ "Time-released": These formulas contain microcapsules that gradually break down into the bloodstream over two to 10 hours, depending on the product. However, there are no reliable studies that show time-released formulas are more efficiently utilized by the body than conventional tablets or capsules.

Chromium We need only a little bit of this mineral, but government surveys show most of us still aren't getting enough. Chromium is critical for proper functioning of insulin, the hormone that regulates blood sugar. **Recommended level:** 25 mcg for women, 35 mcg for men.

Magnesium This is another mineral that comes up short in government surveys. Since magnesium is involved in about 325 metabolic processes including muscle contraction and heartbeat, it's important to get enough. The mineral has also been tentatively linked to protection from diabetes, osteoporosis, atherosclerosis (hardening of the arteries), hypertension, and migraine headaches. **Recommended level:** 310 to 320 mg for women, 420 mg for men.

Zinc Credit this mineral for proper wound healing, tip-top immune function, and shorter bouts of the common cold. Surveys show we're not getting enough from our diets. The amount in most multivitamins will cover the gap. Don't take more than 45 mg, since too much zinc may suppress immunity. **Recommended level:** 11 mg for men, 8 mg for women.

Copper This mineral plays a role in bone and heart health, blood-sugar regulation, and metabolism of iron. **Recommended level:** 900 mcg.

Selenium This antioxidant mineral is sometimes used in the treatment of AIDS, heart disease, and arthritis. It may also help reduce the incidence of and death from lung, colorectal, and prostate cancer. **Recommended level:** 55 mcg.

Swinging Singles

You're taking a multivitamin to fill any nutritional gaps. But could you benefit from other supplements as well? In the case of the three supplements below, probably.

Vitamin C In 2000, new guidelines raised the level for vitamin C to 90 mg for men, 75 mg for women, and for smokers an extra 35 mg. This still may be too low, according to National Institutes of Health research in the U.S., which shows that it takes 200 mg to fully saturate body tissues. Besides its roles in gum and bone health and collagen formation, vitamin C may also play a role in preventing chronic diseases such as cancer and heart disease. If your diet is rich in citrus fruits and other high-C foods such as cantaloupe, cauliflower, green peppers, and broccoli, you may not need to supplement

Choosing a Calcium Supplement

The two leading types of calcium are calcium carbonate and calcium citrate. The latter is better absorbed on an empty stomach (although both are well absorbed when taken with a meal) and may be better for people over 65, some of whom lack sufficient stomach acid to absorb calcium carbonate. Some people find that calcium carbonate causes gas or constipation; for them, calcium citrate is a better choice. For everyone else, calcium carbonate, which is cheaper, is fine. Avoid supplements made from bonemeal, dolomite, and oyster shell, since these contain the highest amounts of lead. If you find those big calcium tablets hard to swallow, look for the new chewable supplements— much like soft candy—or chew extra-strength Tums, which are made from calcium carbonate.

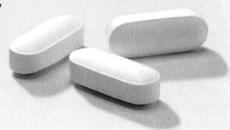

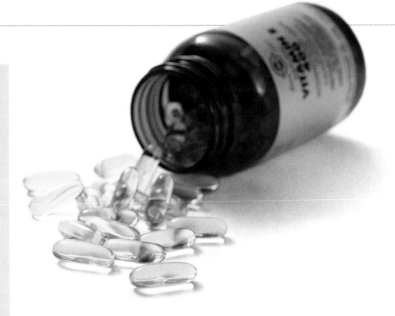

Vitamin E and Heart Disease

If you have heart disease, don't rely on vitamin E to help. While earlier research indicated that the supplements could reduce the risk for heart disease, a more recent, highly regarded study of 9,500 people with arteriosclerosis has found no benefit. It's still possible that the supplements might help healthy people or those in the early stages of the disease. Meanwhile, making lifestyle changes—exercising, watching your weight, eating more fruits and vegetables, and kicking the cigarette habit—are far more important steps to take.

with C beyond the 60 or 90 mg found in most multivitamins. If your diet is lacking in vitamin C, a 250 or 500 mg supplement is sufficient.

Vitamin E The new guidelines for vitamin E are 15 mg daily (22 IU) for men and women. Upper limit is 1,000 mg (1,500 IU). Most multivitamins supply 30 IU of this important antioxidant—still not enough, according to many experts, to provide protection against chronic diseases. Since vitamin E is scarce in a low-fat diet, there's virtually no way to get that amount from food. The vitamin is considered safe at levels up to 1,500 IU, so there's no harm in taking 200 to 400 IU daily—the level many experts recommend.

You'll notice that some brands contain natural vitamin E (d-alpha tocopherol) while others contain the synthetic kind (dl-alpha tocopherol). The natural form is better absorbed by the body than the synthetic form, but manufacturers compensate in the synthetically derived pills by increasing the level of vitamin E. And the synthetic form is usually cheaper.

Calcium Unless you're a big dairy fan, it's not easy to get the recommended 1,000 to 1,200 mg (1,500 mg if you're a postmenopausal woman or a man over 65) of calcium from food. Calcium helps prevent osteoporosis and may help lower blood pressure. Studies show that it may also lower the risk of gum disease, the leading cause of tooth loss in this country and a risk factor for heart disease.

Dairy is the richest source of dietary calcium; an 8-ounce glass of milk contains about 300 mg. Check your multivitamin (they usually contain around 200 mg), and build food sources into your diet. If you're still not getting enough, supplement with 500 to 1,000 mg, taken in two divided doses of 250 or 500 mg a day, one in the morning and one at night with food. Since calcium can't be absorbed without vitamin D, make sure you're getting plenty of D in your diet (fortified milk is the best source), or choose a calcium supplement that also contains D.

Research suggests that a daily dose of 100 to 400 IU of vitamin E may help protect against cataracts and certain cancers and, in people over 60, may boost immunity.

Sorting Out the Other Supplements

More and more of the supplements on the market today are neither vitamins nor minerals, but other substances that supposedly bolster your health. What are they? Here's a brief rundown.

SUBSTANCE	HEALTH BENEFITS	COMMENTS	SUPPLEMENT DOSE

Amino Acids and Similar Compounds
Small organic molecules that help build complex proteins.

SUBSTANCE	HEALTH BENEFITS	COMMENTS	SUPPLEMENT DOSE
Arginine, carnitine, and taurine	■ Effective in the treatment of heart disease and congestive heart failure. May ease angina pain.	■ Take only under supervision of a doctor. Not approved for sale in Canada; may be imported for 3-month supply.	■ The doses needed are quite large—in the range of 15 g a day.
Chondroitin sulfate	■ Relieves arthritis pain and swelling and protects joints.	■ Usually taken together with glucosamine sulfate.	■ 400 mg two or three times a day. You may not feel the effects for up to six weeks.
Glucosamine sulfate	■ Relieves arthritis symptoms and helps protect joints from further damage. May be more effective when taken together with chondroitin sulfate.	■ Glucosamine, a sugar compound, may affect blood-sugar levels. If you have diabetes, talk to your doctor before taking this. May be used long term.	■ 500 mg two or three times a day. You may not feel the effects for up to six weeks.
Lysine	■ Helps prevent cold sores and blisters from herpes virus. May benefit canker sores and shingles.	■ Don't take lysine if you have diabetes.	■ 5,000 mg a day until the flare-up goes away.
SAM-e (S-adenosyl-methionine)	■ Used to treat arthritis, depression, liver and heart disease. It also helps heal damaged cartilage.	■ Made in the body from the amino acid methionine. Not approved for sale in Canada; may be imported for 3-month supply.	■ 400 mg three times a day.

Carotenoids
A group of antioxidant plant compounds that give red, orange, and yellow plant foods their characteristic colors.

SUBSTANCE	HEALTH BENEFITS	COMMENTS	SUPPLEMENT DOSE
Lutein	■ Crucial for protecting eyesight. A shortage could lead to age-related macular degeneration.	■ Found in yellow foods such as egg yolks.	■ Lutein supplements usually contain 6 mg; up to five capsules a day is safe.
Lycopene	■ May lower prostate cancer risk.	■ Found in large amounts in tomatoes. An ounce of tomato sauce contains about 5 mg of lycopene.	■ Supplements usually contain 5 or 15 mg. About 7 mg a day may provide prostate protection.

SUBSTANCE	HEALTH BENEFITS	COMMENTS	SUPPLEMENT DOSE

Enzymes

Proteins that can accelerate or produce a change in certain metabolic processes.

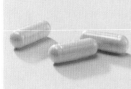

| **Coenzyme Q10 (ubiquinone)** | ■ Considered an anti-aging supplement. May be helpful for heart problems, especially congestive heart failure. Some doctors recommend it if you're taking cholesterol-lowering drugs, which can lower your levels of coenzyme Q10. | ■ A natural substance prevalent in the body and also found in many foods. Supplements should be taken in addition to, not instead of, standard drugs. Be sure to discuss taking it with your doctor before-hand. Expensive. | ■ 50 to 100 mg twice a day. Oil-based gelcaps are better absorbed. |

Essential Fatty Acids

The good fats that you need to stay alive. Since your body can't manufacture them, they must come from your diet.

| **Omega-3 fatty acid (alpha-linolenic acid)** | ■ Supplements may be helpful for arthritis, heart problems, and Crohn's disease. | ■ Found in cold-water fish such as bluefish, herring, salmon, and cod, as well as in flaxseed oil and walnut oil. | ■ One or two capsules a day is usually all that's needed. Your doctor can advise you on a proper dosage. |
| **Omega-6 fatty acids (linoleic acid and gamma-linolenic acid, or GLA)** | ■ Supplements of GLA (a type of omega-6 fatty acid) may help relieve premenstrual and meno-pausal symptoms. GLA is also a medically accepted treatment for fibrocystic breast disease. Widely used in Europe for diabetic neuropathy. | ■ Found naturally in seeds and nuts. 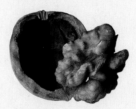 | ■ 3 to 10 g a day, in divided doses. It can take several weeks before you feel any effects. |

Flavonoids

A large group of antioxidant compounds that give fruits and vegetables their characteristic flavors and colors. Flavonoids include carotenoids.

| **Anthocyanins** | ■ Fight free-radical dam-age to tiny blood vessels of the eyes; help prevent hemorrhage and scarring from diabetes. | ■ Found in blueberries, plums, and blue grapes. | ■ One to two 40 mg capsules daily of bilberry standardized to contain 25 percent anthocyanins. |
| **Catechins** | ■ May play a role in preventing blood clots. | ■ Found in tea. 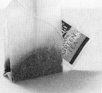 | ■ 240 to 320 mg a day; two green tea extract capsules containing at least 30 percent catechins. |

SUBSTANCE	HEALTH BENEFITS	COMMENTS	SUPPLEMENT DOSE
Grape seed extract	■ Benefits blood vessels and so may cut stroke and heart attack risk, aid poor vascular function in diabetics, and help people with circulation problems (varicose veins, hemorrhoids, easy bruising).	■ Supplements are made from the seeds of red grapes. Pine bark extract contains the same active ingredient (proanthocyanidins) but costs more and isn't necessarily any better.	■ A dose of 50 mg a day is generally considered to be safe and effective.
Quercetin	■ Helps reduce pain and swelling, block allergic reactions, kill viruses, and protect against atherosclerosis.	■ Abundant in onions, scallions, leeks, shallots, garlic, and apples.	■ 500 to 1,000 mg a day.
Resveratrol	■ Helps lower cholesterol, prevent blood clots, and block tumor growth.	■ Found in red wine and purple grape juice.	■ 500 mg a day of supplements made from red grapes or red wine.

Isoflavones

A group of estrogen-like plant compounds.

Ipriflavone	■ Widely accepted natural treatment for osteoporosis, especially when taken with calcium supplements.	■ Can increase bone density.	■ 200 mg three times daily, along with 1,000 mg of daily calcium.
Soy protein	■ For menopausal symptoms such as hot flashes, insomnia, and vaginal dryness. May also help lower cholesterol levels and reduce the risk of heart disease.	■ Found in soybeans, lentils, chickpeas, rice, and oats. Soy contains estrogen-like compounds, and scientists aren't sure whether a diet rich in these compounds may increase the risk of breast cancer in some women. So consider eating soy foods instead of taking supplements or powders.	■ According to the United States Food and Drug Administration, 25 g of soy protein a day is enough to lower your heart disease risk.

Natural Hormones

Chemical substances produced by the body that can regulate or affect the activity of certain organs.

Melatonin	■ May help you fall asleep, although it may not help you stay asleep. Studies are inconclusive regarding its efficacy against jet lag. More research is needed to	■ A powerful antioxidant produced by the pineal gland. Scientists once thought melatonin production declines with age, but a recent study disproved this. Can cause next-day	■ For sleep disturbances, a typical dose is 0.3 to 5.0 mg at bedtime. In some people, taking more than 1 or 2 mg may actually disturb sleep. Supplements don't work

SUBSTANCE	HEALTH BENEFITS	COMMENTS	SUPPLEMENT DOSE
Melatonin (Continued)	assess its value in slowing the aging process.	drowsiness. Long-term safety is unknown. Not approved for sale in Canada; may be imported for a three-month supply.	for everyone, and may not be advisable if your body already produces enough of the hormone.
DHEA	■ Supplementing with this hormone (dehydroepiandrosterone) has become popular because low levels of it have been associated with increased risk of heart disease and other health problems. It is thought to aid general health in older people and boost immune function.	■ Made by the adrenal glands and needed to produce other hormones such as estrogen and testosterone. Don't take DHEA without discussing it with your doctor beforehand. He should determine whether your blood levels are low; if you do supplement, you should be tested periodically. Researchers aren't sure whether increasing your level of sex hormones might raise the risk for prostate, ovarian, and other cancers. It may cause the growth of facial hair in women. DHEA is not approved in Canada. It is a controlled substance (anabolic steroid).	■ 50 to 2,500 mg a day.
Human growth hormone (HGH)	■ Usually prescribed only if your HGH levels are abnormally low.	■ This hormone requires a doctor's prescription. It's expensive and could be dangerous if you don't really need it. Also, be wary of manufacturers' claims that taking supplements of the amino acids your body needs to make HGH (such as arginine and lysine) will boost HGH.	■ Per your doctor's prescription.
"Natural" progesterone	■ Natural creams made from soybeans or wild yam may be an alternative to prescription progesterone for postmenopausal women. Also used for mild depression, fatigue, and breast tenderness.	■ Topical creams containing natural progesterone have not been approved for sale in Canada. Creams actually containing progesterone may be compounded by a pharmacist on a doctor's prescription, or may be obtained from the U.S. via your doctor and the Special Access Program. It is contraindicated in certain cases.	■ Usual procedure is to rub a dab of the cream onto your abdomen daily for two weeks, then take two weeks off. Choose a cream that contains 800 mg of progesterone per 2-oz product. Lower concentrations aren't effective.

Herbs and Your Health

Herbs are an integral part of healing in China and other countries. Learn how they can benefit you, too.

Medicinal herbs have a long history in human healing. Meadowsweet and willow bark, for example, were used to relieve pain and fever for centuries, but it was only in 1899 that salicin, their active compound, was synthesized into the drug aspirin. Plant-based drugs are still an important part of today's medical arsenal. Vincristine and vinblastine, used to treat leukemia, come from a plant in the periwinkle family. The drug tamoxifen, used to treat breast and ovarian cancer, comes from the Pacific yew tree. In all, about a quarter of today's pharmaceuticals come directly from plants, and many more are synthetic versions of plant compounds.

Prescription drugs, whether plant-based or not, can be very effective for treating serious health problems. But for many minor—and sometimes not-so-minor—problems, herbal remedies may work just as well if not better. The relief from herbs isn't usually as fast, but it is often gentler, with fewer side effects.

Choosing Herbs

Choosing a quality herbal product can be a bit tricky. Herbs are variable by nature. Depending on where, when, and how an herb is grown and processed, the strength of its medicinal compounds can vary considerably. Reputable manufacturers now standardize their products to make the amounts of the most active ingredients consistent from one

In China, herbal remedies account for up to half of total medicinal consumption. Now that modern research has proved the healing powers of many herbs, they are becoming a larger part of our arsenal, too.

batch to the next. By choosing standardized products whenever possible, you can be sure you're getting the same dose every time.

Even with standardization, herbal products can vary in quality from manufacturer to manufacturer. To boost your chances of getting a high-quality product, buy herbs and other supplements from a reputable store and choose brands made by national manufacturers.

Using Herbs

The most convenient way to take most herbs is in capsule or tablet form. Provided the herb is standardized, you know exactly how much of the active ingredient you're getting, and you don't have to drink any foul-tasting brews. Some herbs such as goldenseal and echinacea are also sold as tinctures, fast-acting concentrated herbal extracts made with alcohol or glycerin. You generally need to take just a small amount of a tincture, anywhere from a few drops to a teaspoon or so. Tinctures can be mixed with juice to disguise their unpleasant taste.

Mild herbs, especially ones made from leaves or flowers such as chamomile and peppermint, can easily be made into soothing teas using commercial tea bags or dried herbs. Use one prepared tea bag or a teaspoon or so of the dried herb placed in a tea ball or infuser for each cup of boiling water. Let the herb steep for a few minutes before drinking the tea. For a stronger medicinal effect you'll need to make an infusion, a brew that's steeped longer and tastes stronger. Use double or triple the amount of the herb and let it steep for 10 to 20 minutes.

Aspirin Power

There's one simple, safe, and inexpensive supplement that's found in just about everyone's medicine cabinet: aspirin. Recent research strongly suggests that taking a daily low-dose (80 mg) aspirin tablet could have a beneficial and perhaps dramatic effect on your health. Aspirin seems to work by thinning the blood slightly and preventing it from forming the clots that cause heart attacks and ischemic strokes. Taken at the onset of a heart attack, aspirin could save your life.

If you've already had one heart attack, aspirin therapy can sharply reduce your risk of having another. Aspirin can also reduce your risk of having a heart attack or stroke if you have angina. However, it doesn't reduce your overall risk of getting heart disease if you don't already have it.

Still more benefits of aspirin are coming to light. Researchers have discovered that people who take aspirin regularly have significantly reduced rates of cancers of the colon, stomach, and esophagus. Scientists aren't sure why.

Taking aspirin does have possible side effects, such as gastrointestinal bleeding and a slightly increased chance of a stroke from a ruptured blood vessel in your brain (this type of stroke is called a hemorrhagic stroke). Discuss the risks and benefits of aspirin therapy with your doctor before you begin.

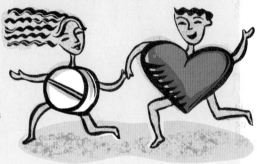

Herb Safety

Before you start taking any herb, be sure you understand what it's for, how much to take, and whether it's safe for you to use. Check with your doctor to make sure it won't interact with any medications you take. A few other tips:

- Unless you're an expert herbalist, don't pick herbs in the wild. You could easily mistake a useless or even dangerous herb for one that's helpful. Moreover, fresh herbs are much less potent than dried ones.
- You may have to take some herbs

WARNING

Never substitute herbs for a drug your doctor prescribes, and always discuss herbal alternatives with your doctor before you try them.

WARNING

Don't take echinacea or goldenseal for longer than eight weeks. These herbs work best when taken at the first sign of illness and continued for only a limited time. Echinacea stimulates your infection-fighting T-cells, but overuse can deplete your reserves and weaken your immune system. Goldenseal has antibiotic properties that can upset the balance of your intestinal flora.

Nonprescription creams containing capsaicin help ease pain from shingles and arthritis.

for days, if not weeks, to feel their effects. Don't exceed the maximum recommended dose in hopes of getting faster results.

● Stop using the herb if you experience upset stomach, diarrhea, headache, skin rash, hives, or other unpleasant symptoms within two hours of taking it.

● If you've taken an herb for the recommended amount of time and you haven't noticed any improvement, stop taking it and consult your doctor.

Herbs That Help

Of the many herbs said to help your health, only a small number have been shown to have measurable, positive effects and to be safe to use. Here's a brief rundown of the most noteworthy herbs for common uses.

For Pain Relief

● **Boswellia.** For relieving the pain and inflammation of arthritis, try this traditional remedy from India. Choose a standardized extract containing 37.5 percent boswellic acids. The usual dose is 400 mg three times a day. It may take four to eight weeks before you feel any benefits.

● **Capsaicin.** This is the substance that puts the "hot" in hot peppers. It helps ease lingering pain after an attack of shingles. It's widely accepted among physicians as an effective treatment for arthritis pain, too. Capsaicin is available in over-the-counter

(OTC) creams sold under various brand names. Rub the cream as directed into the painful area three to four times daily. Be very careful not to get the cream into your eyes, mouth, or other sensitive areas. Never apply the cream to raw or open skin. Relief may require three to four days of use.

● **Turmeric (curcumin) and devil's claw.** These two herbs can be helpful in easing pain from swelling and inflammation due to arthritis, injuries, back pain, surgery, and the like. The turmeric sold in the grocery store as a spice doesn't have enough curcumin to help. Look for a purified version at the health food store and take up to 400 mg three times daily. Devil's claw comes in a standardized extract containing 3 percent iridoid glycosides; take 750 mg up to three times daily.

● **Feverfew leaves.** This herb has been shown to help prevent migraines. It works best if you take 80 to 100 mg of the powdered leaf every day. Taking it *after* a migraine starts won't help.

For Digestive Problems

● **Peppermint and chamomile.** One to three cups of peppermint or chamomile tea is often all you need to soothe mild digestive upsets such as nausea, heartburn, and acid stomach.

● **Ginger.** For preventing motion sickness, try some ginger in capsules, as a tea, or as a spoonful of chopped fresh ginger mixed with a bit of honey. Studies have shown it works better than dimenhydrinate (Gravol) and without the side effects of drowsiness and dry mouth. Ginger works best if you take it about half an hour before your trip begins. Dosage is 500 to 2,000 mg daily.

- **Licorice.** In deglycyrrhizinated form (DGL), licorice root can be helpful for relieving heartburn and ulcer symptoms. Chew two to four 380 mg DGL wafers three times a day. Using the DGL form is important because glycyrrhizin raises blood pressure and may cause water retention. Licorice that does contain glycyrrhizin is beneficial against hepatitis (inflammation of the liver).
- **Milk thistle.** Another herb that's helpful for liver problems is milk thistle, also called silymarin. Choose an extract standardized to contain 70 to 80 percent silymarin and take 100 to 200 mg two or three times daily. Take it between meals for optimal effectiveness.

For Boosting Immunity

- **Echinacea.** Also called purple coneflower, echinacea (pronounced ek ih NAY sha) has been shown to be effective in fighting the viruses that cause colds and flu. The remedy works best if you take it at the first sign of a sniffle or, better yet, at the start of cold and flu season. The tincture form seems to be most effective, perhaps because the liquid is readily absorbed by the lining of the mouth. The usual tincture dose is 3 to 4 ml three times daily, but strengths vary from brand to brand, so follow the label directions. For tablets, the usual dose is 300 mg three times a day.
- **Astragalus.** Used for more than 2,000 years in China, this herb is valued most for fighting colds, the flu, and sinus infections because it prevents viruses from gaining a foothold in the respiratory system. It's used to build up the immune system of people undergoing chemotherapy or radiation treatment. It may help lower blood pressure and prevent angina pain. It also acts as an antioxidant. The usual dose is 200 mg once or twice a day for three weeks, followed by a three-week break.
- **Maitake, shiitake, and reishi mushrooms.** Extracts of these medicinal mushrooms help bolster immunity. Capsules are available that contain all three varieties. Studies suggest that medicinal mushrooms may be powerful enough to help people with HIV infection and AIDS. Reishi extracts also stimulate the production of a substance that kills cancer cells, and studies suggest it can improve survival rates in people with stomach, colon, and lung cancer. Shiitake mushrooms may also help lower elevated cholesterol. Check the labels for dosage information.

For Wounds and Infections

- **Tea tree oil and oil of oregano.** Tea tree oil (made from the sap of an Australian tree) and oil of oregano (from the leaves of the herb) are both natural antiseptics. Taken as directed, they're helpful for minor skin wounds, bug bites, scrapes, and even athlete's foot. To use them on your skin, put just a drop or two of diluted oil on a

Medicinal mushrooms, taken in extract or capsule form, have been shown to boost the immune system. Some have other uses, too. Reishi mushrooms, like the one above, also have anti-inflammatory properties and may help reduce allergy symptoms.

Fast Fact

There isn't really enough ginseng in all the various "energy-boosting" chewing gums, soft drinks, energy bars, and other products to make a difference—and lab tests have shown that some of these products don't really contain any ginseng at all.

Fast Fact

The German Commission E is an independent panel of scientists created by the German government in the late 1970s to study medicinal herbs. The Commission E reports are considered authoritative by doctors and researchers around the world. You can find them, translated into English, in Herbal Medicine, *edited by Mark Blumenthal.*

cotton ball and rub it in. Be careful not to get these oils on your clothes; they'll leave a stain. Taken internally as a few drops of oil in a glass of water, oil of oregano may help treat yeast (candida) and staph infections.

● **Goldenseal.** Although goldenseal has a reputation for helping fight off colds and flu, there's no real evidence that it does. Good studies do show, however, that goldenseal helps heal wounds and may be helpful against bladder infections, sore throats, and mouth sores. For treating a sore throat or mouth sore, use a few drops of goldenseal tincture in half a cup of warm water. Gargle with it or swish it around in your mouth. For urinary-tract infection, use goldenseal capsules. The usual dose is 250 to 500 mg taken three times a day. If you still have symptoms after using goldenseal for a few days, see your doctor.

The Trouble with Ephedra

Ephedra, also called ma huang, is a central nervous system stimulant that is the natural source of the drugs ephedrine and pseudoephedrine. The only Health Canada-approved claim for ephedra is as a nasal decongestant (look for the DIN on the label). Ephedrine-containing products not approved by Health Canada, such as weight-loss teas and energy boosters, are imported into Canada and sold clandestinely in fitness centers.

Ephedra is a relatively safe herb when used in standard doses of 6 to 12 mg. People who take larger doses in search of quick weight loss may experience nervousness, palpitations, and other side effects. Ephedra became the subject of controversy when unscrupulous manufacturers began selling commercial products as a legal "high," an alternative to the illegal drugs called amphetamines. In the U.S., the FDA received many reports of bad reactions and even deaths due to people taking two or three times the safe dosage of the herb. If you have heart problems or high blood pressure, consult a doctor before taking ephedra.

For Heart Health

● **Garlic.** Daily doses of this herb may help ward off heart problems. One of its chemical compounds, ajoene, appears to thin the blood, helping prevent the blood clots that cause heart attacks and some strokes. Other compounds in garlic act as antioxidants and help lower your blood pressure (a single clove a day can help notch it down). A study in 1998 showed that garlic helps keep your aorta (the main artery leading from your heart) flexible as well, which could also help prevent a heart attack. What about lowering your cholesterol level? The results of studies have been mixed.

One to three fresh cloves of garlic a day provide benefits. Supplements seem to work, too. To get the equivalent of three cloves, take 300 mg three times a day of an extract standardized to contain 1.3 percent alliin, one of the active ingredients in garlic. Aged garlic extract doesn't contain alliin and may not work as well. If you want to try it, take up to 7 grams a day in divided doses.

● **Hawthorn flower extract.** This may be helpful for people with heart conditions such as angina and congestive heart failure. The doses needed are fairly large, so talk to your doctor before you try it.

● **Red yeast rice.** The yeast that ferments on this rice acts on the liver to block an enzyme that allows the liver to produce cholesterol. The active ingredient, lovastatin, is the same as that found in some cholesterol-lowering prescription drugs. Don't take this if you're taking a cholesterol-lowering medication or have liver problems. Red yeast rice works best for mildly elevated cholesterol (between 5.2 mmol/L and 6.2 mmol/L).

For Circulatory Problems

- **Ginkgo biloba.** Used for thousands of years in traditional Chinese medicine, ginkgo biloba improves circulation to the brain, heart, and extremities. It is often recommended for varicose veins, hemorrhoids, and poor circulation to the hands and feet. Ginkgo is also helpful for treating dizziness and tinnitus (ringing in the ears). Use an extract standardized to contain 24 percent ginkgo flavone glycosides and 6 percent terpene lactone; the usual dose is two to four 60 mg tablets daily. Warning: Don't take ginkgo if you're also taking a blood-thinning medication such as warfarin (Coumadin).
- **Butcher's broom.** This herb is approved by Germany's Commission E for treating hemorrhoids; it also helps against varicose veins. Look for capsules, ointments, or suppositories standardized to provide a total daily dose of 50 to 100 mg of ruscogenins.
- **Horse chestnut.** This herb increases the strength of veins, which makes it a good choice for varicose veins and hemorrhoids. A typical dose is 300 mg twice a day of an extract standardized to contain 50 mg of escin.
- **Gotu kola.** This Indian herb has proven helpful against varicose veins, probably because it boosts blood circulation. It also appears to strengthen cells in the walls of blood vessels. The usual dose is 200 mg of standardized extract three times a day.

For Better Memory

- **Ginkgo biloba.** Studies have shown that ginkgo improves short-term memory and alertness. It works by increasing blood circulation to the brain. Use an extract standardized to contain 24 percent ginkgo flavone glycosides and 6 percent terpene lactone; the usual dose is two to four 60 mg tablets daily. Warning: Don't take ginkgo if you're also taking a blood-thinning medication such as warfarin (Coumadin).
- **Gotu kola.** Current research supports the notion that this Indian herb helps boost memory and improves learning capabilities, probably by improving blood flow to the brain and aiding the production of neurotransmitters, the brain's chemical messengers. The usual dose is 200 mg of standardized extract three times a day.

For Your Mood

- **St. John's wort (hypericum).** The latest physician guidelines for treating patients with mild depression make it official: St. John's wort works in many cases. It's also much less expensive than the drug fluoxetine (Prozac) and doesn't have its unwanted side effects. Daily doses range from 300 to 900 mg of standardized extract. Start with a low dose and increase it gradually until you feel an effect.

WARNING

Don't take St. John's wort if you are already taking a prescription antidepressant medication. An adverse reaction may result. According to Health Canada, other evidence shows that St. John's wort could affect the metabolism of a variety of prescription drugs, such as anticonvulsants, oral contraceptives, immunosuppressants, and anticoagulants.

An analysis of 23 different studies showed that St. John's wort is as effective as antidepressant drugs for mild to moderate depression, with fewer side effects.

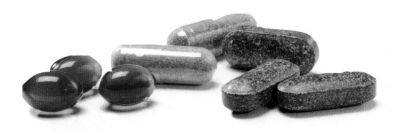

● **Valerian.** This is a safe, nonaddictive sleep aid that won't leave you feeling groggy in the morning. Valerian tea is truly foul-tasting, so take a standardized extract in tablet or tincture form instead. The amount that helps varies from person to person. Follow the instructions on the container and start with the smallest dose.

● **Kava.** This Polynesian root has become popular for relaxing, easing anxiety, and getting to sleep. Skip the tea and take a standardized extract containing 70 percent kavalactones, or look for tablets. A dose of 300 mg before bedtime helps you sleep.

Green Tea: Drink to Your Health

Numerous recent studies have shown that people who drink tea regularly, especially green tea, have lower rates of heart disease, stroke, and cancer than those who don't. The reason is probably the high level of an antioxidant called EGCG—thought by some scientists to be one of the most potent anticancer compounds yet discovered—along with other substances called catechins. Because green tea leaves aren't fermented, as black tea leaves are, all of its antioxidant compounds are preserved. Black tea also offers health protection, although not as much.

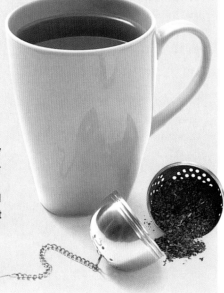

To reap the benefits of green tea, have two to four cups a day if you like it—it's mild tasting and very low in caffeine. If you don't love green tea, even a cup a day may offer some cancer protection, or take green tea capsules. Check the label for the polyphenol content (EGCG is a type of polyphenol), and aim to get 240 to 320 mg of polyphenols a day.

For Energy

● **Ginseng.** One of the most commonly used herbs in China, ginseng is extremely popular in the rest of the world as well. This root has a good reputation as an adaptogen, an herb that acts as a general tonic to help you cope with stress and illness. It's also used as mild, caffeine-free stimulant and energy booster.

There are several types of ginseng, but only Chinese ginseng (*Panax ginseng*) and American ginseng (*Panax quinquefolium*) are true ginseng, and they have similar effects. Siberian ginseng (*Eleutherococcus senticosus*) has a less stimulating effect and may be subject to quality control problems. To be safe, stick to Chinese or American ginseng.

Some people prefer to take ginseng as a tea, but to be sure of getting the dose you want, use capsules standardized to contain 8 percent ginsenoides. Take one to two 150 mg capsules daily, but don't take ginseng continuously for more than two to three weeks. Many experts believe that stopping ginseng for a few weeks will enhance its effectiveness when you resume dosing. Stop if you experience headaches or insomnia.

For Women's Problems

● **Cranberry.** Cranberry is recommended by doctors for treating and preventing bladder infections. Its acidity has an antibiotic effect on the urinary tract. Take 300 to 400 mg in capsules twice a day or drink 8 to 16 ounces of the natural juice daily. Don't use cranberry juice cocktail; it contains too much sugar and not enough cranberry.

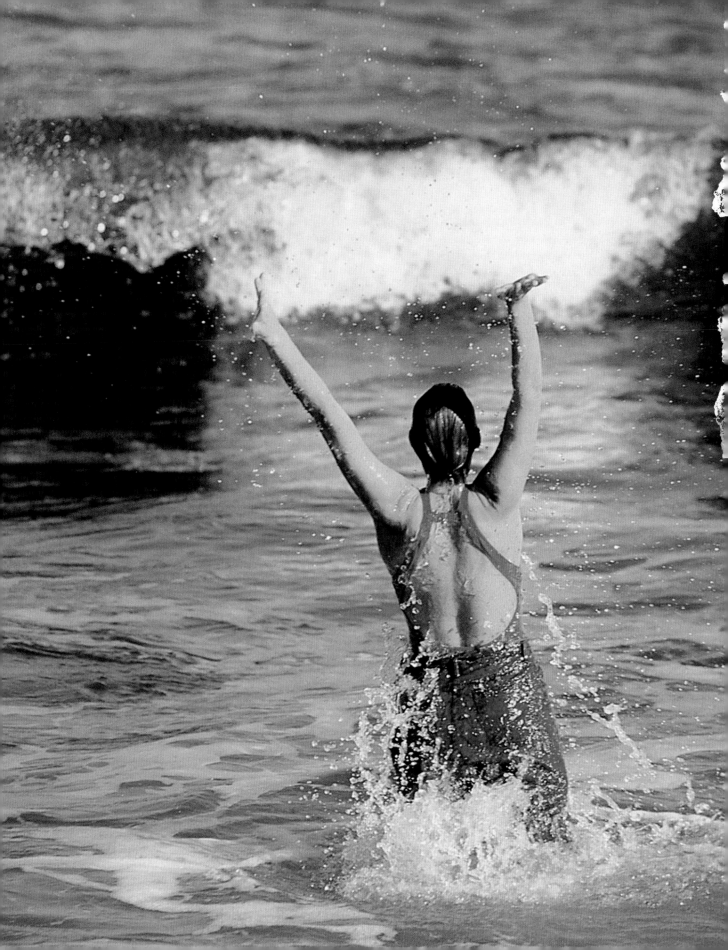

- **Uva-ursi.** Also known as bear-berry, uva-ursi is a natural antibiotic that's effective against bladder infections. It works best if you take it as soon as you feel the first symptoms of an infection (pain during urination, frequent need to urinate, and cloudy urine). Follow the directions on the label and don't use uva-ursi for more than a few days. Daily dosage: 400 to 800 mg.

- **Black cohosh root.** This traditional Native North American remedy has been shown to ease menopausal symptoms such as hot flashes, bloating, depression, and insomnia. Take 8 mg a day of an extract standardized to 1 percent 27-deoxyaceteine or 40 mg a day of the dried root. Take it with meals to reduce the possibility of stomach upset. Warning: Don't confuse black cohosh root with blue cohosh, a potentially dangerous herb.

- **Chasteberry.** Widely used in Europe for relief of menopausal symptoms, chasteberry is also known as chastetree berry and vitex. It's sold in capsules and tincture form. If you use the capsule form, take 20 to 40 mg once a day. Read the tincture label to determine the right dose.

For Men's Problems

- **Saw palmetto.** A major study in 1996 showed that saw palmetto relieves the symptoms of benign prostatic hyperplasia (BPH), or enlarged prostate, just as well as the prescription drug finasteride (Proscar). In fact, the herb could well be the better choice, because it doesn't have any major side effects and doesn't artificially

lower the results of the prostate-specific antigen (PSA) test for prostate cancer. The usual dose is 160 mg twice daily of an extract standardized to 85 percent fatty acids and sterols. Note that the herb does not shrink the prostate.

- **Pygeum.** Made from the bark of an African tree, pygeum is almost as effective as saw palmetto for BPH. The evidence in its favor isn't as strong, however, and pygeum is quite expensive. The usual dose is 50 to 100 mg twice daily of an extract standardized to 14 percent triterpenes.

- **Stinging nettle.** The root of the stinging nettle plant helps to relieve BPH symptoms, although not as well or as quickly as saw palmetto or pygeum. Stinging nettle root is popular in Europe and has been approved for use by Germany's Commission E. The usual dose is 4 to 6 g a day.

- **Cernitin.** A mixture of pollens from three different plants, this herbal formula has been shown to ease symptoms of BPH and chronic nonbacterial prostatitis. A multicenter clinical study showed that a supplement containing cernitin along with saw palmetto, beta sitosterol, and vitamin E provided significant improvement.

Not Worth It

The herb yohimbe, made from the bark of a West African tree, is said to be a male aphrodisiac. It's also the source of a drug called yohimbine that's sometimes prescribed for erectile dysfunction.

As an herbal preparation or prescription drug, yohimbe doesn't work very well, and it often causes unpleasant or even dangerous side effects such as dizziness, nausea, anxiety, and a drop in blood pressure. This is an herb to avoid.

WARNING

Traditional Chinese medicine relies heavily on complex herbal mixtures. It's hard to know exactly what you're getting in these mixtures. For example, in the U.S., the FDA warns that some prepared mixtures and patent medicines imported from China may be contaminated with heavy metals or pesticides. Some contain small amounts of drugs such as diazepam (Valium). In Canada, always look for the DIN on a product label. The presence of the DIN means the product has been approved for sale.

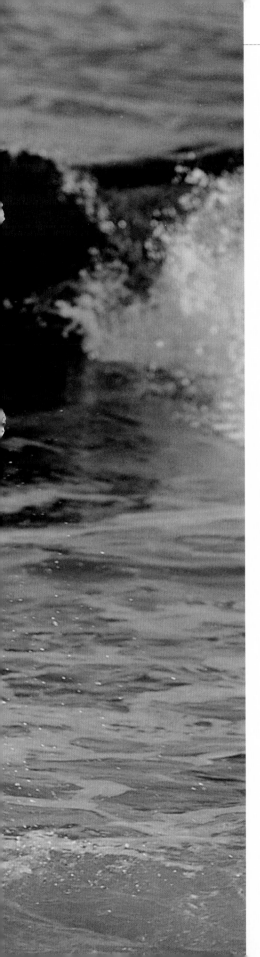

CHAPTER 4

STAYING FIT FOR LIFE

The Exercise Answer

Exercise can cut your risk of every major disease, lengthen your life, and even make you feel happier. Best of all, there's no need to run marathons or even join a gym, since a little activity goes a long way.

We all know that exercise is good for us. But it's time we realized just how powerful an anti-aging tool it really is. Scientists now understand that frailty and many diseases are caused not so much by getting older as by becoming sedentary. Women who stay physically active after age 50 are as fit as—or fitter than—inactive women 20 years younger. They also live longer. And it's never too late to make the move to fitness. In one study, middle-aged men who became fit over a five-year period were 44 percent less likely to die than those who remained unfit.

Exercise is not just an investment in your future; living a more active life makes you feel and look younger today. It makes daily life easier, too. Are you able to carry groceries, lift a bag of cat litter, or pick up a grandchild? Can you rush through an airport or chase after a bus without gasping for breath? Do you have enough energy to tackle a home improvement project after dinner? Aerobic exercise (activities that get your heart pumping hard), strength training (such as lifting weights or doing push-ups), and stretching all dramatically improve your functional fitness—that is, your ability to do daily tasks with ease.

Benefits of Exercise

Immediate Payoffs

Exercise boosts your energy level. If you suffer from a late-afternoon slump, a few minutes of calisthenics or a brisk 10-minute walk will perk you up by getting more blood to your brain. You'll even sleep better if you exercise. Doing so helps you fall asleep faster—and stay asleep. In a Stanford University study, people who walked or did low-impact aerobics for up to 40 minutes four times a week fell asleep twice as fast and slept an hour longer. There's another advantage: As we age, our periods of deep sleep (the most restful kind) tend to shorten, and exercise may be the only way to lengthen them again.

An exercise habit also makes you a calmer person. People who exercise regularly don't experience as much of a rise in blood pressure during stressful situations as couch potatoes do. And in a study done at the University of Texas, people who exercised frequently experienced

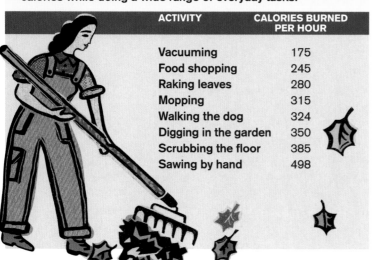

Exercise in Disguise

Can't find the time—or motivation—to exercise? You can burn calories while doing a wide range of everyday tasks.

ACTIVITY	CALORIES BURNED PER HOUR
Vacuuming	175
Food shopping	245
Raking leaves	280
Mopping	315
Walking the dog	324
Digging in the garden	350
Scrubbing the floor	385
Sawing by hand	498

Jump for joy! Exercise fights depression. In one study, 82 percent of people with mild to moderate depression who used weight machines three times a week showed no symptoms after 10 weeks.

37 percent fewer physical complaints during periods of intense stress than those who were least active.

Movement also eases chronic pain and helps relieve menopausal hot flashes. And if you follow a regular exercise program for even a few weeks, you'll feel your self-esteem grow because you've set and met an important goal. Moreover, exercise improves your overall mood, possibly because it triggers the release of endorphins, the body's feel-good brain chemicals.

A Healthier Heart

Almost any kind of physical activity, done consistently, can strengthen your heart—so it pumps with less effort—and keep your artery walls supple, decreasing your risk of heart disease. And moderate to intense exercise (enough to burn 1,200 to 1,600 calories a week) can improve your cholesterol profile by raising your level of HDL—the "good" cholesterol that helps prevent clogged arteries. Regular exercise may also prevent the oxidation of LDL ("bad") cholesterol, a process that encourages it to stick to artery walls.

The American Heart Association and the Canadian Heart and Stroke Foundation have concluded that lifting weights is one of the best things you can do for your heart because it lowers cholesterol levels, reduces blood pressure, and improves overall cardiovascular fitness. It also makes glucose metabolism more efficient and increases your ratio of muscle to fat. Extra muscle mass means a faster

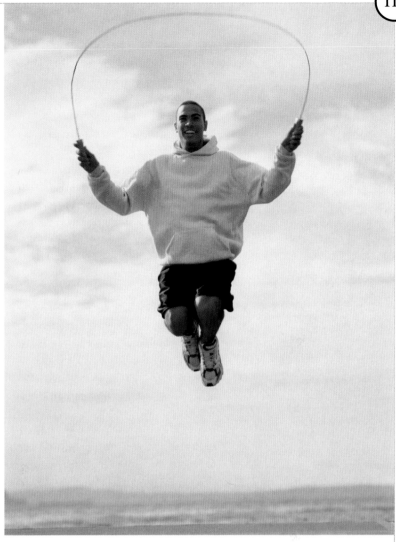

metabolism, since muscle burns far more calories than fat does—even when you're sitting still.

Greater Lung Capacity

Regular aerobic exercise increases your lung capacity, offsetting the 1 percent decline that occurs each year after age 25. This capacity, known as your max VO_2, typically increases by 6 to 20 percent with aerobic training but can climb by as much as 50 percent. When your lung power improves, oxygen enters your lungs more rapidly and carbon dioxide leaves more quickly. The benefit? You're less likely to get winded.

In their own words

Why is fitness important? For Dr. Kenneth H. Cooper, the Dallas physician who set off the fitness revolution with his 1968 book Aerobics, *the rationale is clear: "So I can hike and ski in the mountains above 10,000 feet. You can't do that at 69 unless you're fit. I won't accept mediocrity with my body."*

Fast Fact

One large-scale study of 5,000 women found that inactivity was even more life-threatening than smoking cigarettes.

Stronger Bones

Your bones grow denser with exercise, particularly with strength training and high-impact activities such as jogging. Women over age 50 who strength-train twice a week for one year typically increase their bone density by about 1 percent. Compare that with sedentary post-menopausal women who usually experience a 2 percent bone loss each year, along with a higher risk of falls—a potentially perilous combination.

Reduced Cancer Risk

If you exercise regularly, you stand a good chance of reducing your risk for colorectal cancer, as well as cancer of the lung, breast, prostate, and uterus. In one study, women who exercised moderately at least an hour a day cut their risk of colorectal cancer by 18 percent compared with less active women. In another study of 1,090 women, those who exercised at least four hours a week were half as likely to develop breast cancer as those who didn't work out at all.

Head-to-Toe Benefits

From arthritis to weight gain, exercise plays a role in preventing or managing a wide variety of medical disorders. For instance, strong thigh muscles appear to protect you from developing arthritis in your knees. Doing moderate exercise at least four times a week reduces a woman's chance of developing diabetes by half. And male or female, two to three hours of recreational exercise a week may lower your risk of gallstones by 20 percent.

It's well established that moderate aerobic activity boosts immune system function. One study found that women who walked briskly for 45 minutes five days a week cut their sick days in half. Other studies have demonstrated the positive effects of exercise on the immune system in people as old as 87.

In Short, a Longer Life Span

According to the Cooper Institute for Aerobics Research in Texas, women who are moderately fit are 2.5 times less likely to die prematurely from cancer, heart disease, and other ailments. And you don't have to work out every day to add years to your life. In a 17-year study, people who exercised at least moderately for 30 minutes six or more times a month outlived those who were sedentary by a 43 percent margin. When it comes to longevity, staying physically fit may be even more important than maintaining a healthy body weight. Researchers found that lean sedentary men have higher death rates than men who are overweight but otherwise fit.

Want to cultivate an exercise habit? Gardening counts. According to a University of Arkansas study, gardening once a week strengthened bones more than other activities like walking or swimming. In fact, gardening delivered as great a benefit as lifting weights. Although the study included only women, men benefit, too.

Fitting in Fitness

Your fitness activities needn't be confined to a gym or even done at a set pace. Several studies have found that people who simply add an extra 30 minutes of activity to their day—even the most mundane types of activity, such as yard work or stair climbing—over time reap the same cardiovascular and weight-loss benefits as people who take part in structured exercise programs. So walk instead of taking the car, use the stairs instead of the elevator, and consider using a push-mower instead of a riding mower. Go skating with the grandkids instead of watching.

How Much Is Enough?

In terms of overall health benefits, it doesn't matter what you do to get in shape as long as you burn at least 1,000 to 2,000 calories a week in activity. On the low end, that's equivalent to either a daily 30-minute walk at a 3.5 mph pace or a daily 1.5 mile run in 15 minutes. But aside from walking or jogging, there are countless other ways to accumulate those calorie-burning "points."

Do What You Love

Another way to sneak exercise in your life is to choose an activity you enjoy—one that doesn't feel like exercise, even though it is. Ask yourself, What am I good at? If you play to your strengths, you'll find fitness activities you can enjoy for years. Do you take to water like a fish? Water aerobics, offered at YMCAs around the country, provides a moderate workout that's easy on the joints and is great for people with arthritis. Can't get enough of the great outdoors? Hiking can be enjoyed at any fitness level.

No More Excuses!

Do you find any and every excuse not to exercise? Would you rather do anything else—even sort your socks or clean the oven? Here are a few ways to get you going—and keep you going.

- **Call it by another name.** Substitute any aerobically challenging household activity for the standard exercise routine. If it's something you have to do anyway—like washing the car or planting some bushes in the yard—you'll meet two goals at once.
- **Do it to music.** Sign up for classes in swing dancing—or flamenco, folk, or African dance. All provide a terrific workout and a lot of fun. Or listen to music while you work out; your favorite tunes make the time go faster.
- **Be a bookworm.** Listen to the latest mystery or suspense novel on tape while you exercise. If the book's a page-turner, you'll look forward to that next session to hear the next plot twist.
- **Don't sweat it.** If a damp T-shirt is not your idea of a good time, try gentler forms of exercise such as yoga, tai chi, or ballet-based flexibility classes, offered at many gyms.
- **Partner up.** Exercise is more fun when you do it with a friend. And on days when your motivation is low, you're more likely to stick with the program to avoid disappointing your exercise buddy.
- **Find an electronic coach.** Go online (try iVillage.com or woman.com) and find an Internet buddy to cheer you on to your next fitness goal.
- **Train with an expert.** It's an expense, to be sure, but a personal trainer will help you set goals, design a personalized fitness program, and vary your routine to keep it challenging.
- **Join a club.** Make fitness part of your social routine by joining a running, walking, hiking, biking, or tennis club.

Choose Your Hour

Studies have shown that people who work out in the morning are most likely to stick with a routine. By getting their exercise in before the day starts, they skirt those last-minute scheduling conflicts—and the end-of-day blahs—that thwart the best intentions. What if you're not a morning person? Your best time is whatever works for you. If you're in top form from noon to 1 P.M., aim for a midday or lunchtime workout.

Fast Fact

According to a Johns Hopkins study, you can add two years to your life by climbing stairs for six minutes a day.

YOUR GAME PLAN FOR GOOD HEALTH

Focus on Fundamentals

Before you jump into an exercise program, brush up on the basics. These tips will help you develop a safe, fun routine for the long haul.

Exercise shouldn't be intimidating. By learning the basics—like what to wear, how to warm up, and how to know when you're overdoing it—you'll feel like a pro in no time.

Warm Up and Cool Down

For best results, start each exercise session with a warm-up: 5 to 10 minutes of moderate aerobic activity that heats up your muscles, making them more pliable and less likely to tear. Get your blood flowing by walking at a moderate pace (3 to 4 miles per hour), cycling on an exercise bike (65 to 75 rpm), or circling your arms and marching in place.

End every aerobic session with a cooldown (about half as long as your warm-up) during which you gradually reduce the intensity of your exercise. This prevents blood from pooling in your veins, which could make you dizzy. Follow your cooldown with some stretches designed to loosen up the muscles you've just exercised. (If you stretch cold muscles you'll run the risk of a strain.)

Dress for Success

Choose clothes that allow free movement. Stretchy materials and elastic waistbands are ideal. Don't head out for a walk in street clothes, like jeans, that rub against you as you move. Dress in layers, especially if you're exercising outdoors, so you can remove your outer garments as you warm up. For your first layer, choose something made of a high-tech fabric that wicks moisture away from the body. Avoid cotton, which absorbs sweat, leaving you feeling clammy.

When you exercise, your body loses fluids through sweating, so it's important to keep drinking. For most people, water is ideal. However, if you're an endurance athlete exercising for more than an hour, consider a sports drink; they replenish lost sodium and potassium.

What about sneakers? Certain sports really do require specific kinds of footwear. For instance, aerobic shoes are flexible, moderately cushioned, and have soles that facilitate movement in all directions. Running shoes, on the other hand, are stiff, highly cushioned, and designed for forward movement. If you wear running shoes to an aerobics class, you may have trouble doing side-to-side steps and may raise your risk for ankle sprains. Likewise, if you jog in aerobic shoes, your feet may not feel stable and will get jarred by the impact of running. Cross-training shoes are suitable for several kinds of exercise. Or you can match your footwear to your main activity, whether it's walking, running, tennis, or hiking.

Don't Forget to Drink

Keeping hydrated is important before, during, and after exercise to prevent dizziness, cramps, exhaustion, and even collapse. Drink a tall glass of water at least 20 minutes before your workout, and as you exercise, sip from a water bottle—about two ounces at least every 10 minutes. Don't wait until you are thirsty to drink; by then, you are already dehydrated. Down another glassful of water after your workout.

Start Slow—But Think Big

Many people start out gung ho with an overly ambitious exercise program, push themselves to the point of sore muscles or even injuries, then get discouraged and quit. A better tactic is to think in terms of attainable intermediate goals that build on one another. Work to just beyond your present fitness level, then gradually increase the duration, frequency, and intensity of your activities.

Finding the Right Balance

How do you know when you're challenging yourself enough, but not too much? See where you fit on this perceived rate of exertion scale, sometimes call the Borg scale after its developer, scientist Gunnar Borg. It's not surprising that, according to researchers, your sense of how difficult an exercise is corresponds to physiological indicators of effort, such as your heart rate. If you find an exercise very easy, then you're not challenging your body sufficiently.

THE BORG CATEGORY RATING SCALE

	LEAST EFFORT	
6	Very, very light	
7		
8	Very light	
9		
10	Fairly light	
11		ENDURANCE TRAINING ZONE
12	Somewhat hard	
13		
14	Hard	
15		STRENGTH TRAINING ZONE
16	Very hard	
17		
18	Very, very hard	
19		
20		
	MAXIMUM EFFORT	

The numbers on the left correspond to your estimate of how much effort you're putting out. This is a highly individual matter; only you know how hard a given exercise feels to you. For aerobic activities, aim at first to reach level 11, in which you're working hard but can talk in a breathy way. Work your way up to level 13, in which you're breathing harder but can still speak. Don't work out so hard that you can't talk at all. For strength training, work at level 15 to 17; you should feel that you are approaching your limit.

You might, for instance, have the ultimate aim of improving your cardiovascular endurance by pedaling a stationary bike for 30 minutes almost daily. Set an initial goal of cycling 15 minutes every other day. Once you are comfortable with that level, steadily increase your time in 5-minute intervals—to 20 minutes, then 25 minutes, then 30 minutes. Finally, add sessions one by one until you're cycling 30 minutes, six days a week.

For a simple exercise plan that does the calculating for you, see the walking program on page 122.

Boosting Your Cardiovascular Fitness

Running after a bus—or after the grandkids? You're neither fit nor healthy if your heart and lungs can't keep up.

Cardiovascular fitness (also called aerobic fitness) means you have the stamina to climb a hill or chase after a wind-blown hat without struggling for breath. If you are aerobically fit, your body circulates oxygen-rich blood to the muscles quickly and the muscles use that oxygen efficiently. Also, your heart is strong, so it pumps more blood with each beat and beats less often. (That's why pulse is a good indication of how fit your heart is.) All of this means you peter out less quickly. People at a very low level of cardiovascular fitness can't walk their dogs more than a few blocks and may have trouble carrying laundry up the stairs.

Aerobic exercise—activities that tax the heart, such as brisk walking, jogging, or bicycling—can dramatically postpone the decline in aerobic fitness that usually comes with age. In a study of 1,499 men, the fittest and most active among them experienced almost no decrease in aerobic power between age 30 and 70. Those who were moderately fit and moderately active saw about a 25 percent decline. Those who were sedentary and obese saw their aerobic capacity drop by over 50 percent.

How Much? How Often?

In aerobic training, you continuously exercise your large muscles—your arms, legs, buttocks, and chest—to get your heart beating fast. (You won't get an aerobic workout typing into a personal computer all day.) You know you're working your heart effectively when you feel warm, get sweaty, and breathe heavily (but are not out of breath). For a more precise way to gauge the intensity of your aerobic routine, see "How Vigorous Is Your Workout?" on page 118.

How much of this type of exercise do you need? Experts recommend at least three 20-minute sessions per week, although 30-minute bouts are even better for your health. Either way, this relatively easy prescription is enough to move you from the "sedentary" column to the "active" one. If your main goal is to live longer and feel younger, the 3 x 20 prescription will suffice. If you are preparing for hikes in the mountains, planning a bike trip, or expecting to entertain two energetic grandchildren, you might benefit from more or longer workouts.

Moderate Makes the Grade

Experts used to believe that only the most strenuous exercises, like running or power cycling, were good for the heart. But researchers at Dallas's Cooper Institute for Aerobics Research and elsewhere have determined that even moderate exertion, such as brisk walking, provides significant cardiovascular benefits. Since most people are not ready to make a lifelong commitment to intense exercise, this finding opens the door to fitness for millions.

SimpleSolution

Heart-rate monitors, electronic devices that strap onto your wrist or over your chest, give a highly accurate measure of your pulse without your having to count. The price starts at around $100.

Before You Begin: How Fit Are You?

Are you fit now? Find out by measuring your recovery heart rate, how fast your heartbeat returns to its normal rate after you engage in vigorous exercise—a sign of how efficiently your heart is operating. This test is easier if someone else times you, but you can also time yourself.

Start by doing three minutes of step-ups. Find a sturdy, stable box 12 inches high, or use a bottom stair or step bench. Wearing exercise clothes and shoes, step up with your right foot, then the left, and then step down with right foot and then the left. Repeat, without stopping, for three minutes (set a timer if you need to), keeping an even pace.

Stop. Thirty seconds later take your pulse. Compare the result with the chart at right to judge your fitness. If you are "unfit," make sure you use the beginner's exercise program outlined on page 143. Chart your progress by retesting yourself every couple of weeks.

One important caveat: If you have any history, symptoms, or major risk factors for heart disease (such as smoking, diabetes, or severe obesity) do not take this test or begin any exercise program except under the supervision of a physician.

Gaining Ground

Exercise is more fun when you see steady improvements. This will happen if you gradually make your workouts more difficult by exercising more frequently, for longer periods of time, or at a higher intensity.

The most time-efficient approach to stepping up your routine is to maintain the duration and frequency of your workouts but gradually increase the intensity. Thirty minutes of walking at a leisurely pace burns 85 calories, but 30 minutes at a faster clip burns 136 calories. Calories burned is a good indicator of how much energy you're expending. You'll also burn more calories when you walk, cycle, or jog uphill or set your stationary bike for greater resistance.

Check Your Recovery Pulse Rate

Do three minutes of step-ups (see text at left), pause for 30 seconds, then take your pulse. Compare that figure with the ones below to gauge your level of fitness. Repeat the test every two to four sessions to monitor your improvement.

Women

AGE	VERY FIT	FIT	AVERAGE	UNFIT
30-39	<78	78-99	100-109	>109
40-49	<80	80-100	101-112	>112
50-59	<86	86-105	106-115	>115
60-69	<90	90-108	109-118	>118

Men

AGE	VERY FIT	FIT	AVERAGE	UNFIT
30-39	<84	84-105	106-122	>122
40-49	<88	88-108	109-118	>118
50-59	<92	92-113	114-123	>123
60-69	<95	95-117	118-127	>127

How to Take Your Pulse:
Find your heartbeat by placing your index and middle fingers on either your carotid artery (on your neck in one of the grooves alongside your windpipe) or your radial artery (on your wrist near your thumb). If you have a hard time locating your pulse points, try climbing stairs or jogging in place for a minute or two, then check again. Using a watch with a second hand, count the number of beats in a 15-second period. Then simply multiply this number by four to determine your heart rate per minute.

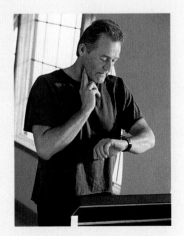

YOUR GAME PLAN FOR GOOD HEALTH

Interval Training

Another way to increase the challenge and burn more calories is to practice interval training, which calls for alternating short, intense bursts of exercise with longer, slower periods of the same activity. For instance, after a 10-minute warm-up, cycle as fast as you can for 30 seconds, then pedal two minutes at a slower pace, then go all out for another 30 seconds, and so forth. As you continue to train, decrease your recovery time, ultimately equalizing your most active and least active intervals.

Interval training is an excellent way to prevent boredom, which is why aerobic equipment found at health clubs almost always includes an electronic program for it. Swimmers often find it's more entertaining to swim a few fast laps, then pause for 30 seconds, then swim another round of fast laps, in sets of four, than to keep a continuous pace. Interval training can also boost performance, possibly because it habituates muscles to working at a high intensity. In one study, it helped competitive cyclists shave two minutes off a 40-kilometer trial.

How Vigorous Is Your Workout?

The best way to gauge the intensity of your workout is to check your heart rate. Your target heart rate is the pulse you're shooting for when you work out. The safe but effective range is between 50 to 85 percent of your maximum rate—the rate you should never exceed. To calculate your maximum rate, subtract your age from 220. If you are 45 years old, your estimated maximum heart rate is 175 (220 minus 45) beats per minute. Your target range is 88 to 149 beats per minute (.50 and .85 times 175). Someone who's been sedentary should aim for 50 to 70 percent of the maximum heart rate. If you're already fit, your target is 65 to 85 percent of the maximum.

The American Heart Association suggests you aim for the following target heart rates:

AGE	TARGET HEART RATE	MAXIMUM HEART RATE
30	95 to 142 beats per minute	190 beats per minute
35	93 to 138 beats per minute	185 beats per minute
40	90 to 135 beats per minute	180 beats per minute
45	85 to 131 beats per minute	175 beats per minute
50	85 to 127 beats per minute	170 beats per minute
55	83 to 123 beats per minute	165 beats per minute
60	80 to 120 beats per minute	160 beats per minute
65	78 to 116 beats per minute	155 beats per minute
70	75 to 113 beats per minute	150 beats per minute

The Importance of Cross Training

Cross training means engaging in a variety of fitness activities. By changing which muscles you work, you help avoid overuse injuries—damage that comes from stressing the same joints and muscles repeatedly. For example, by combining two days of swimming with three days of walking, you mix an exercise that relies heavily on upper-body strength with one that focuses more on the lower body.

The activities need not both be aerobic. Yoga and running are a time-honored combination because yoga helps stretch out the leg muscles that tighten with jogging. It's also more fun to vary your exercise rather than do the same thing day after day.

When Life Gets in the Way

Consistency is key. Think of exercise as preventive medicine. You wouldn't casually quit taking your medicine, so don't just quit exercising. Aerobic fitness doesn't last for long if you stop working out. Within a few weeks, benefits such as a slower heart rate and increased stamina

Cardiovascular Equipment—What's Out There?

The gym versions of these exercise machines are extra sturdy and offer electronic programs that vary the routine, but the simpler at-home models still offer a good workout. Be sure to try out new equipment before buying, and always wear athletic shoes when you use it. Here are some of the possibilities:

Treadmill. The most popular machine both at home and in the gym, it allows you to set your pace, anywhere from a leisurely stroll to a breakneck gallop. More expensive models include an incline feature that

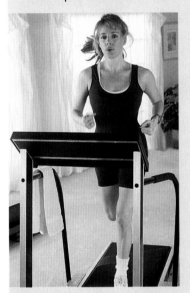

simulates moving uphill and dramatically boosts your calorie expenditure—good for people who want to lose weight but don't want to run. A treadmill is easy to master and very safe. Be warned that hanging on to the front handrail, instead of swinging your arms, reduces your cardiovascular effort and throws off your natural gait.

Stationary bike. An exercise bike has an enormous advantage over most other types of aerobic equipment: Because the machine holds you up, you can read while you're working out. However, since the bike supports your weight, it's difficult to burn a lot of calories except at the highest intensity. Bikes come in two versions, the older uprights and the newer recumbents, which have bucket seats that offer back support (good for people with back trouble). While both models are effective, uprights principally target the upper thighs, while recumbents work the buttocks muscles harder.

Stair climber. Difficult for some beginners, this machine involves stepping on pedals that move up and down but provide resistance. It offers a tough workout that easily reaches the intensity of running. Many people use terrible form on this equipment. When the effort level gets too hard, they put their weight on the handrails, which throws them off bal-

ance and reduces calorie expenditure. It's better to just admit you're on the wrong level and ratchet down the resistance a bit. For tips on form, see page 125.

Rowing machine. This machine can provide a strenuous workout for both the upper and lower body. Sitting on a seat that glides, you pull on a weighted handle (the resistance is adjustable) while the seat slides back and forth and you bend and straighten your legs. Since using proper form will protect your back from strain, be sure to get instructions first. (For tips, see page 125.)

Cross-country ski machine. In a simulation of cross-country skiing, your feet glide on two skis while your arms move a set of cords or poles. Good for working both the upper and lower body, with an emphasis on the lower, this machine can deliver a fairly intense workout. The biggest problem is mastering the coordination required.

Elliptical trainer. This machine looks a bit like a stair climber, but the pedals rotate in a circle as you step on them, creating a movement similar to bicycling standing up. It provides a nonimpact workout that can be gentle or very intense. Some people dislike the sensation of moving their feet through the air or have trouble achieving the balance required.

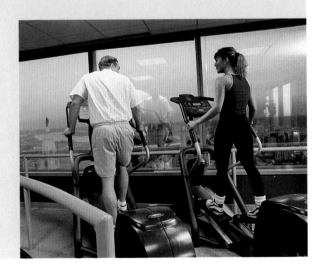

Getting Started: Exercise Your Options

To boost endurance, choose from a huge variety of activities:

For a Moderate Aerobic Workout

- Brisk walking
- Jogging (slow)
- Bicycling
- Low-impact aerobics class
- Step class (with low step)
- Swimming (slow)
- Water aerobics class
- Power yoga (fast-paced yoga)
- Swing dancing
- Stair-climbing machine or elliptical trainer (low resistance)
- Tae bo (beginners version of this martial arts–derived class)

For a Vigorous Aerobic Workout

- Brisk walking uphill
- Race walking
- Hiking with a heavy pack*
- Running (fast)*
- Spinning class (nonstop pedaling on a stationary bike)
- High-impact aerobics class*
- Jumping rope
- Climbing stairs
- Step class (with high step)*
- Rowing (hard)
- Cross-country skiing
- Swimming (fast)
- Water running (running in water with a flotation device that keeps you erect)
- Tae bo (advanced version)*
- Stair-climbing machine or elliptical trainer (high resistance)
- Racquetball*
- Squash*
- Handball*

*If you have any orthopedic problems, get your doctor's okay before trying these high-impact activities.

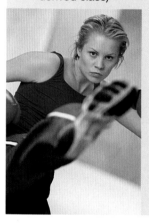

Fast Fact

Walking can help relieve some of the symptoms of osteoarthritis. Research suggests that people with arthritis of the knee who exercise in moderation have less pain and disability than those who don't exercise.

---

start to disappear. Since it takes a lot more effort to attain a level of fitness than to maintain it, never quit for long periods of time. If you find that you can't work out at your usual level, try to do half. Studies say that this rate of exercise will nearly sustain your present fitness level for about 12 weeks. Once you're able to, gradually increase the intensity, duration, and frequency of your routine until you're back where you left off.

Walk Yourself Fit

Walking is one of the best exercises around. It doesn't require special skills, costly equipment, or complicated instruction. It's free, and you can do it almost anywhere, almost any time. Compared to running, walking is relatively easy on the joints and bones. When you run, the force of each foot landing is about three to four times your body weight, which puts your knees, ankles, and shins at risk for injury. The stress from walking is only about half as great. For most people, the biggest danger is a twisted ankle from walking on uneven ground—an injury that heals much faster than the damaged knees and shin splints that plague runners. In fact, many runners turn to walking in middle age because they want to avoid further damage to their bodies.

Walking strengthens your muscles and your heart and lowers your blood pressure. It also helps build bone. It's so good for you that it can even lengthen your life. According to recent research, walking vigorously for 30 minutes just six times a month may lower your risk of premature death by 50 percent.

Strolling, Brisk Walking, and Race Walking

Walking to boost cardiovascular fitness is different from a casual stroll. While any kind of movement improves your health, fitness walking, also known as power walking or brisk walking, requires moving at a pace that will bring your heart rate into the target zone (see page 118)—a pace fast enough that you're breathing hard, but not so fast that you're out of breath.

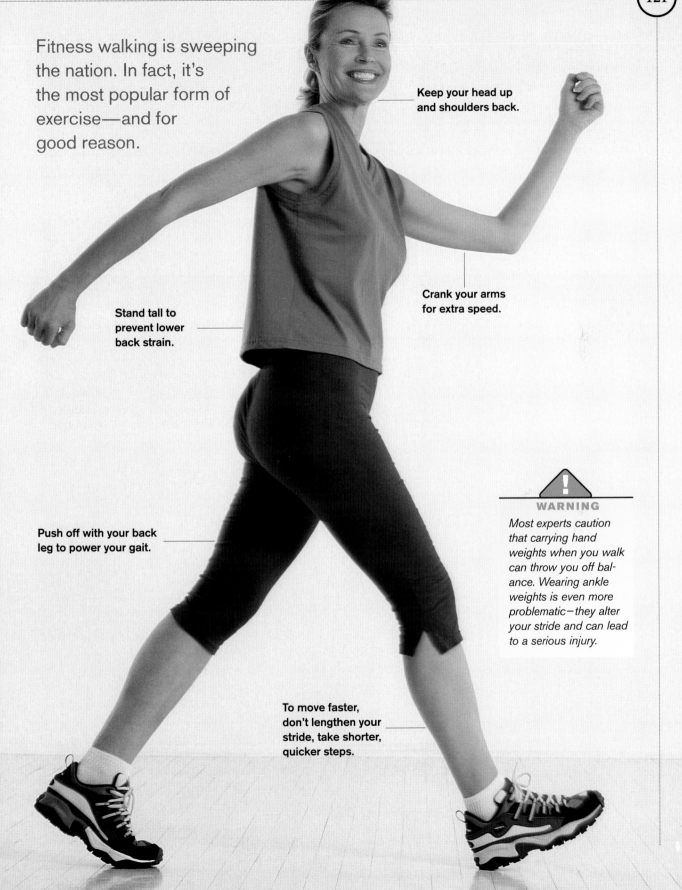

Fitness walking is sweeping the nation. In fact, it's the most popular form of exercise—and for good reason.

Keep your head up and shoulders back.

Crank your arms for extra speed.

Stand tall to prevent lower back strain.

Push off with your back leg to power your gait.

To move faster, don't lengthen your stride, take shorter, quicker steps.

⚠ WARNING

Most experts caution that carrying hand weights when you walk can throw you off balance. Wearing ankle weights is even more problematic—they alter your stride and can lead to a serious injury.

12-Week Walking Program

This program requires you to monitor your heart rate and build to a certain level of intensity. If you prefer, you can measure yourself against the Borg scale (see page 115). By the eleventh week, you should be walking up and down hills or climbing stairs to boost your workout.

WEEK	FREQUENCY	WARM-UP	WALK	COOLDOWN
1	5 times a week	5 minutes slow walking	10 minutes at 50-60% maximum heart rate	5 minutes slow walking
2	5 times a week	5 minutes	15 minutes at 50-60% max heart rate	5 minutes
3	5 times a week	5 minutes	20 minutes at 50-60% max heart rate	5 minutes
4	5 times a week	5 minutes	20 minutes at 60% max heart rate	5 minutes
5	5 times a week	5 minutes	20 minutes at 60-70% max heart rate	5 minutes
6	5 times a week	5 minutes	20 minutes at 60-70% max heart rate	5 minutes
7	5 times a week	5 minutes	25 minutes at 60-70% max heart rate	5 minutes
8	5 times a week	5 minutes	25 minutes at 70% max heart rate	5 minutes
9	5 times a week	5 minutes	30 minutes at 70% max heart rate	5 minutes
10	5 times a week	5 minutes	35 minutes at 70% max heart rate	5 minutes
11	3 times a week	5 minutes	35 minutes at 70% max heart rate	5 minutes
	2 times a week	5 minutes	30 minutes at 70% max heart rate, including 5 minutes of hills or stairs	5 minutes
12	3 times a week	5 minutes	35 minutes at 70% max heart rate	5 minutes
	2 times a week	5 minutes	30 minutes at 70% max heart rate, including 10 minutes of hills or stairs	5 minutes

123

Easy Ways to Work in a Workout

Small changes in your daily routine can add up to big health benefits. Here are some ways to put more exercise in your life:

- Play ball with your kids or grandchildren.
- Cancel your newspaper delivery and walk to the store every morning to buy it instead.
- Take your dog out for an extra walk every day, or change your route to cover hillier terrain.
- Dust off your bicycle and take it for a weekend spin through the neighborhood.

- Take two extra full turns around the mall whenever you go shopping.
- Choose the farthest parking spot and let your legs do the rest.
- Walk the golf course rather than taking a cart.
- Rake leaves by hand instead of using a blower.
- Stretch and strengthen your ankles and lower-leg muscles while you watch TV. First, alternately flex and extend your feet. Then make circles in the air with your feet, rotating your ankles clockwise, then counterclockwise.

WARNING

If you have high blood pressure, skip the coffee or cola before heading out for your walk. Moderate walking temporarily elevates your systolic blood pressure by 12 to 18 points. Caffeine can raise it another seven points or so.

Fitness walking is not as quick as race walking. Race walkers, who have an unusual gait that involves swaying the hips back and forth, can easily walk 12-minute miles, faster than some people jog. But for most people, fitness walking, in which 14- to 15-minute miles are common, is more comfortable.

Watch Your Form

You already know how to place one foot in front of the other, and your gait is probably fine for fitness walking. But how is your posture? Many people slump over when they walk which, over time, can lead to problems such as muscle strain and pain in the neck, lower back, and hips. As you walk, point your chest straight ahead. And tuck in your belly, which is doing a lot of the work in holding up your back. Every five minutes or so, do a mental scan of your posture. Are you standing straight? If not, pull yourself back into alignment.

What are your arms doing while you walk? If you hold them still, or swing them without bending them, you're slowing yourself down. Here's a better option: Bend your arms at a 90-degree angle and swing them in sync with the opposite leg. This motion will not only feel more natural, but it will also add speed and power to your walk.

Speeding Up

Many people try to walk faster by lengthening their stride. Big mistake. This movement—known as over-striding—puts you off balance without quickening your pace. Since the power in your gait comes from pushing off your back leg and foot, it's more effective to take short, quicker steps when you want to move faster. Also concentrate on pumping your (bent) arms fast, which will help speed up your legs.

Don't overdo it, however. Reduce your pace if you can't speak easily while walking or if it takes more than six minutes for your pulse to normalize after a fitness walk.

SimpleSolution

Want company? The American Volkssport Association holds non-competitive group walks all over North America. Call 800-830-WALK (or access their Internet site at www.ava.org) to find a club near you.

Aerobics, the Safe Way

Week after week you feel your endurance building. Then—wham!—you twist an ankle or pull a muscle, and you're back in front of the TV set. Nothing throws a wrench into a fitness plan as fast as an injury.

Play it smart. One key to exercising safely is the warm-up phase. For 6 to 10 minutes, do a low-intensity version of the activity you're about to perform to loosen up your muscles and make you less prone to injury. Paying attention to technique also protects you. Here, activity by activity, are some of the most common aerobic pitfalls and how to avoid them.

Cycle Right

When cycling, pay special attention to your seat height. Position the seat so that when you extend one leg fully on the down pedal, with your foot flat, that knee is slightly bent. If the seat is too low, you'll stress your knees. If it's too high, you'll place undue force on your lower back. But when the seat is properly positioned, you'll work the intended muscles—the quads (on the fronts of the thighs) and the gluteals (in the buttocks).

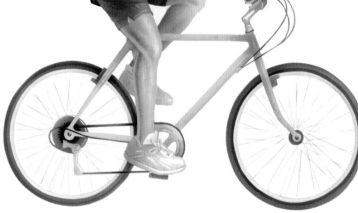

Feet First

When you walk, jog, or run, strike the ground first with your heel, then with the ball of your foot, and finally push off from your toes. This heel-ball-toe pattern helps prevent shin splints and shin pain. For activities that involve jumping, such as rope jumping or step aerobics, the pattern is reversed: toe-ball-heel. Sport-specific footwear is designed to absorb impact at those parts of the foot that strike the ground most directly. For example, aerobic dance shoes are most padded at the ball of the foot, while running shoes have more cushioning at the heel.

Row, Row, Row

If you're working out on a rowing machine, maintain proper posture by always keeping your shoulders aligned directly over your hips. Avoid the common mistake of sliding your seat backward before you move your arms. Instead, slide back and pull at the same time. Otherwise you risk straining your lower back. To protect your joints, never lock your knees or elbows.

Posture Perfect

If you're using a stair climber, avoid overstressing your knees by keeping your extended leg slightly bent and both knees aligned behind your toes; this may require you to lean back a bit. Also, avoid the common mistake of resting your forearms along the handrails for support. People have developed elbow tendinitis and carpal tunnel syndrome from overextending their elbows and wrists while on a stair climber.

In the Swim

Take a few swimming lessons if you haven't done so recently. New techniques help prevent shoulder problems and allow you to swim more efficiently. The S-patterned stroke at right gives you more thrust because your arms push against still water, not their own choppy wake. As shown below, keep your head down except to breathe; turn it just until your mouth is out of the water. Keep your shoulders higher than your legs, and kick from your hips, not your knees. Don't arch your back.

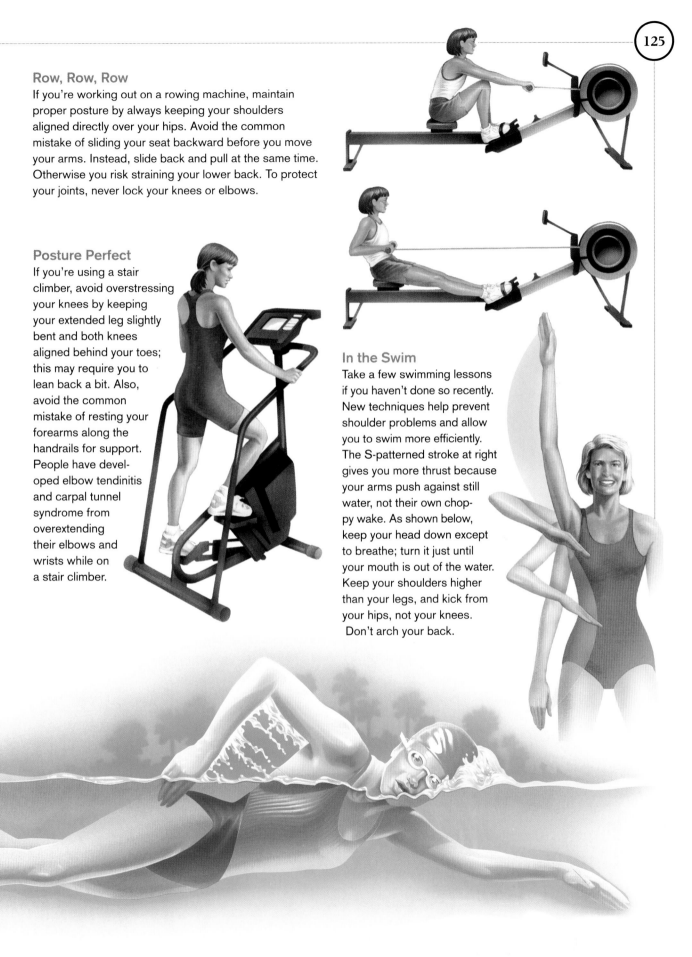

Building Muscle Strength

Building muscle is one of the best ways to stay younger longer. It will help boost your metabolism, offset bone loss, and give you more energy to boot.

Do you have trouble carrying heavy bags of groceries, moving furniture, or unscrewing a tight lid? If so, you probably wish you had the strength you used to take for granted. The expression "use it or lose it" perfectly describes how muscles are maintained. They become stronger (and bigger) when they're subjected to greater force than they're used to, but they decline in strength (and size) when they're underutilized.

Muscle mass peaks around age 30 and decreases very gradually until your fifties, when the decline becomes much more pronounced.

If you're active, the rate of decline is considerably reduced. Older adults who've engaged in strength training for 15 years or more are as strong or stronger than inactive 20-year-olds, according to a Johns Hopkins study. And it's never too late to start. In a Tufts University study, when volunteers in their nineties followed an eight-week strength-training program, some increased their strength threefold.

Progressive Resistance

If you want stronger muscles, you have to tax them a bit more than usual, a concept known as the overload principle. Don't overdo it though. If you suddenly try to pick up a sofa, for instance, you're asking for trouble.

After your muscles adjust to a new load, increase the load again if you want to move to the next strength level. Following this principle, a traditional strength-training program calls for adding more weight as you get stronger, doing more repetitions, working out more often,

Free Weights or Machines?

Should you use free weights or weight-training machines? It's a matter of personal preference. Each option has its advantages. Machines are designed to give you a proper workout on targeted muscles. Once you get into position, minimum coordination is required. The machine supports your body weight as you move the mechanical parts.

Free weights are more difficult because you must balance and align your body while working out, which means you end up working more muscles at once. Free weights are more versatile, however. You can do hundreds of exercises with one set of 5- or 10-pound weights, and you can work out in your living room rather than having to go to a gym.

or some combination of these three factors. You may, however, be happy with a certain level of development and decide to maintain it.

How Much? How Often?

To burn fat, tone existing muscle, and build new muscle, the American College of Sports Medicine recommends two to three sets of 10 to 12 repetitions ("reps" in gym lingo) for each major muscle group two to three times a week. Reps are the number of times you perform a specific exercise.

By the last two or three reps of each set, the muscle you're working should be near exhaustion—an indication you're challenging it sufficiently. If you've been working out for some time and want to increase the challenge, do three or four sets of 8 to 10 reps, or increase the amount you're lifting by two to five pounds.

Rest for 40 to 75 seconds between sets. This allows your blood to clear away the lactic acid that builds up inside your muscles when they work to their limit.

To avoid damaging your muscles, give them at least one full day of rest between strength-training sessions. The downtime is crucial to allow your muscles to rebuild in response to the stress.

Maintain Good Form

If you're new to weight training, it's very important to have someone check your form. Many exercises are easy to do incorrectly, and it can be difficult to check your own posture. Check with your local gym— it may offer weight-training instruction—or consider hiring a personal trainer for one or two sessions.

In general, while you're moving weights, remember to keep your back straight and stable rather than arched. Never sway back and forth to generate power. Instead, lift and lower weights slowly so that your muscles—not momentum or gravity—do the work. Focus on using only the muscles that you are trying to work. Periodically scan your body to see if you're clenching your jaw or tensing your neck; you could create soreness that has nothing to do with building muscles.

Always exhale as you exert force to help power your movement. Inhale as you relax. If you're doing push-ups, for example, inhale as you lower your body to the floor, and exhale as you straighten your arms (the hardest part of the exercise). Don't hold your breath; it's a common mistake, and one that can temporarily raise your blood pressure.

When Will You See Results?

Your body contours should change within a month of consistent weight training. (If not, check in with a pro for some corrections.) Don't expect big results, though—that will take three to six months of steady work. Some muscles grow stronger much faster than others; in general, large muscles like the chest, back, and buttocks develop first. Don't worry about bulking up too much. It takes hours of work per day to build huge muscles; they don't happen by accident.

As your strength improves, your aerobic workouts will get easier. And that's not the only extra benefit. By lifting weights and building lean body mass, you're increasing your basal metabolism. That's because you burn more calories per minute maintaining muscle weight than fat weight—even at rest.

Fast Fact

Women who weight-train twice a week can boost overall strength by as much as 75 percent, according to recent research out of Tufts University. And when compared with sedentary women, the weight trainers had better flexibility and balance and increased self-confidence, and they were less likely to suffer from insomnia.

In their own words

"I only became aware of the way...little energy expenditures were burdening me when, as my muscle tone and general level of strength improved, they lightened. I didn't think I needed to be strong. Then I noticed—when, for example, I spent a day at yard work— that it was useful to be strong all day long. I began to enjoy that, secretly."

—John Jerome, describing how he became a competitive swimmer for the first time at age 47, in Staying with It: On Becoming an Athlete

Strengthening Your Lower Body

These exercises will strengthen your legs, buttocks, and hips. They rely on your body weight to provide resistance. As you grow stronger, you can increase resistance by adding leg weights or using elastic resistance bands, sold in sporting-goods stores. Start with two to three sets of 10 to 12 repetitions of each exercise.

Adduction

Adductors (inner thighs)

- Lie on your right side with your left leg angled in front of you and the inside edge of your left foot resting on the floor. Keep your right leg straight without locking your knee. Your ankle, knee, hip, and shoulder should form a straight line.
- Raise your right (lower) leg as high as you comfortably can. Hold for one second, then lower it slowly to within one inch of the floor. Hold, then repeat. Your lower leg should not touch the floor until the end of the set.
- After each set, switch sides.
- **To step it up**
  Add ankle weights to the leg you're lifting. If you have knee problems, place the weights above your knee.

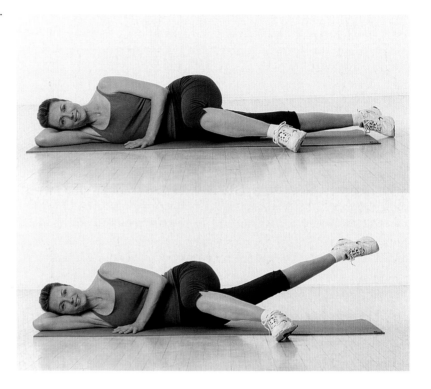

Abduction

Abductors (outer thighs), and gluteals (buttocks)

- Lie on your right side with your right knee and hip each bent at a 45-degree angle. Keep your upper leg nearly straight, and keep your torso straight to avoid stressing your lower back.
- Raise your upper leg as high as you comfortably can. Hold for one second, then slowly lower it until it is almost touching your lower leg. Your upper leg should not touch your lower leg until the end of the set.
- At the end of each set, switch sides to work the other leg.

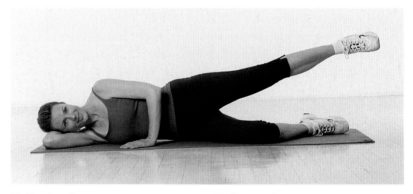

- **To step it up**
  Add ankle weights to the leg you're lifting. If you have knee problems, place the weights above your knee.

- **Expert tip**
  In any strengthening exercise, mentally focus on the muscles you're targeting. It helps you maintain proper form and reduces your reliance on other muscles.

Squats

Quadriceps (fronts of your thighs), gluteals, hamstrings (backs of your thighs)

- Stand in front of a chair with your feet about hip-width apart. Keep your body erect and your chin raised slightly throughout this exercise.
- Slowly lower your hips toward the chair as if you're about to sit. Just before your body touches it, return slowly to a standing position. Keep your back straight, your knees behind your toes, your weight centered over your midfoot and heels (not over your toes), and your feet flat on the floor.
- If you need help with balance or flexibility, place a small board, ½- to 1-inch thick, under your heels.

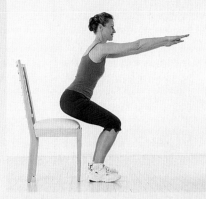

- **To step it up**

  Remove the chair and lower your hips until the tops of your thighs are parallel to the floor. As you get stronger, increase resistance by holding dumbbells at your sides or in front of your chest.

Lunges

Quadriceps, gluteals, and hamstrings

- Start with your feet hip-width apart or slightly closer. Raise your chin slightly throughout this exercise.
- Take a large step forward with your right leg, planting your foot firmly on the floor with your toes pointed forward or slightly inward. Align your right knee over your right foot. Throughout this exercise, keep your back straight and your knee behind the toes of your forward foot.
- Bring your left knee straight down until it is an inch or two from the floor. To raise yourself, press firmly into the floor with your right foot while extending your right knee.
- Return to the initial standing position and repeat with your left leg forward.
- **To step it up**
  Hold dumbbells at your sides.

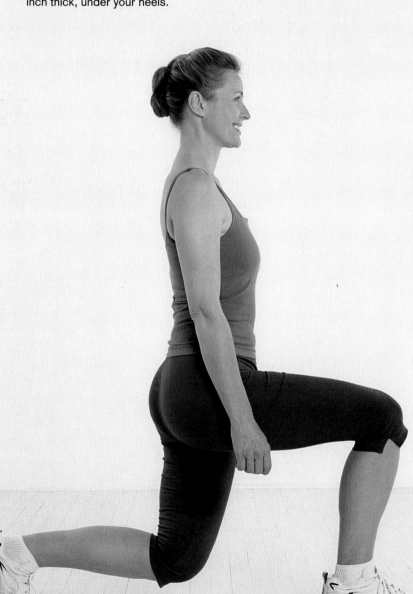

Strengthening Your Upper Body

These exercises will give you the strength to polish the car, carry a suitcase, and shovel snow. They will also boost your performance in many sports, including golf and tennis. They are especially important for women, who tend to lack upper-body strength. Start with two to three sets of 10 to 12 repetitions of each exercise.

Chest Press

Pectorals (large muscles in your chest), deltoids (shoulders), and triceps (backs of your upper arms)

■ Lie faceup on a bench. (You can also do this exercise on the floor, but your range of motion will be limited.) Keep your feet on the bench, knees bent, to support your lower back. Hold a pair of dumbbells at your chest as shown, your palms facing your knees.

■ Exhale as you press the weights upward, bringing them close together but not touching, and extending your elbows almost fully.

■ Inhale as you lower the weights slowly, reversing the movement. Keep your wrists aligned with your elbows throughout the exercise. Lower your elbows to just below torso level.

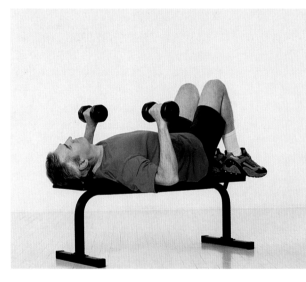

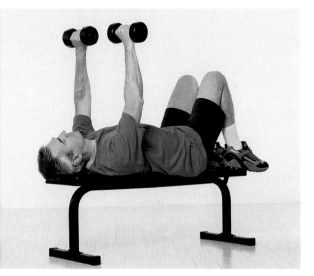

One-Arm Dumbbell Row

Latissimus dorsi (two muscle groups that connect your shoulder blades to your hipbones)

■ Rest your left knee and hand on the edge of a bench or firm chair or sofa. Bend your right knee slightly so your weight is distributed evenly on both legs. Lightly grasp a dumbbell with your right hand, and let it hang straight down by your side. Keep your working arm close to your body. Keep your back straight and your shoulders level.

■ Exhale as you pull the dumbbell upward toward your waist, stopping when it almost touches your torso.

■ Inhale as you lower it slowly to the original position. At the end of each set, switch sides.

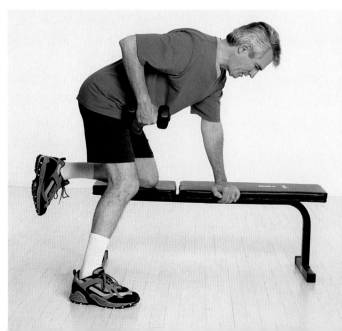

Kickback

Triceps

- Rest your right knee and right hand on a bench or chair and extend your left leg behind you, your left foot flat on the floor. Grasp a dumbbell lightly in your left hand, your elbow at your side, your arm bent at a 45-degree angle.
- Exhale as you straighten your left arm almost fully. Keep your elbow at your side and move only your forearm.
- Pause, then inhale as you lower your arm to its original 45-degree angle. After each set, switch to work your other arm.

Curl Twist

Biceps (front upper arms)

- You can sit or stand for this exercise. If you stand, keep your feet hip-width apart and bend your knees slightly. Lightly grasp a pair of dumbbells, keeping your arms straight at your sides, your palms facing your legs.
- Exhale as you raise the weights toward your shoulders, gradually turning your wrists so your palms face your shoulders. Pin your elbows at your sides so that only your forearms move. Tense your abdominal muscles for support.
- Without resting, inhale as you lower your arms slowly to the original position.

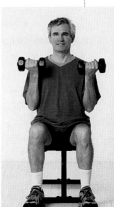

Lateral Raise

Deltoids

- You can sit or stand for this exercise. If you stand, keep your feet hip-width apart and bend your knees slightly. Lightly grasp a pair of dumb-bells and let them hang down at your sides while bending your elbows slightly. Tense your abdominal muscles for support during this exercise.
- Exhale as you raise your arms outward until they are parallel to the floor. Your wrists, elbows, and shoulders should be in a straight line. Don't lock elbows.
- Inhale as you lower your arms until they nearly touch your sides.

Strengthening Your Midsection

Strong muscles in your core—your torso—stabilize your body, allowing you to sit for long stretches without slumping or rake leaves (your arms move while your trunk provides leverage). Strong abdominal and back muscles help prevent back strains and also help power your golf swing and your swimming stroke.

GREAT FOR YOUR BACK

Reverse Crunch

Lower abdominals, some upper abdominals

- Lie faceup on a mat or carpet with your knees bent. Raise one leg at a time, straightening each leg so that the soles of your feet face the ceiling. Raise your head from the floor slightly, placing your palms behind your head to provide neck support.
- As you exhale, contract your abdominal muscles (abs) to pull your legs back about 30 degrees toward your head. Use your abs, not your leg muscles, to accomplish this.
- Inhale as you relax your abs to slowly return your legs to their original position.
- Do two sets of 15 reps.

GREAT FOR YOUR BACK

Oblique Twist

Obliques (the diagonal muscles that run along the sides of your waist)

- Lie faceup on a mat or carpet with your knees bent. Place your left ankle across your right knee and your left hand palm up on the floor perpendicular to your body. Place your right palm behind your head to provide neck support.
- Exhale as you raise your upper body, bringing your right shoulder toward your left knee.
- Pause briefly, then inhale as you slowly lower your upper body to the mat. Your right hand should not pull your head forward, but simply support it. Switch sides.
- Do two sets of 15 reps, each side.

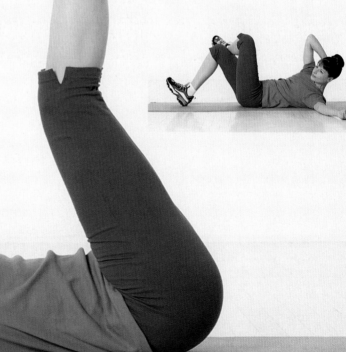

Crunch

Upper abdominals

- Lie faceup on a mat or carpet with your knees bent and your feet on the floor. Point your toes up to provide extra back support. Place both hands under your head with the index fingers and thumbs of each hand touching. Don't interlock your fingers or pull on your head, which can result in strained neck muscles. The effort should come from your abs, not your arms. Throughout this exercise, keep your lower back pressed into the floor and avoid bouncing or jerking movements.
- As you exhale, curl your upper body toward your thighs about 30 degrees. Pause briefly, then inhale as you slowly lower yourself.

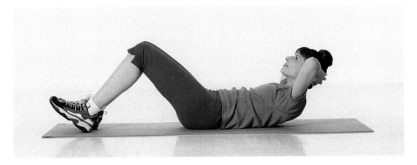

- Do two sets of 15 reps each.
- Expert tip

  When working any muscle group, exercise your larger muscles first. If you work your small muscles first, they'll be too tired to support your larger muscles during their workout. Using this strategy, do your abdominal exercises in this order: Reverse Crunch, Oblique Twist, Crunch.

Lower Extension

Lower back extensors

- Lie facedown on a mat with your arms resting at your sides.
- As you exhale, keep your upper body in contact with the mat and raise your legs upward as high as you comfortably can. Inhale as you lower your legs slowly toward the floor. Allow your legs to tap the floor momentarily between each repetition.
- Start with a goal of one set of 10 to 15 reps, then as

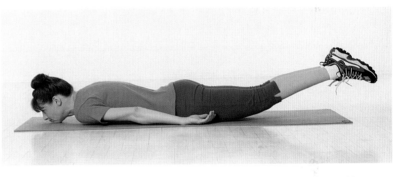

your back becomes stronger, do two sets, with a brief stretch between sets.

Upper Extension

Upper back extensors

- Lie facedown on a mat with your arms resting at your sides.
- Exhale as you raise your upper body slowly off the floor as high as you comfortably can.
- Inhale as you lower yourself slowly toward the floor. Allow your chest to tap the floor momentarily between each rep.
- Start with a goal of one set of 10 to 15 reps. As your back muscles become stronger, perform two sets of up to 15 reps each, with a brief stretch between sets.

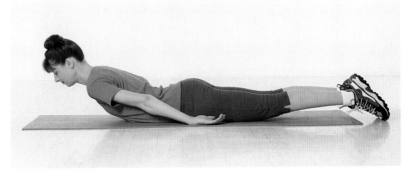

- To step it up

  Place both hands behind your head while you do this exercise.

Stretch Your Limits

Many adults can't touch their toes. Are you one of them? Getting limber again can help ease an aching back and prevent injury, too.

Children bend like rubber bands, but adults—especially those who sit at a desk all day—tend to lose their full range of motion. For instance, the hip flexor and lower back muscles shorten, throwing off your posture. Lack of flexibility also paves the way for muscle pain—especially back, neck, and shoulder stiffness—and injury.

Following a stretching routine can keep tendons, ligaments, and joints limber and help relieve muscle tension and arthritis pain.

All the stretches on the following pages are particularly effective when combined with the strength-building exercises that work the postural muscles (see pages 130 and 132-133).

Once you've fully extended a muscle, hold the stretch for a few seconds. Never bounce. Stretch only after warming up to avoid damaging muscles and tendons.

Lower Body

These stretches are especially important if you spend a lot of time sitting. Perform each one four or more times.

Quad Stretch

Quadriceps
- With your left hand on a chair back for balance, bend your right knee and grasp your ankle with your right hand.
- Pull slightly, producing a strong stretch across the front of your thigh. Exhale as you contract your buttocks and hamstrings. Hold two to four seconds, then inhale and release. Switch legs and repeat.

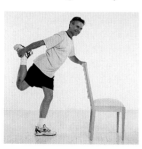

Across-the-Knee Raise

Abductors and gluteals
- Lie on your back with both knees bent and your feet flat on the floor, your arms out to your sides. Place your right ankle across your left knee.
- Exhale as you bring your left leg toward your chest, carrying your right ankle with it. If needed, use your arms for support. Hold the stretch two to four seconds. After several reps, switch legs and repeat.

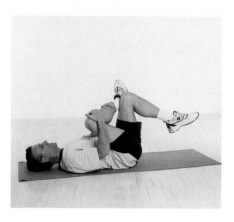

Straight-Leg Stretch

Hamstrings
- Lie on your back, both knees bent, and feet flat on the floor. Extend your left leg upward until nearly straight.
- With both hands behind your thigh, exhale, pulling your leg gently toward your chest to feel the stretch in your hamstring. Hold two to four seconds.
- Inhale as you return your leg to its original position. After several reps, change legs.

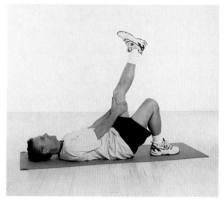

Upper Body

These stretches are easy to do anywhere, any time—and they feel great. Aim to stretch two or three days a week. With any stretch, you should feel tension but not pain.

Behind-the-Neck Stretch

Triceps and deltoids

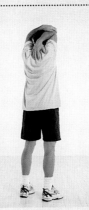

- While standing or sitting, bend your right elbow, grasp it with your left hand, and reach your right hand down toward your left shoulder blade.
- Pull on your right elbow slightly until you feel a stretch along the back of your upper arm. There is very little range of motion with this exercise. After two or three reps, switch arms and repeat.

Straight-Arm Extension

Biceps

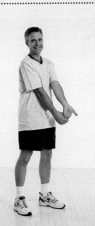

- While standing, fully extend your left arm so your palm is facing forward. Grasp it with your right hand.
- Exhale as you press gently against that palm, bending your wrist back until you feel a stretch across the inside of your left elbow. Hold, then release. There is very little range of motion with this exercise. Perform two or three reps, then repeat with your right arm.

Extended-Arm Pull

Latissimus dorsi, trapezius (triangular muscle in your upper back), and deltoids

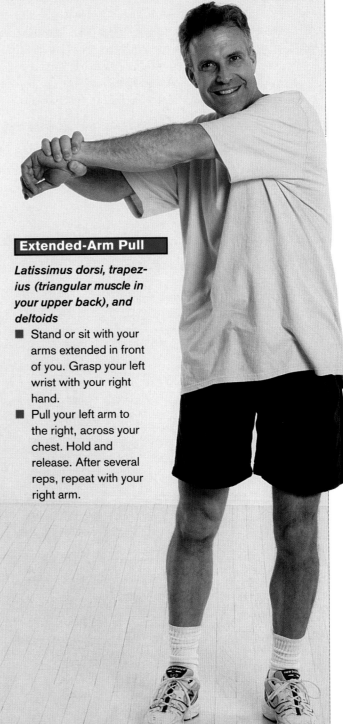

- Stand or sit with your arms extended in front of you. Grasp your left wrist with your right hand.
- Pull your left arm to the right, across your chest. Hold and release. After several reps, repeat with your right arm.

Hand-on-Wall Stretch

Pectorals and deltoids

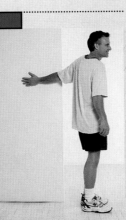

- Stretch your left arm behind you, palm against a wall, elbow slightly bent.
- Exhale as you turn slowly to the right, maintaining the bend in your elbow, until you feel a stretch across your left shoulder and chest. Hold, then release. Repeat several times, then switch arms.

GREAT FOR YOUR BACK

Core Body

Perform your core body stretches before and after every workout—two reps of each exercise before, and three to five reps of each afterward.

Knee Hug

Lower back

- Lie on your back with your knees bent and your feet flat on the floor.
- Exhale as you use your abs and hips to pull your knees toward your chest. Place your arms behind your knees with your palms on your elbows. Use your arms to pull your knees closer to your chest.
- Hold for two to three seconds, then release your legs, lowering your feet slowly to the floor. Repeat.
- To increase this stretch, raise your chin to your knees as you hug your knees to your chest.

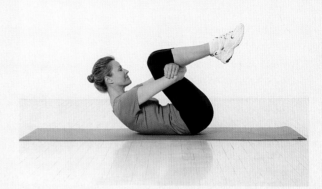

GREAT FOR YOUR BACK

Cobra (Press-ups)

Abs and lower back

- Lie facedown on the floor with your hands near your shoulders, palms against the floor.
- Exhale as you start to straighten your arms to raise your upper body, keeping your elbows tucked close to your sides. Keep your hips and lower body relaxed and on the floor.
- Stop when you begin to feel a stretch in your lower back or waist. Hold for two seconds before lowering yourself to the original position. Repeat.

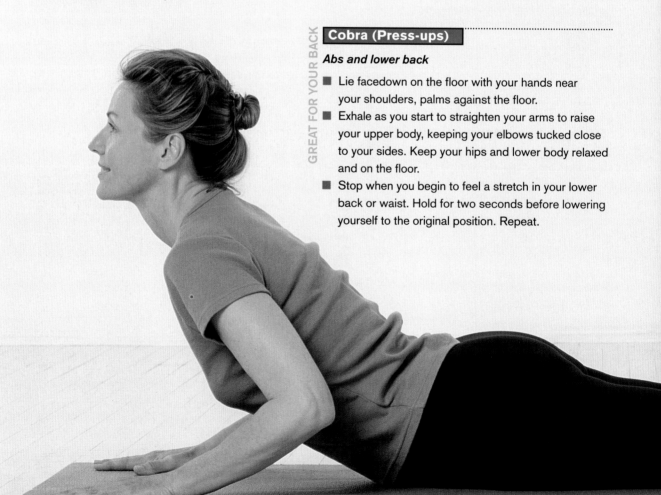

Side Twist

Entire side-muscle groups, from outer thighs and hips to upper back

■ Lie on your back, your arms out to the sides, your knees bent, and your feet flat on the floor.

■ Exhale as you lower both legs slowly to the left, keeping your knees together and bent. With your left hand, gently press down on your right leg until you feel a strong stretch along your right side.

■ Inhale as you raise your legs toward center. Repeat for two to four reps, then switch sides.

■ To intensify this stretch, bring your upper leg slightly forward as you lower your legs to the side.

Cat's Back

Upper and lower back and spine

■ Rest on your hands and knees, keeping your back flat.

■ Exhale as you curl your back upward and lower your head until you're looking at your abdomen. Hold for a moment.

■ Inhale as you lower your back slowly until it is arced as far as comfortable, raising your head so you're looking up toward the ceiling. Repeat.

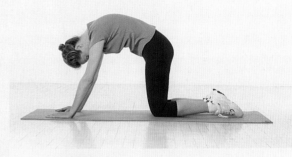

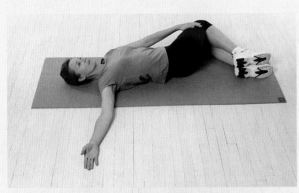

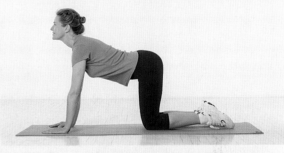

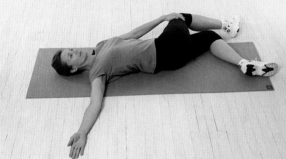

Activities for Improving Flexibility

● Swimming
● Tai chi
● Yoga
● Fencing
● Ballet and modern dance
● Pilates classes and training (a technique originally developed for dancers and now available on videos and in health clubs)
● Group fitness classes with a stretching segment
  ● YMCA "healthy back" classes
    ● Feldenkrais technique (a low-intensity method for improving alignment)

Balancing Acts

Kids bounce; adults don't. To avoid dangerous falls, it's time to fine-tune your sense of balance.

For reasons that are not yet clear, balance tends to decline with age. It's a serious problem, given that balance-related falls account for more than half of accidental deaths in the elderly.

To some extent, your ability to stay balanced is a function of how strong you are. Even if your sense of balance is okay, you can't stand on one leg very long if that leg is weak.

So staying strong or becoming stronger can certainly help keep you upright.

The strength and flexibility exercises described on pages 128-137 can help you maintain balance and coordination. But as you grow older, it becomes more important to include some exercises specifically aimed at improving your balance.

Basic Balance Moves

Here are three exercises to get you started on the road to better balance. Do your balance workout in bare feet or socks (on a nonskid floor) to help you develop the muscles in your feet.

Backward Leg Lift

- Stand alongside a chair with your feet about six inches apart. Rest your hand lightly on the chair back, and maintain a slight bend at the knees.
- Shift your weight to your right leg and lean forward slightly as you slowly press your left leg back (top photo), squeezing your right gluteal muscles (buttocks). Hold for one second before returning to the starting position.
- Repeat with the right leg. Alternate legs for 10 to 15 reps.
- **To step it up**
  Hold your leg in the back position for a longer count, do more reps on each side, and/or remove your hand from the chair.

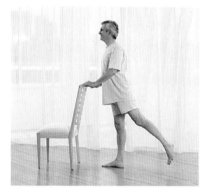

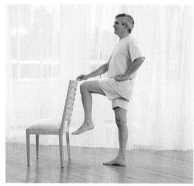

Bent Leg Lift

- Stand alongside a chair with your feet about six inches apart. Rest your hand lightly on the chair back and maintain a slight bend at the knees.
- Shift your weight to your right leg and slowly raise your left knee up toward your waist (bottom photo), flexing your knee and hip joints. Hold for one second before lowering your leg.
- Repeat with the right leg. Alternate legs for 10 to 15 repetitions.
- **To step it up**
  Hold your leg in the up position for a longer count (up to four seconds), gradually increase consecutive repetitions on each side, and/or remove your hand from the chair.

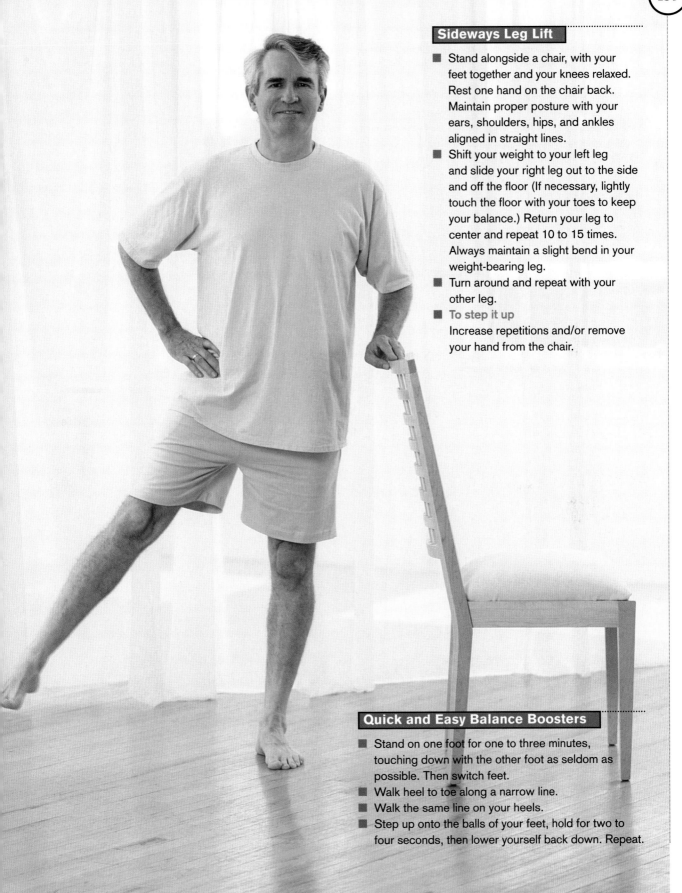

Sideways Leg Lift

- Stand alongside a chair, with your feet together and your knees relaxed. Rest one hand on the chair back. Maintain proper posture with your ears, shoulders, hips, and ankles aligned in straight lines.
- Shift your weight to your left leg and slide your right leg out to the side and off the floor (If necessary, lightly touch the floor with your toes to keep your balance.) Return your leg to center and repeat 10 to 15 times. Always maintain a slight bend in your weight-bearing leg.
- Turn around and repeat with your other leg.
- To step it up
  Increase repetitions and/or remove your hand from the chair.

Quick and Easy Balance Boosters

- Stand on one foot for one to three minutes, touching down with the other foot as seldom as possible. Then switch feet.
- Walk heel to toe along a narrow line.
- Walk the same line on your heels.
- Step up onto the balls of your feet, hold for two to four seconds, then lower yourself back down. Repeat.

Taking Balance Further

For better balance, try yoga! The following poses develop not only balance, but also concentration, coordination, and strength. Each pose is begun and sustained with deep, slow, rhythmic breathing. Hold the pose for 15 seconds, or to a point that's comfortable for you. Then release, switch sides, and repeat.

Tree

- Stand with your shoulders relaxed, your spine straight, your hands in prayer position at your heart, and your feet six inches apart.
- Bend your left knee and place your left foot as high on your right leg as is comfortable.
- Raise your arms overhead and straighten your elbows.

Stick

- Stand with your shoulders relaxed, spine straight, arms by your sides, and feet six inches apart.
- Raise your arms overhead close to your ears, your hands together with index fingers pointed and other fingers interlaced.
- Raise your right leg slowly, balancing over your left foot. Pivot over your hip, keeping your arms, spine, and right leg in a straight line. As you progress, that line should be parallel to the floor.

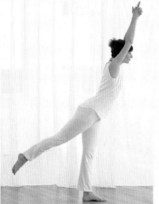

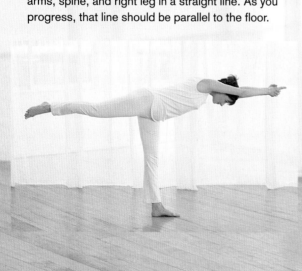

Warrior I and II

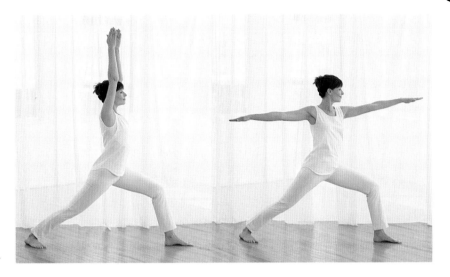

- Stand with your shoulders relaxed, spine straight, feet six inches apart.
- Raise your arms overhead with palms facing.
- Step out about four feet with your left foot, bending your left knee directly over your ankle. Straighten the knee of your right leg, and drop your heel to the floor.
- For Warrior II, drop your arms parallel to the floor, and gaze over your forward hand.

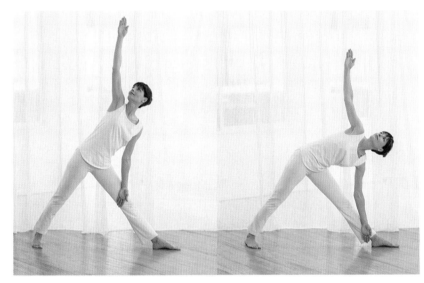

Triangle

- Stand with your shoulders relaxed, spine straight, feet six inches apart.
- Step out about four feet with your left foot, and raise your arms to shoulder height. Reach and lean to the left.
- Drop your left hand to your knee, raise your right arm overhead, and keep your shoulders in alignment.
- Slide your left hand toward your ankle, point your right hand up, and gaze at your extended hand.

Advanced Balance Workouts

Looking for an even more challenging balance workout? Consider buying an exercise device that forces you to use your "neutralizers" and "stabilizers"—small muscles involved in balance that usually aren't targeted in aerobic or strength-training workouts. The first two devices focus on torso muscles; the last two work torso and leg muscles. All usually come with suggested exercises.

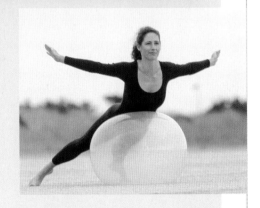

1. Stability ball. Sit on or lean against this sturdy, oversize beach ball.
2. Biofoam roller. Use this solid foam cylinder during floor exercises.
3. Wobble or rocker board. Place this wooden board over a special ball or cylinder, and stand on it while exercising.
4. Soft-cushioned balance pad or air-filled pillow. Use these to add an extra dimension to standing exercises.

The Fastest Way to Fitness

Experts say the best way to establish a new habit is to practice it, without fail, for three weeks running. Start an exercise habit with one of these programs.

New to regular exercise? Don't be daunted. You're in for big payoffs. If you haven't exercised in a while—or ever—even small amounts of physical activity will make a difference. For instance, 20 minutes on a stationary bike can lower your levels of stress hormones for at least two hours, according to an Indiana University study. And one low-intensity session of weight lifting can reduce stress, anger, and fatigue for up to three hours according to another report. After a few weeks, you'll see your muscles grow stronger and your aerobic power improve. You might even sleep better.

A Six-Week Starter Program

To follow the beginner program outlined on page 143, begin by working on your cardiovascular endurance with fast walking, pedaling on a stationary bike without resistance, or slow swimming. Warm up and cool down before and after by doing the same activity at a slower pace for a few minutes. Beginning at week 3, add two strength-training sessions, doing two or three sets of the exercises described on pages 128-133. You can do them immediately after your endurance workout or on alternate days. Immediately after each workout segment, stretch the muscles you used while they're still warm. Always give yourself at least two days of rest a week. You can stay at this level indefinitely or move on to the intermediate stage.

Intermediate Routine

With the intermediate-level routine, your goal is to build up to 30-minute cardiovascular and strength-training

9 Picks in Exercise Videos

Exercise videos add variety to your workouts and help you stay motivated and entertained.

Beginner Level

- *Leslie Sansone's 2-Mile Walk:* For rainy days, a "walk" in front of the TV with simple steps like marching in place, kicking, and tapping.
- *Karen Voigt's Pure & Simple Stretch:* A relaxing series of static and moving stretches.
- *Buns of Steel: Starting Simple–Toning:* A no-frills routine tailor-made for novices.

Intermediate Level

- *Donna Richardson's Donna-Mite:* An unintimidating aerobics workout with oldies tunes and a very enthusiastic instructor.
- *Karen Voigt's Yoga Sculpt:* Combines muscle toning and flexibility training, with an emphasis on improving your core strength.
- *Kathy Smith's Secrets of a Great Body:* Toning exercises very clearly explained in separate videos for upper and lower body.

Advanced Level

- *Super Callanetics:* Without using weights or any other equipment, this challenging workout promises fast results.
- *AeroJump Ultimate Jump Rope Workout:* A high-impact workout with jump ropes led by a former middleweight boxing champion.
- *Reebok Intense Moves Gin Miller:* The choreography is simple, but the high-intensity interval training makes this workout a challenge.

sessions. Add minutes to your strength-training sessions by increasing the number of sets you do (up to four sets of each of the exercises described on pages 128-133) and by adding in new exercises that address your particular needs. Increase the weight load as you get stronger.

In week 5, increase the intensity of your endurance workout by adding hills to your walking routine, increasing the resistance on your stationary bike, or speeding up your swimming. This is also a good time to start cross training (see page 118) by taking up a second aerobic activity.

You can combine the aerobic and strength-training workouts into one session or do them on separate days. Make sure you begin each session with a warm-up and follow it with a cooldown and at least five minutes of stretching. Two days of rest per week should provide adequate time for your muscles to recover.

In the Groove: An Advanced Program

The advanced routine assumes you're already comfortable with half-hour sessions of aerobic exercise and strength training. The goal now is to ratchet up your workouts.

In week 2, you start weight training three times a week instead of two. By week 6, your strength-training sessions stretch to 40 minutes. Your aerobic exercise holds steady at three 30-minute sessions per week, but the intensity increases at week 5 with the addition of interval training (see page 118). Warm up and cool down as before, and make sure to stretch all the muscles you targeted. Allow at least one day of rest per week for muscle recovery.

Six-Week Fitness Programs

No matter what your fitness level, you can find an exercise program that's right for you below. During the endurance exercise segment, work in your target heart-rate range (see page 118).

	WEEK	EXERCISE TYPE	FREQUENCY	DURATION
BEGINNER	1	Endurance	2 to 3 times a week	15 minutes
	2	Endurance	2 to 3 times a week	20 minutes
	3	Endurance	2 to 3 times a week	20 minutes
		Strength training	2 times a week	15 minutes
	4,5	Endurance	3 times a week	20 minutes
		Strength training	2 times a week	15 minutes
	6	Endurance	3 times a week	20 minutes
		Strength training	2 times a week	20 minutes
INTERMEDIATE	1	Endurance	3 times a week	20 minutes
		Strength training	2 times a week	20 minutes
	2	Endurance	3 times a week	25 minutes
		Strength training	2 times a week	20 minutes
	3	Endurance	3 times a week	30 minutes
		Strength training	2 times a week	20 minutes
	4,5	Endurance	3 times a week	30 minutes
		Strength training	2 times a week	25 minutes
	6	Endurance with increased intensity	3 times a week	30 minutes
		Strength training	2 times a week	30 minutes
ADVANCED	1	Endurance	3 times a week	30 minutes
		Strength training	2 times a week	30 minutes
	2,3	Endurance	3 times a week	30 minutes
		Strength training	3 times a week	30 minutes
	4	Endurance	3 times a week	30 minutes
		Strength training	3 times a week	35 minutes
	5	Endurance	3 times a week (once or twice with interval training)	30 minutes
		Strength training	3 times a week	35 minutes
	6	Endurance	3 times a week (once or twice with interval training)	30 minutes
		Strength training	3 times a week	40 minutes

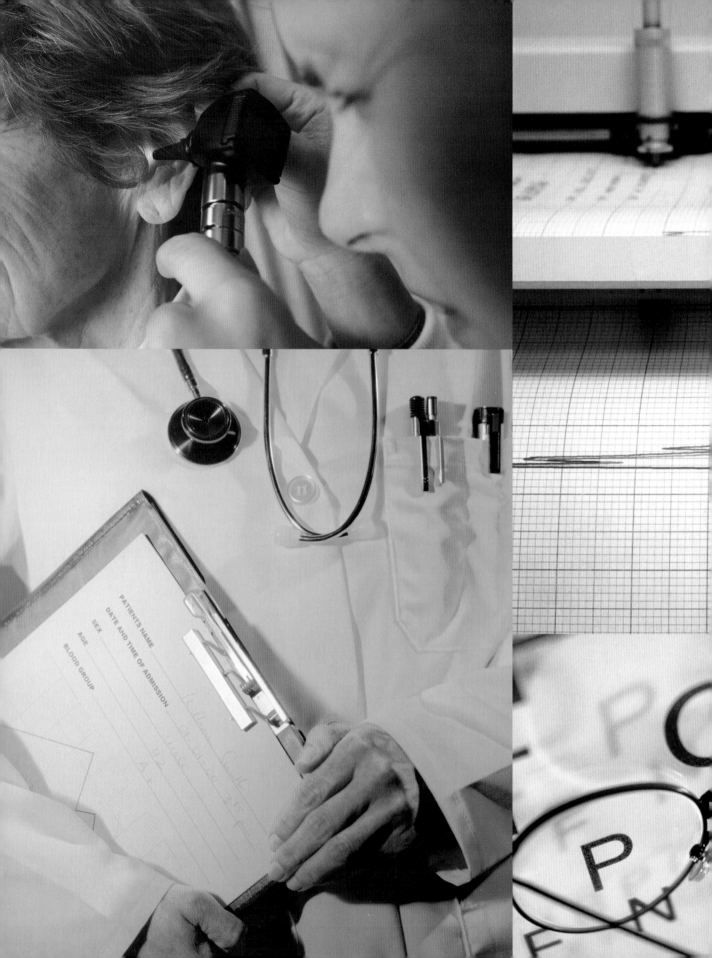

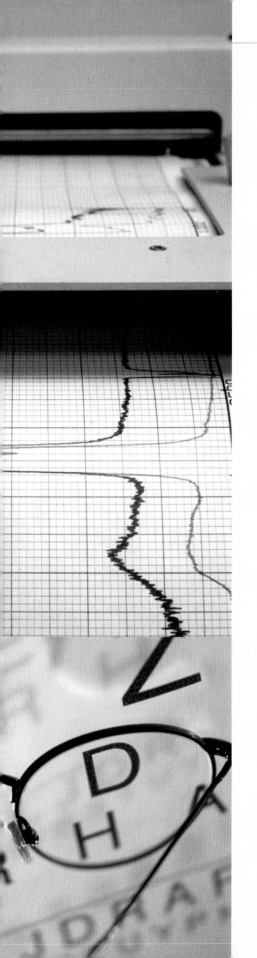

CHAPTER 5

MEDICAL TESTS THAT CAN SAVE YOUR LIFE

Sensible Surveillance

Your early warning system for serious health problems, medical screening tests are gifts from modern science—so why not take advantage? Your life could depend on it.

"It can't happen to me." That's not just the foolish refrain of teenagers who don't know any better; it's also the unfortunate mind-set that causes many adults to forgo simple medical screening tests that could save their lives. As a result, thousands of people die each year from diseases that could have been treated if caught early on. Consider these findings:

- In 2000, among Canadian men, prostate cancer continues to be the most frequently occurring cancer. Starting in 1994, the number of new cases of prostate cancer began to decline after increasing rapidly for several years. These trends were likely due to the swift increase in the use of early detection techniques such as the prostate-screening test known as PSA (prostate specific antigen).

- According to the Canadian Cancer Society, the number of new cases and death rates for colon cancer continues to decrease in this country. Evidence suggests that lifestyle changes such as diet have contributed to the decline. Screening may have contributed to the reduction in death rates.

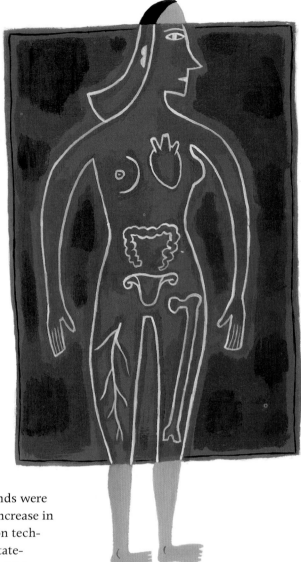

Gone is the annual physical. Now doctors use periodic preventive exams and screening tests as needed based on your age, medical history, and risk factors.

- Deaths from cervical cancer have declined steadily for the past three decades in Canada, due in large part to the widespread use of regular Pap test screening.

- Controlled trials indicate that a 30

SimpleSolution

Kill two birds with one stone: If you're going to the doctor for any kind of follow-up visit, ask if he or she can squeeze in any medical screening tests you're due for. It doesn't take much time to have blood drawn for a PSA or thyroid-function test, for instance, and it will save you another trip to the doctor.

A Shot of Prevention

Immunizations aren't just for kids. Health Canada's Immunization Guide recommends the following shots to protect adults—especially those over age 65—from a small number of infectious diseases that can pose big health problems.

SHOT	WHEN	WHY	WHERE TO GET IT
Tetanus-diphtheria booster	▪ Every 10 years (that is at ages 25, 35, 45, 55, 65 and so on).	▪ Tetanus is an acute infectious disease of the nervous system caused by microorganism. Although it is rare, more than 60 percent of cases occur in people over age 60.	▪ Your doctor's office, local health department, and local hospital public clinic.
Influenza (flu) vaccine	▪ Yearly (in Ontario, for everyone. All other provinces, for people age 65+ or for those in high risk groups).	▪ More than 90 percent of influenza deaths occur in older people. While the vaccine may not always keep you from catching the flu, it will keep you from becoming seriously ill.	▪ Your doctor's office, local health department, and local hospital public clinic.
Pneumonia vaccine	▪ One time, at age 65—additional vaccines not recommended except for people at risk, such as organ transplant recipients and people with kidney failure.	▪ Some 6,000 people die from pneumonia each year in Canada, and fatalities are most common in older people.	▪ Your doctor's office, local health department, and local hospital public clinic.
Hepatitis B vaccine	▪ Any time, particularly if you are sexually active, if you live with someone who has the virus, or if you have a job, such as nursing, that raises your risk of exposure.	▪ Hepatitis B causes a serious acute illness, and in 10 percent of cases, the infection becomes chronic and can lead to liver failure.	▪ Your doctor's office, local health department, and local hospital public clinic.
Varicella zoster (chicken pox) vaccine	▪ Any time after you confirm that you've never had chicken pox; lots of people make it to adulthood without being exposed. If you're not sure whether you've ever had chicken pox, get a blood test for varicella antibodies.	▪ Chicken pox is no picnic for children, but it's truly dangerous to adults. It can cause extremely high fever, brain inflammation, and nerve damage.	▪ Your doctor's office, local health department, and local hospital public clinic.

percent reduction in breast cancer death rates can be expected in women age 50 to 69 in which at least 70 percent of the women are screened every 2 years.

Don't be afraid of what your doctor might discover through a medical screening test; the prospect of having a disease and not knowing it until it's too late to treat it is far more frightening. And don't wait for your doctor to suggest a test—especially if a certain disease runs in your family. Ask to be screened.

SimpleSolution

Do you always put off important tests like your annual Pap smear or skin-cancer screening? See if you can schedule your appointments for these tests on approximately the same day every year for the next five years, and choose a date you'll remember— an anniversary, for instance. Advantage: You'll always know when your appointment's coming up. Also, you're less likely to cancel an appointment you've already made than to "forget" to schedule one at all.

Getting Down to Basics

Health experts say the complete yearly physical—the one in which you disrobe, give blood and urine, and gaze at the wall while your doctor taps, prods, and listens to your body—is unnecessary. In the 1970s, the Canadian government established a task force to evaluate routine medical tests. Their recommendations included tailoring tests according to the needs of the individual, and eliminating many routine procedures, such as chest X-rays and electrocardiograms. Scientific studies now show that these tests were not effective in preventing disease.

In general, healthy adults age 40 to 65 should have a checkup (not a complete physical) every one to three years, and those over age 65 should go yearly. The checkup should include any screening tests for which you're due. If it's time for a mammogram, your doctor will refer you to a radiologist or breast-imaging center. Your doctor should ask about your risk factors for major diseases and discuss appropriate lifestyle changes.

Confused About the Flu Shot?

Here's the straight story:

MYTH Flu shots don't really work.
FACT The shot is about 70 to 90 percent effective. You might avoid the flu without one, but why take the risk? Each year, up to 75,000 hospitalizations are flu-related, and 500 to 1,500 deaths are due to the flu or its complications. That's why Health Canada urges everyone over 65 to get an annual flu shot.

MYTH The shot will give you the flu.
FACT You won't contract the flu, because the vaccine is made with inactive viruses. However, the shot may leave your arm sore, trigger mild muscle aches and fatigue, and make you temporarily feverish.

MYTH You don't need a yearly shot.
FACT You should get a flu shot annually because each year a new flu strain hits. The Laboratory Center for Disease Control (LCDC) and other organizations predict which strain will be active and develop a new vaccine against it.

Ready, Set, Checkup!

According to _Consumer Reports_, the average patient spends only about 18 minutes with the doctor during a regular checkup—that is, an appointment not to address a specific problem, but to assess overall health and take appropriate screening tests.
To make the most of that time:

- **Tell your doctor about all the medications, supplements, herbs, and over-the-counter drugs you're taking.** Also share information about any specialists or alternative health-care practitioners you are seeing.
- **Be honest and open.** Don't be afraid to discuss embarrassing topics. If you don't reveal certain symptoms, for instance, the doctor may fail to diagnose a condition.
- **Ask for clarification.** If you're confused by what your doctor says, ask for a simple explanation. The doctor may have article reprints or patient information brochures on topics that concern you.
- **Take notes.** Write down the doctor's advice on self-care measures. Record the exact names of recommended supplements or over-the-counter drugs. If he suggests a weight-loss, exercise, or smoking-cessation program, ask which he thinks is best. Also jot down possible aftereffects of any tests or immunizations you've just had.

Important Exams: Your At-a-Glance Reminder

Make a photocopy of this chart and post it on your fridge or another place where you'll see it often.
In the last column, log the date of your most recent screening test or medical exam.

HOW OFTEN	TYPE OF TEST	WHO NEEDS IT	DATE PERFORMED
Once a month	Breast self-exam	Women	_____
	Testicular self-exam	Men	_____
	Skin self-check	Both	_____
Twice a year	Dental checkup	Both	_____
Yearly	Blood pressure check ■	Both	_____
	Cholesterol check ■ ■	Both	_____
	Pap test and pelvic exam ■ ■ ■	Women	_____
	Clinical breast exam	Women	_____
	Mammogram ■ ■ ■ ■	Women, age 50+	_____
	Digital rectal exam	Both, age 50+	_____
	Prostate specific antigen ■ ■ ■ ■ ■	Men, age 50+	_____
	Fecal occult blood test ■ ■ ■ ■ ■ ■	Both, age 50+	_____
	Skin check by physician	Talk to your doctor	_____
Every three years	Fasting blood glucose ■ ■ ■ ■ ■ ■ ■	Both, age 45+	_____
Every three to five years	Thyroid-stimulating hormone (TSH) test	Both, age 50+, in presence of symptoms	_____
Every five years	Flexible sigmoidoscopy ■ ■ ■ ■ ■ ■	Both, age 50+	_____
Every decade	Colonoscopy ■ ■ ■ ■ ■ ■	Both, age 50+	_____
At least once	Electrocardiogram	Both, after age 40	_____
Varies by risk factors	Bone-density test ■ ■ ■ ■ ■ ■ ■ ■	Both	_____

■ Every other year beginning at about age 20, and at every doctor's visit
■ ■ Baseline test at age 35 to 40 for men, age 40 for women. Begin testing earlier if you have a family history of heart disease or risk factors such as smoking. People with healthy cholesterol levels need testing every five years
■ ■ ■ Every year or every third year after two consecutive normal tests. Discuss with your doctor
■ ■ ■ ■ Women at risk should consider having a mammogram at a much younger age. Talk to your doctor
■ ■ ■ ■ ■ Men with a family history of prostate cancer or symptoms should start testing at a younger age. Talk to your doctor
■ ■ ■ ■ ■ ■ Start testing earlier if a family member has colorectal cancer or if you have risk factors. Discuss with your doctor
■ ■ ■ ■ ■ ■ ■ Yearly if you are obese, have elevated cholesterol, or have an immediate family member with diabetes
■ ■ ■ ■ ■ ■ ■ ■ Determine when to begin bone-density testing with your doctor

Dental, Vision, and Hearing Tests

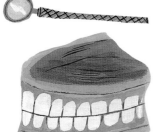

After age 35, about three out of four people have some form of gum disease, and many of them don't even know it. Regular brushing, flossing, and professional cleaning can help prevent it.

Fast Fact

Recent studies show that routine panoramic dental X rays may detect more than just gum disease; they can also help spot cardiovascular disease by revealing blockages in the large arteries that run along the neck. Such blockages indicate an increased risk of stroke and heart attack.

Dental Exam

Aging affects the teeth and mouth in several ways: Saliva, a natural dental protectant, becomes less abundant, allowing cavity-causing bacteria to thrive. Pearly white teeth lose their sheen, sometimes taking on a dingy, gray hue. Old fillings may break. But the most worrisome age-related dental problem is periodontal, or gum, disease—a major reason some 30 percent of people over 65 lose all of their teeth. To detect periodontal disease before it does serious damage, you need regular dental care.

Who needs it The Canadian Dental Association recommends, as a general rule, regular checkups every six months to make sure your gums and teeth stay healthy.

How it's done The dentist does a visual exam of your mouth, looking not just for cracked and decayed teeth, but also for growths and sores on the tongue, palate, and mucous membrane that lines the cheeks and covers the gums. Some dentists now use intra-oral cameras, tiny video cameras placed inside the mouth to project greatly enlarged images on color monitors. Dental X rays, however, are still necessary to detect hidden problems, particularly below the gums. The scheduling of X-ray exams is individualized for each patient. Your dentist may also use a pointed probe to measure the depth of your gum pockets. This quick exam can help determine whether you're beginning to show any signs of gum disease.

What the results mean If your dentist finds cavities, cracked teeth, or broken fillings, he'll determine the best option for repair (filling, crown, root canal, extraction). He will recommend careful flossing and regular use of an antiseptic mouthwash and may refer you to a periodontist or oral surgeon if you have severe or rapidly advancing gum disease.

Eye Exam

Farsightedness affects just about everyone over age 40, so if you do much reading—or anything else that requires you to focus on something close to your face—you'll probably need prescription glasses. Other age-related vision problems such as glaucoma, cataracts, and macular

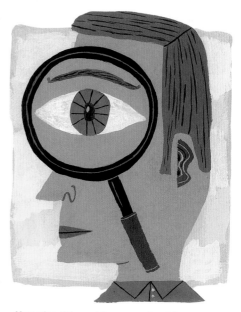

If you're 65 or older, you should see an optometrist every year to check for cataracts and other eye problems.

degeneration develop gradually. Regular eye exams can detect these potentially serious conditions in their early stages.

Who needs it The Canadian Association of Optometrists recommends eye exams every year or two between ages 20 and 64 and yearly exams at age 65 and older. If you wear contact lenses, have a known eye disease, or have diabetes, you'll need to visit the doctor more often.

How it's done The doctor examines the outside of your eyes for problems like swelling or infection, then checks your retina with an ophthalmoscope (a small device that shines light into your pupil) to detect any damaged blood vessels. He may give you eyedrops that dilate your pupils to get a better view. Every exam should include a test for glaucoma, a serious condition in which pressure builds up inside the eye. This painless test is done with a tonometer, which measures pressure in the eye.

What the results mean If an optometrist or primary-care physician detects a serious eye problem, you'll need to see an ophthalmologist, a medical doctor with advanced training in the diagnosis and treatment of eye diseases.

Hearing Test

Impaired hearing is a problem for one in three people over age 65. The most common cause is presbycusis, caused by the gradual deterioration of the structures that conduct sound waves through the ear.

Who needs it There's no official recommendation about how often you should have a hearing test. In general, though, if you have to strain to hear normal conversations or contin-

ually turn up the radio or TV, an evaluation is in order.

How it's done A thorough hearing test is usually done in a soundproof booth. With headphones on, you're asked to indicate in which ear you hear sounds of different pitches and volumes. You may also be asked to listen to and repeat a series of words presented at different volumes.

What the results mean A below-normal result on a hearing test may mean only that you have excess earwax or a mild middle-ear infection, both easy to treat. After your doctor rules out these causes, she may recommend that you see an ear, nose, and throat specialist for further testing.

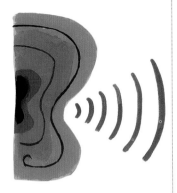

At first, hearing loss may involve only higher-pitched sounds. Consonant sounds may drop out, making it hard to distinguish between "fish" and "dish."

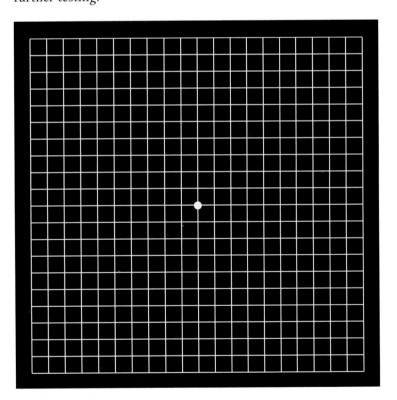

Your eye doctor may use the Amsler Grid, above, to test for signs of macular degeneration: 1. Hold the grid approximately 12 inches from your eyes. 2. First, test your right eye by covering your left eye. Then repeat the procedure with your right eye covered. 3. Look at the center dot. 4. If you notice any waves, distortions, or blind spots in the grid-lines, contact your eye doctor.

Cardiovascular Tests

Blood Pressure Check

This test measures how forcefully your heart pumps blood through your arteries. It should be performed at every checkup.

Who needs it A blood pressure check is mandatory every other year beginning around age 20. After age 65, many doctors feel you should be checked yearly.

How it's done An inflatable cuff is placed around your upper arm. The cuff is pumped up until it squeezes your arm snugly (to cut off your blood supply). Then it's allowed to deflate while the person administering the test listens with a stethoscope placed below the cuff for when the sound of your heartbeat appears and disappears.

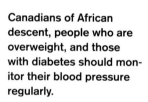

Canadians of African descent, people who are overweight, and those with diabetes should monitor their blood pressure regularly.

What the results mean Blood pressure is reported in two numbers, 130/85, for example. The top number (called the systolic reading) is the pressure exerted when your heart beats, while the bottom number (called the diastolic reading) is the pressure exerted when your heart rests between beats. Blood pressure varies throughout the day, so don't panic if you get one high reading. To get a true picture, your doctor may average several readings.

Ideally, the top number is around 120, and the bottom number falls between 70 and 80. You're in the "normal" range if your top number is between 120 and 129 and your bottom number is between 80 and 84. "High-normal" ranges from 130 to 139 and 85 to 89. Any reading above 140/90 is considered high blood pressure, which can weaken your arteries, increasing your chance of heart attack and stroke. Low blood pressure (any reading significantly

Getting Better Results

To get more accurate readings from your blood pressure and cholesterol tests, follow these tips.

Blood Pressure

- Don't have the test when you're frazzled. Stress can send your readings higher.
- Don't have the test right after smoking, drinking caffeine or alcohol, or eating a large meal.
- Don't talk, chew gum, or cross your legs during the test.
- Empty your bladder, sit comfortably, and try to stay calm. Anxiety about being in the doctor's

office can cause a temporary increase in blood pressure called "white-coat syndrome." Blood-pressure tests should be administered after you've been quiet and relaxed for at least five minutes.

Cholesterol

- If possible, sit and relax for 5 to 15 minutes before the test. Lying down or standing up can cause inaccurate results.
- Don't exercise strenuously the day before the test or drink alcohol for two days before; you'll temporarily raise your HDL levels.

lower than 120/70) is hypotension; it usually isn't a problem unless it causes fainting or light-headedness.

Cholesterol Test

This test measures fats in the bloodstream. One of these fats, cholesterol, is produced naturally by the liver to make cell membranes and some hormones. A little goes a long way—too much can block blood vessels, causing a heart attack or stroke.

Who needs it A baseline cholesterol test is recommended for men age 35 to 40 and women age 40. Adults whose levels are normal should be screened every five years. If you have high cholesterol or other risk factors for heart disease (see page 360), you should be tested yearly.

How it's done A fingerstick blood sample is sent to a lab for analysis.

What the results mean A total cholesterol below 5.2 millimoles per liter (mmol/L) is desirable; 5.2 to 6.2 mmol/L is borderline high; 6.2 mmol/L and over is high. For a more sensitive indicator of heart disease risk, however, you need measurements of low-density lipoproteins (LDL) and high-density lipoproteins (HDL), substances that carry cholesterol through the bloodstream. Alone or in combination, a high total cholesterol, a high LDL level, or a low HDL level can indicate likely heart disease. A healthy LDL reading is less than 3.4 mmol/L. A good HDL reading is over 0.9 mmol/L.

A triglyceride reading of less than 2.3 mmol/L is considered normal; over 2.3 mmol/L requires a change in lifestyle and diet. Medication may be needed. High readings are linked to coronary artery disease and untreated diabetes in some people.

Electrocardiogram (ECG)

This test records in graph form the electrical impulses that make your heart beat. It is performed whenever heart disease is suspected. It's also used to evaluate the effectiveness of heart drugs and determine the heart's condition after a heart attack.

Who needs it A baseline ECG is recommended for people over age 40 who have more than two heart attack risk factors (see page 360) or are starting an exercise program after being sedentary for a long time.

How it's done You either lie down (resting ECG) or walk on a treadmill (exercise ECG, also called a stress test) with small metal contacts called electrodes taped to your chest and possibly your wrists and ankles. The electrodes connect to a machine that records your heart's activity.

What the results mean The test detects any abnormalities in heart rhythm and any cardiac damage (evidence of a heart attack) or heart enlargement or inflammation.

Fast Fact

A magnetic resonance imaging (MRI) may detect heart disease more accurately than an exercise ECG. In this test, a form of adrenaline is injected into your blood, increasing your heart rate to the point you'd reach by running on a treadmill. The MRI machine then produces an image of the heart and the coronary blood vessels to reveal any blockages.

An exercise ECG can detect damage caused by a heart attack. It shouldn't be performed on anyone with uncontrolled high blood pressure.

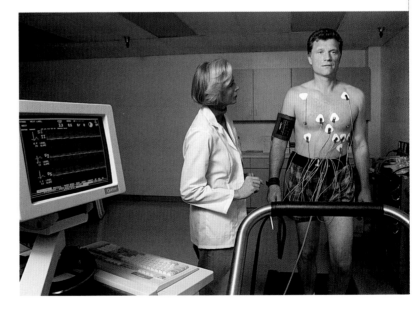

Cancer Screening Tests

Mammogram

The risk of breast cancer increases with age, so it's unfortunate that older women are less likely to have mammograms. In one survey, more than 50 percent of women between ages 75 and 85 had never had one.

If you're frightened by the radiation exposure during a mammogram, consider this: A woman getting a single dose of radiation for treatment of breast cancer receives several thousand rads (units of energy from radiation). A woman getting a mammogram every two years between ages 50 and 69 receives about 2 rads total. **Who needs it** The Canadian Cancer Society recommends that women ages 50 to 69 have a mammogram every two years in combination with a breast exam by a trained health professional. High-risk women may require more frequent mammograms. **How it's done** A female technician places your breast between two metal plates on the X-ray machine. She compresses the breast for a few seconds and takes an X ray from above and one from the side. The compression feels uncomfortable and your breasts might ache for a few minutes.

Some doctors now use digital mammograms, which provide a clearer image—one that can be stored electronically and adjusted for over- or underexposure. Another new tool is a specialized magnetic resonance imaging test called a Rodeo MRI. When used in conjunction with mammograms, this MRI can detect tumors in women with dense (thick) breasts or in those who have breast implants. **What the results mean** Any masses or white spots that suggest cancer may require a biopsy. (Your doctor will refer you to a specialist who will remove a small piece of breast tissue for testing.)

Getting the Best Mammogram

If you're still menstruating, have your mammogram in the middle of your cycle, when your breasts are less tender. Avoid caffeine for a week before the test because it may increase breast tenderness in women with fibrocystic breasts. And don't use deodorant, perfume, or powder the day of the test; their residue may show up on the X ray as suspicious markings, contributing to a false-positive reading.

Pap Tests

Ever since the Papanicolaou (Pap) test—a lab analysis of cells scraped from the cervix—was developed, it has remained the standard way of detecting cervical cancer. **Who needs it** The Canadian Cancer Society recommends that all women who have become sexually active have a Pap test, no matter what their age. Even if you are no longer sexually active, you should still have regular Pap tests. If you have had your uterus surgically removed, you should discuss with your doctor

The Breast Self-Exam

Women discover nearly 80 percent of breast cancers through self-exams. You should perform a self-exam once a month, about a week after your period ends. If you're past menopause or have irregular periods, perform the exam on the same date each month.

Here's how:

- Lie down, slip a pillow under your right shoulder, and tuck your right arm behind your head. (Some women check their breasts in the shower or bathtub, because wet, soapy fingers glide more easily.)
- Pressing firmly, feel your right breast with the fingers of your left hand. Work in a circle (from the center out), or in an up-and-down pattern, until you've covered the entire breast.
- Now move the pillow under your left shoulder, tuck your left hand behind your head, and check your left breast with your right hand.
- Next stand in front of a mirror with your hands on your hips, then raised overhead, and look for any visible lumps, skin puckering, dimpling, or nipple changes. Gently squeeze each nipple to check for discharge.

If you feel a lump, don't panic—it's not necessarily a tumor. It may simply be a noncancerous hardening of tissue called a fibrous breast lump or a benign cyst (a fluid-filled sac in the breast that can be painful). Call your doctor as soon as possible.

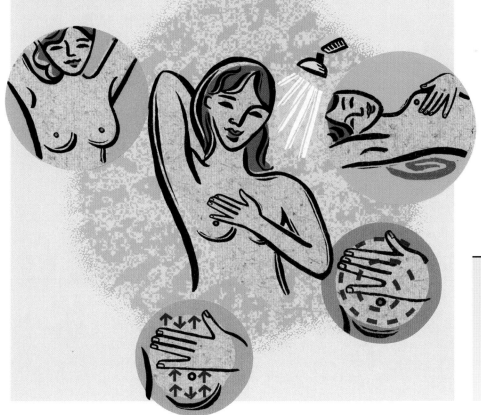

In their own words

Addressing the U.S. Congress about cervical cancer, Sharyn Lenhart, M.D., past president of the American Medical Women's Association, said: "The majority of deaths from cervical cancer are unnecessary and preventable. Two-thirds of cervical cancers occur in women who have not been screened."

WARNING

Although it's rare, men can get breast cancer, too. Early symptoms include a painless lump, skin ulceration, and nipple changes like retraction and discharge, which may be bloody.

whether you still need Pap tests and how often.

A surprising number of Canadian women do not regularly have a Pap test. In a recent study, 15 percent of women reported they had never been tested. And about 30 percent hadn't been screened in the last three years. In 2000, there were 1,450 cases and 430 deaths due to cervical cancer in Canada.

How it's done The gynecologist inserts a metal device called a speculum into the vagina, then passes a swab through it to obtain a sample of cells from the cervix and endocervical canal. The sample is spread on a glass slide and sent for analysis.

Sometimes, after a routine Pap test, the results are uncertain. The typical procedure is to repeat the Pap test in six months, with another repeat if that test result is uncertain. Eventually your doctor will arrange for a colposcopy, a procedure that gives her a magnified view of the cervix and allows her to remove a sample of tissue for further analysis. However, with the new human papil-

loma virus (HPV) test, when a woman's Pap result is uncertain, there is no need to wait months to repeat the Pap test. Instead, the woman's doctor takes a sample for HPV analysis (HPV is present in some 99 percent of all cervical cancers). If the result is positive, then the woman can proceed directly to the colposcopy and then a biopsy. This could speed up the time to diagnose cervical cancer or rule it out by six months. The cost of the HPV test is probably not covered by your provincial insurance or territorial health plan. But supplemental insurance plans may pay for it.

What the results mean If your Pap test is positive for abnormal cells, it doesn't necessarily signal cancer. Mild dysplasia, or early noncancerous cell changes confined to the thin layer of tissue that covers the cervix, sometimes progresses to cancer if left untreated, but often returns to normal. Severe dysplasia involves almost the full thickness of the epithelium and indicates late-stage precancerous cell changes. Either condition calls

---

Testing Your Testes

The testicular self-exam is to men what the breast self-exam is to women: a way of familiarizing yourself with your body and detecting any changes early on. It should be done once a month. Testicular cancer is most common in men age 20 to 25, but since it often causes no symptoms until it spreads to the lymph nodes and lungs, older men should also examine themselves.

Here's how:
● Use both hands to examine each testicle separately. Put your index and middle fingers underneath and your thumbs on top.
● Gently roll each testicle between your fingers and thumbs. It should feel smooth and rubbery. Feel

for hard, pea-sized lumps and changes in shape, size, or texture.
● Also check your penis for lumps or sores.

If you notice anything suspicious, see your doctor. He can perform an ultrasound to help determine if there is a lump—and if so, what's causing it. Painful lumps or an enlarged testis may be caused by testicular cancer. Inflammation may also be caused by a bladder infection or a collection of blood that can develop after injury to the scrotum. Small sores on the testis or penis may be caused by skin cancer or, more commonly, by sexually transmitted diseases such as herpes, syphilis, and the human papilloma virus (HPV), which causes genital warts.

for close monitoring during more frequent checkups. If the test suggests a malignancy, your doctor will arrange for a colposcopy.

Digital Rectal Exam

This manual exam of the anus and rectum is a quick, inexpensive way to detect abnormalities. In men, it's used to screen for prostate enlargement or nodules; in women, for growths in the uterus and bladder. **Who needs it** Everyone after age 50 should have one annually. **How it's done** The doctor first inspects the skin around the anus for any abnormality. Then with a lubricated, gloved finger, he probes for abnormal growths or inflammation. **What the results mean** Swollen tissues in the rectum and anus could signal hemorrhoids. Tears, abscesses, or inflammation may indicate an infection that can be cleared up with antibiotics or surgery, if necessary. A lump may indicate cancer. In men, if a prostate abnormality is found, the doctor may order a prostate-specific-antigen test (see *Is a PSA Worth It?* at right). To confirm a diagnosis of prostate cancer if the rectal exam and PSA suggest it, your doctor may order X rays, blood and urine tests, or an ultrasound. A small tissue sample may be taken for analysis.

Colorectal Cancer Tests

The following tests are used to detect early signs of colorectal cancer, the third most common cancer in men and women and the second leading cause of all cancer deaths. It can occur in the colon or rectum and is one of the most easily prevented cancers. If caught early, the

Is a PSA Worth It?

In 1997, more than 3,600 men died of prostate cancer, most of them over the age of 70 (prostate cancer is rare in men under age 50.) These men with prostate cancer all have high levels of substances called prostate specific antigens (PSAs). (Antigens are substances recognized as foreign by the body's immune system.) The problem is that many men who have a noncancerous enlargement of the prostate also have high levels, which is why the PSA test is controversial as a screening test for prostate cancer. The test yields a false-positive result in as many as three out of four cases.

Some doctors recommend a PSA every year for all men over age 50. Others advise it only for men in high-risk groups. Still others use it only to check for recurrences of prostate cancer in men who've already been treated for it. The best advice? Talk it over with your doctor so you can make an informed decision.

cure rate is over 90 percent. In Canada, guidelines are currently being developed for mass colorectal screening. Until then, however, the Canadian Cancer Society recommends that everyone age 50 to 75 should talk to their doctor about colon screening tests. People with a family history of colorectal cancer, should talk to their doctor about screening at an earlier age.

The Fecal Occult Blood Test

One of the most important basic screening tools for colon cancer, this test detects hidden ("occult") blood in the stool. In a study recently published by the *Journal of The National Cancer Institute*, researchers found that people who had the test annually were 33 percent less likely to die of colon cancer, and those who took the test every other year were 21 percent less likely to die of the disease. **Who needs it** Starting at age 50 talk to your doctor about this test. If you have a family history of colon cancer, discuss testing at an earlier age. **How it's done** Your doctor either

In their own words

"Some people find that procedures like stool tests, flexible sigmoidoscopies, and colonoscopies aren't appealing. I can tell you firsthand they are much more appealing than dying of this disease... I am gratified that in the U.S., Medicare now covers colon cancer screening for people 65 and over. It is incumbent that we convince seniors to take advantage of this fact. Had Charles Schulz, for example, been screened, he and we would still be enjoying his beloved Peanuts.*"*

—*Katie Couric, testifying before the U.S. Senate's Special Committee on Aging*

> **Fast Fact**
>
> *Colorectal cancer responds best to treatment when it is diagnosed and treated as early as possible. Treatment is most effective before the disease spreads.*

takes a stool sample during a rectal exam or gives you a kit so you can give the sample at home. Most kits require you to collect samples from three different bowel movements.

To get the most accurate results possible, don't provide a stool sample during your menstrual period or if you have bleeding hemorrhoids. Limit alcohol consumption and avoid turnips, horseradish, beets, citrus fruits, and red meat for three days prior to the test. Avoid drugs, such as aspirin, that irritate the stomach. **What the results mean** Blood in the stool can be caused by cancer, with and without polyps—mushroom-shaped growths on the intestinal wall. It calls for a more intensive test such as a flexible sigmoidoscopy or colonoscopy.

The Flexible Sigmoidoscopy

During this test, the doctor inserts a long, flexible tube into the lower third of the colon, where 65 percent of cancerous growths occur.
Who needs it Starting at age 50, talk to your doctor about this test. If you have a parent, sibling, or child with colorectal cancer or other bowel disease, talk to your doctor about testing at an earlier age.
How it's done You'll need to stick to

a clear liquid diet for 12 to 24 hours before the test and perform an enema that morning. During the test, you lie on your side, knees bent. The doctor inserts a lighted viewing tube called a sigmoidoscope into the rectum and lower colon. The 10- to 20-minute procedure is relatively painless. You may, however, feel pressure and mild cramps when the scope is inserted and have gas and bloating for a few hours afterward.
What the results mean Most disorders of the anus or rectum—from hemorrhoids and inflammation to infection and cancer—can be diagnosed with this test. If your doctor finds an abnormal growth, he'll send a tissue sample to a lab for analysis.

The Colonoscopy

Similar to a sigmoidoscopy, this test uses a longer tube and examines the full length of the colon. It's usually done only for people at high risk of colorectal cancer and those who have gotten positive results on their fecal occult blood test or sigmoidoscopy.
Who needs it Starting at age 50, talk to your doctor about having this test. If you have more than one first-degree relative with colorectal cancer or other bowel disease, talk to your doctor about testing at an earlier age.

One More Colon Test

A double-contrast barium enema is another option for colon cancer screening. You take a laxative and enema beforehand. A chalky barium sulfate material, through which X rays cannot pass, is placed into the anus. You change positions until the barium is directed to the colon, then X rays are taken. The barium shows up white on the X ray, revealing contours, polyps, tumors, or other structural abnormalities.

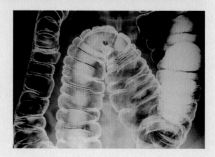

How it's done You'll be on a clear liquid diet for 48 hours beforehand, drink a laxative solution the prior night, and use an enema in the morning. You'll receive an IV containing pain medication and a sedative. After the doctor inserts the colonoscope, images appear on a TV monitor for the doctor to examine. The test takes about 30 to 60 minutes. You'll need to rest for an hour or two afterward until the sedative wears off.

Some doctors now use a new technology called virtual CT colonography to detect tumors. The technique, which is less invasive, requires no sedative and takes only about 10 minutes. The clean colon is inflated with air by means of a small, soft-tipped tube inserted into the rectum. Then you hold your breath while you are moved through a CT scanner, which produces digital images of the entire colon. Although researchers have found results to be 90 percent accurate, a positive diagnosis for cancer is usually followed up with a standard colonoscopy anyway.

What the results mean Any polyps (benign growths) the doctor finds may be removed during the exam with a device inserted into the colonoscope. Another device may be used to obtain cell samples from any suspicious lesions for biopsy.

Skin Tests

Forty years ago, we didn't know sun exposure causes skin cancer. Now baby boomers and their parents are paying for hours spent on the beach or on the slopes without sun protection. Even today, 50 percent of Canadians do not adequately protect themselves from the sun, although they know they should, according to a study. About 68,000 Canadians will get non-melanoma skin cancer this year. Skin examinations can catch it before it spreads.

Who needs it Anyone who's been in the sun, particularly people at high risk for skin cancer (those with fair skin, light hair, freckles, and who have skin cancer in the family). If you're over age 40, check your own skin monthly and have a dermatologist check it at least once a year.

How it's done Here's what you should look for in a self-exam:

- Any ulcer or skin wound that doesn't heal within six weeks
- Any lump or growth that bleeds persistently
- Any suspicious, shiny, firm, or raised skin growth (especially if it seems to have enlarged since your last check)
- Any red, scaly, encrusted surface of the skin that itches and doesn't seem to be healing
- Any mole that itches, is tender, or has changed in size, color, or shape

Do this **ABCD** check for all moles:

- **A**symmetry: The two halves don't match
- **B**order irregularity: The edges appear to be jagged
- **C**olor: The color isn't uniform
- **D**iameter: It's more than one-quarter inch wide

Check yourself in front of a full-length mirror, using a hand mirror to view your back. Use a blow-dryer to separate your hair so you can check your scalp.

What the results mean If you notice anything suspicious, see a dermatologist right away. He or she can examine your entire body, remove any suspicious growths, and send the tissue to a lab for examination.

Mole Check

If a mole looks like one in the left column, it's probably safe. If it resembles one in the right column, have a dermatologist examine it as soon as possible.

NORMAL	HAVE YOUR DOCTOR EXAMINE

Shape

REGULAR   IRREGULAR

Surface

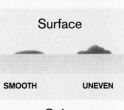

SMOOTH   UNEVEN

Color

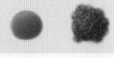

CONSISTENT   MOTTLED

Three More Important Tests

Osteoporosis and osteopenia (decreased bone density) can now be detected and treated early, thanks to rapidly improving technology such as the DEXA scan.

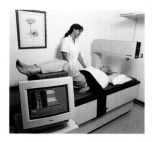

Bone-Density Tests

The Osteoporosis Society of Canada reports that some 1.4 million Canadians suffer from osteoporosis. The cost of treating the disease and the bone fractures it causes is estimated to be $1.3 billion each year. Osteoporosis can strike at any age, and many cases go undiagnosed. The disease can progress slowly, without your knowledge—unless you get tested for it. Without testing, osteoporosis may be discovered only after much of the damage is done—when a sudden strain, bump, or fall results in a fracture, or when a "dowager's hump," caused by compression fractures of the spine, has already formed.

Who needs it No single cause for osteoporosis has been identified. However, certain risk factors seem to play a role. The Osteoporosis Society of Canada suggests that you evaluate your own risks by reviewing the risk factors (see *Common Risk Factors* at right), and determining which ones apply to you. The more risk factors you have, the greater your chances of developing osteoporosis. Specifically if you have four or more of the common risk factors listed, discuss being tested for bone loss with your doctor.

Common Risk Factors

Some people have risk factors that increase their likelihood of developing osteoporosis (note that people with no risk factors may still develop the disease). You're at greater risk if you:

- Are female
- Are age 50 or older
- Are past menopause
- Have had prolonged sex hormone deficiencies
- Have had your ovaries surgically removed or have had menopause before age 45
- Do not get enough calcium
- Have limited exposure to sunlight or insufficient vitamin D in your diet
- Have had a previous fracture with minimal trauma
- Do not get enough exercise
- Have a family history of osteoporosis
- Are thin, small-boned
- Are Caucasian or Asian
- Are a smoker
- Drink caffeine (consistently more than 3 cups a day of coffee, tea, or cola)
- Drink alcohol (consistently more than 2 drinks a day)
- Use certain medications for extended periods or in high doses (corticosteroids, anticonvulsants, thyroid hormone, aluminum-containing antacids)

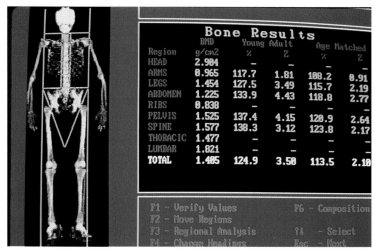

		Bone Results				
	BMD	Young Adult			Age Matched	
Region	g/cm2	%	Z		%	Z
HEAD	2.904	–	–		–	–
ARMS	0.965	117.7	1.81		108.2	0.91
LEGS	1.454	127.5	3.49		115.7	2.19
ABDOMEN	1.225	133.9	4.43		118.8	2.77
RIBS	0.838	–	–		–	–
PELVIS	1.525	137.4	4.15		120.9	2.64
SPINE	1.577	138.3	3.12		123.8	2.17
THORACIC	1.477	–	–		–	–
LUMBAR	1.821	–	–		–	–
TOTAL	1.405	124.9	3.50		113.5	2.10

F1 – Verify Values   F6 – Composition
F2 – Move Regions
F3 – Regional Analysis   ↑↓ – Select
F4 – Change Headings   Esc – Next

How it's done Two tests commonly used to evaluate bone density are the dual energy X-ray absorptiometry (DEXA) and the ultrasound scan. The DEXA is the most accurate test and is used for diagnosis and for assessing treatment, but it may also be used for screening. The test, which emits low levels of radiation, measures bone density at the spine, hip, and/or wrist—considered to be the most reliable areas for measurement. The ultrasound scan, on the other hand, is used only for screening. It emits no radiation, and measures bone density in the wrist or heel.

What the results mean If an ultrasound shows osteoporosis, the doctor will usually order a DEXA. DEXA scores compare your bone mass to the standard. A score of -1 to -2.5 indicates osteopenia (decreased bone density). A score of -2.5 or lower means you have osteoporosis. Any scores higher than -1 indicate healthy bone mass.

Thyroid-Stimulating Hormone (TSH) Test

Experts estimate that about 1 million Canadians have problems with their thyroid gland—a small gland that lies just under the skin near the trachea (windpipe) in the neck. It secretes a hormone, thyroxine, that helps regulate growth, metabolism, digestion, and body temperature. Many thyroid problems go undetected, even though screening is as simple as taking a blood test.

Who needs it While there are no Canadian guidelines for screening, some experts recommend that women age 65 and older have tests every three to five years, and men age 65 and older get tested regularly.

Do-It-Yourself Medical Tests

A large number of home medical tests are now available in drugstores. They provide quick, accurate results without a visit to the doctor. Although they can't substitute for professional medical care, a suspicious test result may motivate you to get to the doctor quickly. Experts advise consulting a health professional when you get your home test results; she can help you interpret them and advise you if any further action is necessary.

Be sure to check the expiration date before using any of these products, since an expired test kit may yield inaccurate results.

Blood Pressure Monitor:
There are three at-home options: aneroid units (which require the use of a stethoscope), electronic monitors with manual inflation, and electronic monitors with automatic inflation. Some units you use around your arm, and others allow you to track your blood pressure through your finger or wrist. All take about two to five minutes to give results. Prices range from $60 for basic units to $175 for more high-tech models.

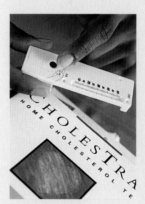

Cholesterol Check:
You prick your finger and fill a tiny blood reservoir on a thermometer-like device to check blood levels. Then you compare the readings to government guidelines. It takes about 15 minutes to complete. These tests measure total blood cholesterol but do not distinguish between good (HDL) cholesterol and bad (LDL) cholesterol. Cost: about $30.

Glucose Test:
You prick your finger with a disposable lance, drop the blood on a chemically activated test strip, then place the strip in a meter that reads your glucose level. Prices range from $34 to $115 for the monitoring kit (a one-time purchase) and disposable strips cost about $1 each. Other less-expensive glucose tests check your urine.

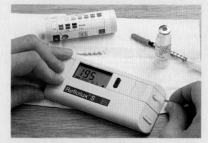

You dip a stick in your urine stream and get results (by the color of the stick) within 90 seconds. These tests may be less accurate than the blood tests.

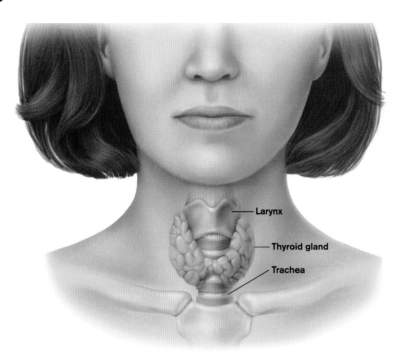

The thyroid gland in the throat produces thyroid hormone in response to another hormone, called thyroid stimulating hormone (TSH), which is secreted by the pituitary gland in the brain.

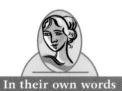

In their own words

"Diabetes can creep up silently over the years. Most people think it's just a nuisance, but it's a serious disease, and more and more people are developing it," said JoAnn Manson, M.D., an endocrinologist at Brigham and Women's Hospital in Boston and professor of medicine at Harvard Medical School, reporting for the National Women's Health Resource Center.

How it's done For 24 hours prior to the test, you'll be asked to avoid drugs that can affect the results, including aspirin, corticosteroids, and iodine-containing drugs and vitamins. Blood is drawn and sent to a lab to check levels of thyroid-stimulating hormone (TSH).

What the results mean Low levels of TSH may indicate hypothyroidism, which can cause such symptoms as fatigue, weight gain, and constipation. If you have hypothyroidism, your doctor will probably prescribe a thyroid replacement drug. High TSH levels, which are less common, may indicate hyperthyroidism, which can cause symptoms such as a fast heartbeat, weight loss, and dizziness. Treatment may involve antithyroid medicines, radioactive iodine treatment, or surgery to remove all or part of the thyroid gland.

Diabetes Tests

More than 2 million Canadians have diabetes, a disorder in which the body doesn't produce enough insulin (the hormone needed to extract glucose from the blood) or is resistant to the action of insulin. It can be diagnosed early on with a fasting plasma glucose (FPG) test or an oral glucose tolerance test (OGTT). The sooner you detect diabetes, the more quickly you can treat it and prevent serious complications such as heart attacks, strokes, and kidney problems.

Who needs it The Canadian Diabetes Association recommends routine screening every three years for everyone age 45 or older, and screening every year for those with other risk factors, such as having a parent or sibling with the disease.

How it's done Your FPG reading is taken from a blood sample usually drawn in the morning, before you've eaten. If you are having an OGTT, bring a book, since the whole exam can take more than two hours. You'll be instructed to fast for eight hours (overnight) before the test and to avoid certain drugs, such as acetaminophen and oral contraceptives, which can affect the results. You'll be asked to drink several ounces of a glucose (sugar) solution, then blood and urine samples will be taken after one hour and again after two hours.

What the results mean Normal level of glucose in the blood ranges from about 3.8 to 6.1 millimoles per liter of blood (mmol/L). If your blood sugars measure higher than 7.0 mmol/L, you have diabetes. If your blood sugars are below 3.5 mmol/L, you may have hypoglycemia, a condition that produces sudden severe hunger, headaches, anxiety, sweating, and confusion.

Got It Covered!

Most of the vaccines or tests below are covered by provincial and territorial health plans according to frequency and guidelines determined by medical authorities. Check with your doctor.

VACCINE OR TEST	FOR WHOM	HOW OFTEN
Flu shot	■ Ontario: Everyone All other provinces and territories: everyone age 65+ or those in high risk groups	■ Yearly
Pneumonia vaccine	■ Everyone at age 65. Additional vaccines not recommended except for people at high risk, such as those with kidney failure	■ One time
Hepatitis B vaccine	■ For all at risk, especially health-care workers or those living with an infected person	■ One time
Routine mammogram	■ All females over age 50. Earlier if warranted by family history or health problems	■ Every 2 years
Pap test	■ All females over age 18 until age 70	■ Yearly, or every 3 years after 2 consecutive normal tests
Pelvic exam	■ All females	■ Yearly
Tests for colorectal cancer	■ For people age 50+	■ As ordered by your doctor
Tests for prostate cancer	■ Males	■ As ordered by your doctor
Bone-density tests	■ Females and males at risk	■ Discuss with your doctor

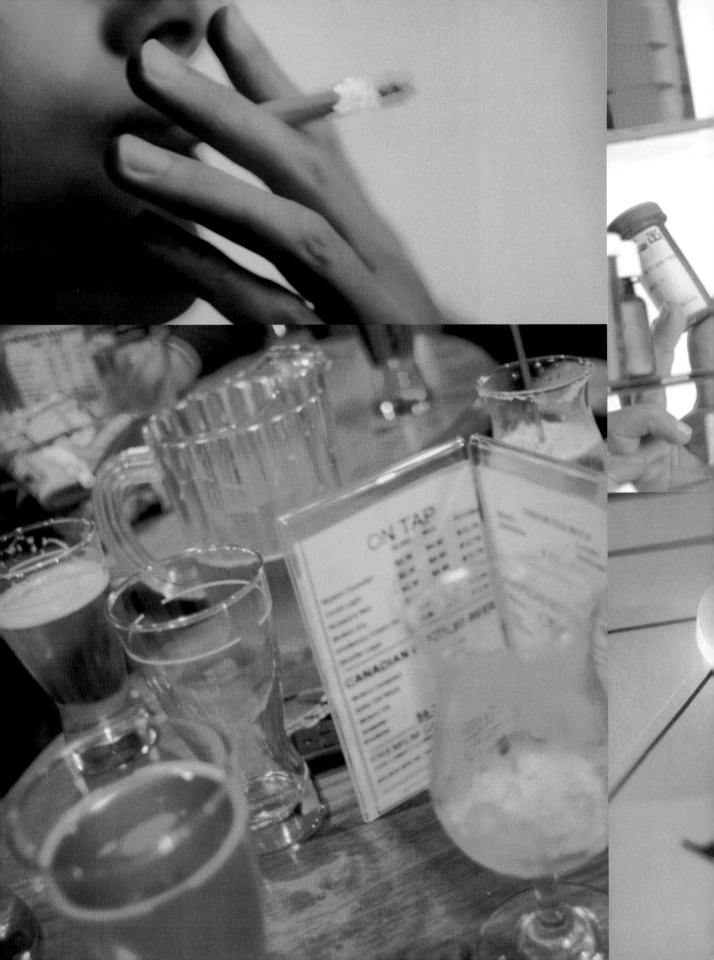

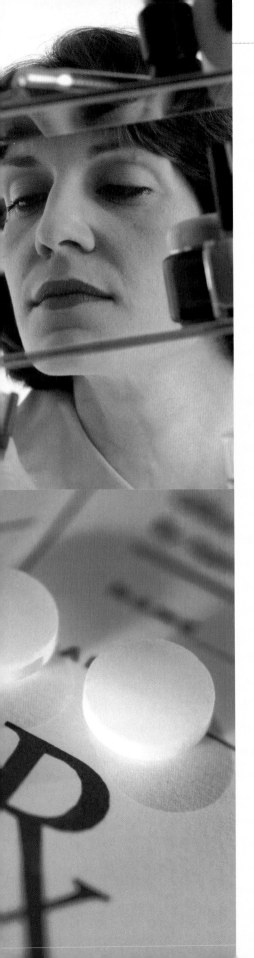

CHAPTER 6

AVOIDING COMMON HEALTH TRAPS

Is Your Health Going Up in Smoke?

Smoking is the single worst thing you can do for your health. Fortunately, it's never too late to reap the benefits of quitting.

Even if you follow every tip in this book, you're not looking after your body if you still smoke. The fact is, smokers do more harm to their body than if they ate pepperoni pizza every day and never got off the sofa. If you've tried to quit before and failed, it's time to summon your resolve and try again.

Lung cancer is the leading cause of death from cancer. It causes almost a third of cancer deaths in men and 25 percent in women. Eighty-five percent of lung cancer is related to tobacco use. But long before smoking kills you, it ages you. You can see for yourself that smoking accelerates the drying and wrinkling of the skin. But there are less obvious effects as well. Smokers' arteries, for example, show serious thickening from the buildup of plaque. In one study, the carotid (major neck) arteries of smokers had thickened as much as those of nonsmokers who were ten years older. Indeed, smoking takes years away from your life. Nearly half of all chronic smokers die an average of 20 to 25 years before their time.

Besides an early death from cancer or heart disease, smoking can cause such lung disorders as emphysema and chronic bronchitis. People who smoke over a pack a day have almost triple the risk of contracting pneumonia than that of nonsmokers.

By lowering levels of estrogen in men and women, smoking speeds bone loss. If a woman smokes a pack of cigarettes every day, she'll enter menopause with 5 to 10 percent less bone mass than a nonsmoker. In men, smoking can also affect sexual performance. It's scientifically proven that smoking can clog penile blood vessels in the same way that it clogs cardiac vessels, leading to impotence.

Pipe Dreams and Cigar Stories

You don't hear much about the dangers of pipes and cigars, but the fact is, they are every bit as lethal as cigarettes. All tobacco smoke contains the same cancer-causing chemicals. Cigars and pipes use black (air-cured) tobacco, which carries a greater risk of cancer of the esophagus than the tobacco in cigarettes. Cigars can contain seven times more tar and four times more nicotine than cigarettes. In fact, a large cigar can pack as much tobacco as an entire pack of smokes.

Despite its resurgence in popularity spurred by sports figures, smokeless tobacco (such as snuff and chewing tobacco) isn't safe either. It's still loaded with nicotine, which is readily absorbed by tissue in the mouth, along with a number of cancer-causing chemicals.

The Benefits of Quitting

The good news is that no matter what your age or how long you've smoked, you'll live longer if you quit today. The Coronary Artery Surgery Study in the U.S. examined nearly 2,000 long-term smokers over age 54. Those who quit had substantially lower death rates six years later than those who didn't. Even the oldest ex-smokers had a higher survival rate.

Not only will you live longer if you quit, you'll feel better, breathe easier, and find that you have more energy. You'll have fewer respiratory infections, headaches, and stomach-aches. What's more, you'll save money. Your clothes and breath won't reek any longer. And your habit won't aggravate—or threaten the health of—the people who live and work with you. Best of all, you'll stop being a slave to tobacco and take back control of your life.

What Are Your Chances of Success?

Your chances of quitting skyrocket if you have help of some sort. Most smokers are better off with a combination of medication (such as nicotine-replacement gums, patches, or drugs) and behavior-modification help (such as a support group or self-help tape). See page 171 for more details on nicotine-replacement products and prescription drugs your doctor might recommend.

PERCENTAGE OF SUCCESS

Nasal spray (not yet available in Canada)	30%
Prescription drug (bupropion)	28%
Replacement nicotine + behavioral therapy	27.5%
Inhalers (not yet available in Canada)	19%
Behavioral therapy	15%
Gum	14%
Patch	8%
Self-help only	4%

Source: CDC Office on Smoking and Health

How Dangerous Is Secondhand Smoke?

Living or working with a smoker can be deadlier than smoking. Why? The smoke that most smokers breathe is filtered. But people nearby breathe smoke that comes from the burning end of the cigarette (or cigar or pipe) without the benefit of filtration. It has much higher concentrations of tar, nicotine, and the other gases in tobacco smoke, raising the risk of not only heart attack and lung cancer but, as scientists have recently discovered, also stroke. According to an Australian study, secondhand smoke from a spouse can double your risk of stroke. Secondhand smoke poses an even greater risk for people who already have a respiratory problem or heart condition. Think about these facts the next time someone beside you lights up. Secondhand smoke…

- contains more than 4,000 chemical compounds, including carbon monoxide, formaldehyde, ammonia, nickel, zinc, and acetone, lead, benzene, arsenic, and dioxin. More than 40 of these may cause cancer
- aggravates symptoms of hayfever and asthma
- causes more than 300 deaths in nonsmokers from lung cancer each year in Canada. In addition to lung cancer, secondhand smoke has been linked to leukemia and lymphoma, as well as cancer of the sinuses, breast, brain, uterus, cervix, and thyroid.

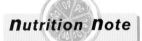

Nutrition note

Smoking depletes vitamin C levels—one possible reason why smokers are more prone to cataracts and macular degeneration. Until you quit, eat plenty of citrus fruits, strawberries, kiwi, dark leafy greens, broccoli, and red peppers, and consider taking a supplement.

Preparing to Quit

Before you try to kick the habit, lay some groundwork to boost your chances of success.

There is no one magic bullet to help you stop smoking. In fact, research has proved that you're more likely to succeed if you combine several strategies. No matter which ones you choose, talk to your loved ones, friends, and co-workers before you start. Tell them you'd like to count on their help. Ask people not to smoke when you're around. If you can, find someone to quit with.

As you start to think about quitting, visualize yourself as healthier, more attractive, sexier. Picture yourself in control of your smoking, and hold on to the image.

When you're ready to get serious, schedule an appointment with your doctor. Discuss nicotine and non-nicotine aids (see the chart on page 171), as well as other strategies you're considering. If you haven't had a physical recently, now is the time to have one. It will give you a "before" picture to compare with your new non-smoking self.

If you've tried to quit before, review any successes you've had. What worked, even if only for a short time? Consider meeting with a counselor; he or she can help you deal with your feelings and fears more openly and learn the coping skills you'll need to become a successful quitter.

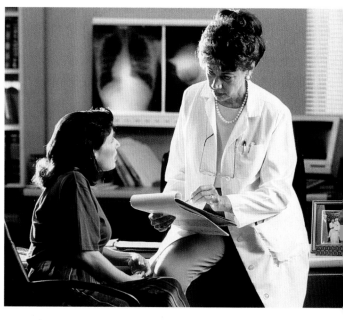

Talk to your doctor about quitting. Besides prescribing nicotine-replacement products, she can help you tailor a stop-smoking program to fit your needs.

Finally, many insurance plans support a variety of smoking cessation efforts. Check your plan's coverage. Your benefits administrator can help.

Set a Date

Pick your quit date. Tell your friends, family, and co-workers. Make the date close enough to take seriously, yet far enough away to allow preparation time. Some people choose a vacation day, when they're away from usual routines. Others prefer the structure of their regular schedule. Don't pick a day when you anticipate being under stress.

Before the date arrives, try to picture the problems you might

---

Fast Fact

Fewer than 5 percent of smokers who try to quit on their own are successful. But in studies around the U.S., 40 to 60 percent of smokers who combined prescription drugs, nicotine replacement, and counseling remained smoke-free a year after completing their cessation program.

Timetable to Recovery

The longer you stay smoke-free, the more you'll realize what "recovery" really means. Although some damage (to your lungs, for example) may be permanent, your body has an amazing ability to repair itself. This chart gives you an idea of how soon you'll notice the benefits of quitting.

ELAPSED TIME SINCE QUITTING	EFFECTS ON YOUR BODY
20 minutes	■ Your blood pressure goes down, your pulse drops, and your hands and feet get warmer.
8 hours	■ The carbon monoxide level in your blood drops to normal and the level of oxygen in your blood increases to normal.
24 hours	■ Your chance of having a heart attack begins to fall.
72 hours	■ Your lung capacity has already improved.
Within 1 week	■ Your senses of taste and smell improve. Your breath, hair, and fingers are noticeably cleaner.
2 weeks to 3 months	■ Because your lung function and circulation are improving, it's easier to walk. As the hairlike structures lining your airways recover, they remove more mucus from your respiratory passages, which you'll cough up at first as your lungs and sinuses clear.
1 month to 9 months	■ You notice less coughing, congestion, fatigue, and shortness of breath.
5 years to 15 years	■ Your risk of heart attack and stroke are back to normal.
10 years	■ Your risk of lung cancer falls to half that of continuing smokers. Your risk of other associated cancers drops.
15 years	■ Your risk of dying prematurely is now nearly equal to that of people who've never smoked.

encounter and think of solutions ahead of time. Also, find ways to remove temptation from your path.

● **Plan activities** that make you feel good, healthy, and energetic during your first few weeks of quitting. They can both distract and reward you. Take your grandkids to the zoo. Treat yourself to a half day at a spa; it's a much better use of the money you've been spending on cigarettes.

● **Start an exercise program.** More people succeed in quitting if they exercise. Exercise increases your energy and also boosts your metabolism, helping you avoid weight gain, which can easily throw a wrench into your resolve. It may also take the edge off withdrawal symptoms such as irritability, headaches, and lethargy.

● **Improve your diet.** Besides curtailing weight gain, eating right will

In their own words

After failing four times, I quit the fifth time for good—20 years ago. Now, when I teach stop-smoking classes, I pass along this advice:

First, plan ahead. Know what you'll do when the urge to smoke arises. People use sunflower seeds, gum, knitting needles, popcorn (a kernel at a time), swizzle sticks, toothpicks, bags of vegetables, or ice water (this is very popular). I used thin pretzel sticks, because I found that when I bit off both ends I could drag on them like a cigarette. When they got soggy I ate them.

Second, stop the triggers in their tracks. Change your morning routine so you sidestep your usual trigger to smoke (try drinking tea instead of coffee, or sit in a different chair to read the paper, for example). Change your route when you go out so you don't pass by your usual stop where you replenished your smokes.

—Roseanne Joseph

WARNING

Never smoke while using a nicotine-replacement product. Doing so may result in an overdose that can trigger a heart attack.

help you replenish antioxidant vitamins and minerals and boost your protection against free radicals created by tobacco smoke. Drink at least eight glasses of water a day to help flush toxins from your system and thin sinus and lung congestion. And store a stash of raw vegetables in the refrigerator for those oral cravings you're bound to have.

● **Pick a readily accessible buddy** who's willing to be available whenever you need to talk.

● **List your reasons for quitting.** Post the list where you'll see it often and read it at least once a day.

Take the Easier Way

Experts know you're more likely to go back to smoking within three months if you haven't changed your routines and behaviors. Nicotine-replacement products can buy you time to make those changes. They also boost your overall chances of success. By sending a controlled amount of nicotine to your brain via your bloodstream, they satisfy your body's craving without the drawbacks of tobacco. See the chart at right for help in choosing the product that's best for you.

Should you worry about becoming addicted to the nicotine replacement itself? Here are the facts:

● Most people gradually reduce their use of nicotine-replacement products until they've completely stopped.

● Few people use them for longer than the recommended three to six months.

● Replacement nicotine won't damage your lungs, and it's not known to cause cancer by itself.

● Since it's considerably less harmful to your body to get nicotine through a gum or patch than through tobacco, some doctors may permit long-term use of these products.

Don't Go It Alone

Research shows that the most successful approach to quitting is using nicotine-replacement products and seeking some kind of support in order to change your behavior. Quit for Life is a smoking cessation program offered by Health Canada (www.hc-sc.gc.ca/english/tobacco. htm). Other sources are Canadian Lung Association (www.lung.ca/ smoking), National Clearinghouse on Tobacco and Health (www.ncth.ca). Check your phone book for stop-smoking programs. Look for a group with a trained leader that meets in regular sessions (20 to 60 minutes) over at least a two-week period.

Try listening to audiotapes to help you over the rough spots. Log onto www.quitsmoking.com for an idea of what's on the market.

Should You Quit Cold Turkey?

Most smokers who successfully quit do it cold turkey. The problem with quitting gradually (sometimes called "fading") is that it makes it harder to stop by lengthening the period of withdrawal.

If you're a heavy smoker, however, it may not be realistic to stop all at once, since you're accustomed to large doses of nicotine. You may want to reduce your smoking to less than a pack a day before you quit cold turkey. Talk to your doctor about how you can do this more easily, perhaps with the help of the drug bupropion (Wellbutrin). This antidepressant helps balance the levels of certain brain chemicals associated with mood and mental state. You can also help wean your body off nicotine by smoking less often, inhaling fewer times with each cigarette, and inhaling less deeply.

Great Aids to Get You Through

Nicotine-replacement products come in several forms, so become familiar with everything on the market, and discuss what's best for you with your doctor. Antidepressant drugs may also be an effective addition in some cases.

NICOTINE AID	KEY FACTS
Nicotine Patch	■ No prescription required. ■ Available in several strengths. ■ Delivers nicotine into the bloodstream through capillaries at the surface of the skin. ■ Levels out blood nicotine levels throughout the day to eliminate cravings. ■ Side effects may include insomnia (if so, take it off at night and put it back on in the morning) and skin irritation (if so, use alternate sites). ■ Generally used for 6 to 12 weeks.
Nicotine Nasal Spray	■ Not yet available in Canada. ■ Absorbed into the bloodstream through nasal mucous membrane within 5 to 10 minutes. ■ Side effects may include nose and throat irritation, watery eyes, sneezing, and coughing. ■ Reduce use after 8 weeks. ■ May irritate the nose and cause coughing and sneezing.
Nicotine Inhaler	■ Not yet available in Canada. ■ Absorbed through the mouth, throat, and lungs; effect peaks in 20 minutes. ■ Side effects include coughing, mouth and throat irritation.
Nicotine Gum	■ No prescription required; available in two strengths. ■ To use, chew just enough to release a small amount of nicotine (peppery taste). "Park" it between your cheek and gum to allow nicotine to be absorbed. When taste disappears, chew again until taste reappears. Park it again. Discard after about 30 minutes. (It takes 20 minutes for the nicotine to be fully absorbed.) ■ Many people chew too few pieces per day, and for too few weeks, to gain the maximum benefit. Many doctors recommend a fixed schedule of one piece every one to two hours for one to three months. ■ Side effects can include hiccups, upset stomach, sore jaw, burning sensation in the mouth (often a result of chewing it the wrong way).

NON-NICOTINE AID	KEY FACTS
Bupropion (Wellbutrin)	■ Prescription required. ■ Raises blood level of dopamine (same brain chemical affected by nicotine) to create a feeling of well-being. ■ Can be used in combination with nicotine replacement therapy. ■ Start one week before you quit and continue for 8 to 12 weeks. ■ Side effects include insomnia, agitation, anxiety, dry mouth, headache, and skin rash.
Other Antidepressants	■ Serotonin-enhancing drugs such as Zoloft and Prozac are being tested for effectiveness.

Six Weeks to Success

The following game plan is based on a quit date three weeks away. If the date you choose is sooner or later, you can adapt the program to suit your own time frame.

WEEK 1

Take a Look at Your Smoking Habits

Start a smoking diary. Each day, every time you smoke, briefly record

- the time
- what you're doing
- why you're using tobacco this time
- how you feel afterward.

At the end of each day, review your smoking patterns. What triggers your tobacco use? Is it boredom, anger, fatigue, nervousness, or certain social situations? Look for other ways to cope with these feelings or circumstances.

WEEK 2

Change Some Habits

Tell friends, family, and co-workers your quit date. Ask them to help. Review your reasons for quitting at least once a day. Change your routines so it's less convenient to smoke:

- Buy cigarettes by the pack, not the carton.
- Skip the afternoon coffee break (when you would normally smoke) and go for a walk or drink a glass of juice instead.
- If you normally smoke in heavy traffic, stock the car with sugarless gum or hard candy and reach for that instead.
- Stay away from smoky environments.
- Delay your first smoke of the day. Try to push it an hour later every three or four days.

Aim to get your smoking down to less than a pack a day before your quit date. Your doctor might prescribe the antidepressant bupropion to help you accomplish this more easily.

Fast Fact

It usually takes three or four attempts for a smoker to quit for good.

WEEK 3

Start the Countdown!

Remind folks that your quit date is nearly here. Continue to put off your first smoke of the day. Also:

- Try going smoke-free for one day.
- Remove the lighter from your car.
- Confine your smoking to one room.
- Hold your cigarette in the other hand.

The night before your quit date, soak your remaining cigarettes in water and throw them in the trash. Get rid of all ashtrays, lighters, and matches. Have your nicotine-replacement products or other aids ready. Before bedtime, review your reasons for quitting. Visualize yourself victorious over tobacco, smoke-free, and healthy.

WEEK 4

Your Quit Date

Take this week one day at a time. When you wake up, reread your reasons for quitting. Repeat to yourself: "I can do anything for one

---

If You Stumble Along the Way

Be prepared for possible relapses before you quit for good. Relapse usually occurs the first week after you quit, when withdrawal symptoms are at their peak. If it happens:

- Stop what you're doing. Throw out the tobacco product.
- Take a break. Go for a walk or do something to boost your spirits fast, such as buying yourself some flowers.
- You can stop—you've proven it. Consider the tar and nicotine you spared your body and the expense you spared your wallet while you stopped.
- Review your reasons for quitting. Talk over your setback with a friend or professional. Devise a new strategy for coping with whatever was behind your setback.
- Decide to return to your program. Remember, the only way to fail is to stop trying.

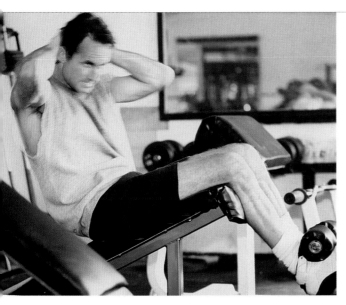

Exercise can distract you from the urge to smoke and helps offset any weight gain that quitting may trigger.

Worried About Weight Gain?

You're not necessarily going to gain weight when you give up tobacco; not everyone does. But the average smoker who quits gains 5 to 8 pounds, at least over the short term. Here's why.

First, nicotine suppresses your appetite. You simply don't feel like eating as much when you smoke. Second, like a pep pill, nicotine speeds up your metabolism, so you burn more calories. Given the same amount of activity and the same diet, you burn 200 more calories a day when you're using tobacco than when you're not.

But you can burn those 200 extra calories a day by increasing your activity level (even vacuuming for a half hour and doing some light gardening would do it). Or you could begin cutting back on high-calorie snacks (just an ounce and a half of potato chips equals about 200 calories).

Remind yourself often that a few extra pounds are much less damaging to your health than smoking. And 5 to 10 pounds are a lot less noticeable to other people than yellow teeth, bad breath, wrinkled skin, and smelly clothes.

day." Record your feelings in your diary. Use your nicotine replacement or other aid as planned. Avoid alcohol and caffeinated drinks, which can increase your desire for nicotine. Stay away from social situations that may cue your smoking habit.

Remember, craving is a normal part of withdrawal. Each craving usually lasts just a few minutes. When you have the urge to smoke, take some deep breaths and then drink a glass of water, or do some jumping jacks. Keep handy a pack of gum, some carrot sticks, or cinnamon sticks to suck on. Your goal today: No tobacco use.

You may feel restless and have trouble concentrating. Hate nicotine for that. If you have trouble sleeping, eat a few spoonfuls of yogurt or drink a glass of warm milk before bed—they contain chemicals called tryptophans that are soothing and may help you nod off.

Did you make it through the day? If so, great! And tomorrow will be easier. If you didn't, don't feel guilty; it doesn't mean you're a failure. Quitting is a process, not a single event.

WEEK 5 Hang in There!

Enjoy the sharper sense of smell and taste you've acquired. If nicotine withdrawal still causes sleep problems, try the deep-breathing exercise on page 202. When temptation rears its ugly head, go

places (like the movies) where you're not allowed to smoke. Get lots of exercise. Use the nicotine-replacement products or prescription drugs. Continue your diary.

Before you go to bed each night, celebrate being free of the nicotine demon that day. When you wake up in the morning, take a deep breath and smell the air. You are already healthier than you were last week.

WEEK 6 You're Getting There!

Continue with your game plan—it's working! Consider joining a health club. (Use the money you would have spent on tobacco.) Take a good look at yourself in the mirror. Notice the cleaner teeth, healthier skin, brighter hair.

Beware of the subtle opportunities for relapse: an argument with your spouse, heavy traffic, meeting that friend you haven't seen in a while for a drink. Take it one day at a time. At the end of the week, celebrate your success, but keep your guard up. For some people it takes years to lose the craving for nicotine.

Rethinking Drinking

There's been great news about the health benefits of alcohol in recent years. But drinking too much takes away the potential benefits —and adds plenty of risks.

You've probably heard the reports that moderate drinking can actually be good for your heart. But before you stock up on beer, wine, or liquor for "medicinal purposes," read the fine print.

Alcohol and Aging

Many experts define moderate drinking as no more than a drink a day for most women and no more than two drinks a day for most men. But even moderate drinking may be ill-advised as you get older.

Research shows that as you age, you absorb alcohol more readily and are more sensitive to its effects. So the number of drinks you could tolerate years ago may be too much for you now. Why? First, your body's ratio of water to fat falls as you age, so there's less water to dilute the alcohol. Second, you have less blood flow to the liver and less efficient liver enzyme

action, so your body doesn't metabolize alcohol as readily.

Chances are you're also taking more drugs now, both prescription and over-the-counter. These can pose dangerous interactions when mixed with alcohol, so be sure you read the labels. (See the chart on page 179 for more details.) Alcohol compounds the risk of falls and other accidents, too.

Women need to be especially careful, since most women can't tolerate as much alcohol as men can. One reason is that they are generally smaller, and smaller people have less blood

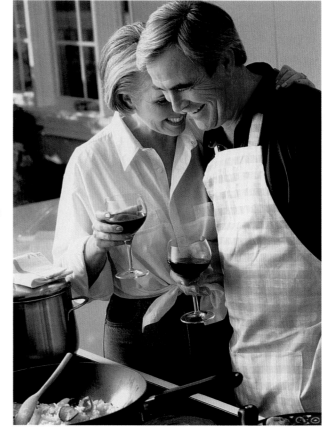

Dinner anyone? Drinking with meals slows the rate at which alcohol is absorbed into the bloodstream, and you're more likely to drink moderately if you drink while you eat.

Fast Fact

According to The Center for Addiction and Mental Health in Canada, older adults should not have more than 8 standard drinks a week and should not drink every day.

volume, so a little alcohol goes a longer way. Women also produce less of the enzyme that breaks down alcohol in the stomach before it is absorbed into the bloodstream. And they have a higher proportion of body fat, which does not absorb alcohol. The result? Drink for drink, women have 75 percent more alcohol in their bloodstream than men do.

The Pros

Despite the caveats, there's no doubt that, for many people, limited amounts of alcohol can help you live longer and decrease your risk of heart disease. Those who may be at risk for heart disease or stroke and those who are diabetic appear to benefit most from moderate alcohol intake (one or two drinks per day) over the course of their lifetimes.

For example, in a University of Wisconsin study of diabetic men and women with an average age of 69, the risk of death from coronary heart disease was significantly lower among moderate drinkers compared to abstainers. The death rate for those who had a drink a day was less than half of that for those who didn't drink at all.

Alcohol consumed in modest amounts may help
- raise your level of HDL ("good") cholesterol
- prevent blood clots
- lower your risk of heart attack, heart disease, adult-onset diabetes, and ischemic stroke.

By raising your level of HDL cholesterol, alcohol inhibits the buildup of plaque in the blood vessels, since HDL carries "bad" cholesterol (LDL) out of the body. Alcohol also appears

Who Shouldn't Drink?

Researchers say you shouldn't consume any alcohol if you:

- have high blood pressure
- have high triglyceride levels (check your cholesterol report)
- have liver disease
- have ulcers or severe stomach acid reflux
- have sleep apnea
- plan to drive, operate machinery, or do something else that requires your attention or skill
- are a recovering alcoholic
- are trying to become a father
- are trying to conceive or are pregnant or breast-feeding
- are taking medications that interact with alcohol (check with your doctor or pharmacist, and see some examples in the chart on page 179).

to have a slight blood-thinning effect, which offers some protection against heart attack and stroke.

In the U.S. Physicians' Health Study, men who drank one alcoholic beverage a day had a significantly lower risk of death compared with those who rarely or never drank. This lower death rate can be attributed mostly to a reduced incidence of coronary heart disease in people age 50 to 60. Don't overdo it, however. Death rates rise significantly with three or more drinks a day.

The Cons

Does all this mean you should start drinking alcohol if you don't already drink? Not at all. One reason is that no one can predict who might be at increased risk for alcoholism. And of

WARNING

Drinking alcohol with carbonated beverages (rum with Coke, for instance) speeds the emptying of the stomach into the small intestine, where alcohol is absorbed more quickly.

What's in a Drink?

A **"drink of alcohol"** delivers .5 ounce of pure ethanol. Each of the following is considered one drink:

- 1.5 ounces of 80-proof distilled spirits (105 calories)
- 12 ounces of beer (150 calories, 100 calories for light beer)
- 3.5 ounces of table wine (85 calories)
- 3.5 ounces of dessert wine, like port or sherry (140 calories).

course, if you drink too much, any potential benefits of alcohol will be offset by the dangers inherent in alcohol-related disease.

Those dangers are considerable. Even light alcohol consumption has been linked to cirrhosis and cancer of the liver, a number of other cancers (of the breast, mouth, throat, and esophagus), as well as high blood pressure, hemorrhagic stroke, osteoporosis, and depression. Here are some of the findings:

- The risk of cirrhosis can jump dramatically with two to three drinks a day and may even increase in some cases with one or two drinks a day.
- Alcohol can increase the risk of breast cancer beginning at just a few drinks a week. One study showed that breast cancer was 50 percent more likely to develop in women who consume three to nine drinks per week than in women who drink fewer than three drinks a week.
- Alcohol has been linked to cancers of the mouth, pharynx, larynx, and esophagus at less than one drink a day.

WARNING

Postmenopausal women who are taking estrogen-replacement therapy should be extra careful not to drink too much alcohol. Some studies suggest the combination compounds your risk of breast cancer. The relative risk increases approximately 10 percent if you have one drink per day.

- Two drinks a day can increase a woman's risk of hip fracture by shrinking her bone mass.

Alcohol has a number of other negative effects. You probably know that it can dull a person's mental edge, judgment, coordination, reaction time, and memory. Drinking can also disturb blood sugar levels, impair sexual functioning, and even interfere with normal sleep patterns, making it more difficult to stay asleep and suppressing up to 20 percent of rapid eye movements (REM) in the restorative stage of sleep. And heavy, prolonged drinking can actually cause the brain to shrink.

The Bottom Line

Since alcohol can be potentially good and bad for your health, how are you to know how much is helpful or harmful? For some people, one drink a day may be okay; others should set the limit at two or three drinks per week. If you're in doubt, talk it over with your doctor. You can't make a sound decision unless you consider your health history and current health risks. In the meantime, here are the general rules of thumb:

- If you don't drink, don't start. The risks that come with frequent drinking—impaired judgment, memory, reasoning, and self-control—outweigh the benefits.
- If you do drink, limit yourself to one drink a day (five to seven drinks a week) to stay on the safe side. A study by Harvard University of 22,000 men found that, in terms of heart health, the ideal number of drinks for men is two to four per week. Men who had two or more drinks a day had a

SELF TEST

Are You Drinking Too Much?

Dependence on alcohol is a serious problem that requires professional help. If you think you might have a problem, take the Alcohol Use Disorders Identification Test (AUDIT) below, developed by the World Health Organization.

These questions pertain to your use of alcoholic beverages during the past year. A drink is defined as a bottle of beer, a wine cooler, a glass of wine, a cocktail, or a shot of hard liquor. The points for each answer are listed after the answer. Add the points for all your answers to get your score.

◀ **1.** How often do you drink alcoholic beverages?
Never	0
Once a month or less	1
2 to 4 times per month	2
2 to 3 times per week	3
4 or more times per week	4

◀ **2.** How many alcoholic beverages do you have on a typical day when you are drinking?
1 to 2 drinks	0
3 to 4 drinks	1
5 to 6 drinks	2
7 to 9 drinks	3
10 or more drinks	4

◀ **3.** How frequently do you have 6 or more drinks on one occasion?
Never	0
Less than once a month	1
Once a month	2
Weekly	3
Daily or almost daily	4

◀ **4.** How often in the past year have you been unable to stop drinking once you had started?
Never	0
Less than once a month	1
Once a month	2
Weekly	3
Daily or almost daily	4

◀ **5.** How often in the past year have you been unable to do what was expected of you because of drinking?
Never	0
Less than once a month	1
Once a month	2
Weekly	3
Daily or almost daily	4

◀ **6.** How often in the past year have you needed a drink in the morning after a night of heavy drinking?
Never	0
Less than once a month	1
Once a month	2
Weekly	3
Daily or almost daily	4

◀ **7.** How often in the past year have you felt guilty after drinking?
Never	0
Less than once a month	1
Once a month	2
Weekly	3
Daily or almost daily	4

◀ **8.** How often in the past year have you been unable to remember the events of the previous evening because of drinking?
Never	0
Less than once a month	1
Once a month	2
Weekly	3
Daily or almost daily	4

◀ **9.** Have you or someone else ever been injured because of your drinking?
Never	0
Yes, but not in the past year	2
Yes, during the past year	4

◀ **10.** Has a relative, friend, or health-care professional ever expressed concern about your drinking?
Never	0
Yes, but not in the past year	2
Yes, during the past year	4

If you scored 8 or more, you probably have a drinking problem. In fact, according to most experts, if you wonder whether you have a drinking problem, you do.

Where to Get Help

◀ Alcoholics Anonymous: check your phone book for local chapters. There are more than 5,000 groups in Canada.

◀ Al-Anon: www.al-anon.org

◀ Women for Sobriety, a self-help group for women: www.womenforsobriety.org

◀ Centre for Addiction and Mental Health: log on to www.camh.net, or call 1-800-463-6273 (toll-free in Ontario only) or 416-595-6111.

Just because you can buy a drug over the counter doesn't mean it's safe to drink while taking it.

death rate 63 percent higher than that of men who didn't drink.

- Don't "save up" your drinks and have several at a time. There are no health benefits from binge drinking—only a significantly higher risk of premature death. Concentrated drinking (more than three drinks per occasion for women, or more than four for men) can be more dangerous than a steady alcohol intake. It can cause an irregular heartbeat, which can lead to blot clots and possibly trigger a heart attack. And remember, more than two alcoholic drinks a day elevates your blood pressure, which raises your risk of heart disease and stroke.

- In general, if you're temperate in your drinking and are in good health, you may not experience any negative effects of alcohol. You may even gain some benefits.

Alcohol and Drugs Don't Mix

Alcohol is a drug—a central nervous system depressant that acts like a sedative or tranquilizer. When it's mixed with other drugs, it can spell serious trouble. And don't think the problem is only with prescription drugs. Just because you can buy a drug over the counter doesn't mean it's safe to drink alcohol while taking it. Acetaminophen (Tylenol), for example, can cause serious liver damage when paired with alcohol. So can aspirin and ibuprofen. See *Common Drug and Alcohol Interactions,* right, for more information.

Demystifying the "French Paradox"

You've probably heard of the so-called French paradox—the phenomenon in which people from France have lower rates of heart disease despite their affinity for cigarettes and foods high in fat. Scientists speculated that another habit of the French—their love of red wine—made the difference. Specifically, an antioxidant substance in red wine called resveratrol was the focus of much attention. But there might be more to the story.

Although the antioxidants and other plant chemicals in wine may indeed protect the cardiovascular system, it's probably not these compounds that have the greatest impact on your heart. Researchers now believe that the alcohol itself—any alcohol—helps the heart by raising levels of HDL, or "good," cholesterol. HDL carries cholesterol out of the body and inhibits blood clotting, which can lead to heart attacks and strokes.

The French also have other habits that may contribute to their heart health. For instance, they tend to consume more fresh fruits and vegetables, serve smaller portions of meat, and cook with monounsaturated fats, such as olive oil. And they aren't as hooked on high-fat, high-sodium snack foods as we are.

Common Drug and Alcohol Interactions

Even aspirin can be dangerous when combined with alcohol. Talk to your doctor and pharmacist about how alcohol affects all the medications you take, both prescription and over-the-counter. When in doubt, avoid alcohol if you're taking any drug. Below are some common drug-alcohol interactions.

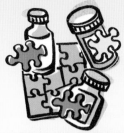

DRUG	INTERACTIONS WHEN TAKEN WITH ALCOHOL
Over-the-counter (OTC) Drugs	
Acetaminophen (such as Tylenol, Tempra)	■ May cause serious liver problems.
Antihistamines (such as Benadryl, Chlor-Tripolon, and many OTC cold medications)	■ Increase drowsiness.
Aspirin (such as Bayer)	■ Increases risk of bleeding in the stomach and intestines. May cause liver problems.
Ibuprofen (such as Advil, Motrin IB)	■ Damages stomach lining. May cause liver problems.
Prescription Drugs	
Certain antibiotics (such as cefotetan, and metronidazole)	■ May cause nausea, vomiting, cramps, headache, and flushing. Do not take with alcohol.
Antidiabetic drugs (such as Glucophage, Diamicron)	■ Large doses may increase the risk of low blood sugar and may also cause nausea or headache.
Narcotic pain relievers (such as Darvon-N, Demerol, Tylenol #3, and cough syrups with codeine)	■ Can cause excessive depression of the central nervous system. Do not take with alcohol.
Anti-anxiety drugs (such as Valium, Xanax, and BuSpar) and certain antidepressants (such as Elavil, Wellbutrin, and Prozac)	■ Can cause excessive depression of central nervous system. Do not take with alcohol.
Sedative-hypnotics (such as Dalmane, Halcion, and Nembutal)	■ Increase the sedative's depressive effects. Do not take with alcohol.
Warfarin (Coumadin)	■ Increases risk of bleeding.

⚠ WARNING

You are more likely to become dependent on alcohol if you have
- *a history of poor family relationships (possibly including violence or inconsistent parenting)*
- *siblings who abuse alcohol or drugs*
- *a father who is dependent on alcohol.*

Minding Your Medicines

Some of the most common risks to your health come in pill form. Follow the right precautions to make sure the drugs you take don't do more harm than good.

Arthritis pain…indigestion… high blood pressure…high cholesterol…. The older we get, the more drugs we're likely to take for our ills. Older North Americans are thought to take an average of six medications each day. Individuals age 60 and over use about three times as many prescription drugs as the general population, and even more over-the-counter (OTC) drugs.

Older people are also more sensitive to medications and more prone to side effects. That's because as we age, our liver and kidneys become less efficient, so we metabolize drugs more slowly. As a result, we may need less of a certain medication than we did before.

Here's a guide to taking drugs safely and avoiding some of the most common drug pitfalls.

Avoiding Drug Interactions

By far the biggest problem in taking drugs is the danger of interactions. Drugs can interact with other drugs and also with food. They can also interfere with diseases or conditions you have (other than the one for which you're taking the drug).

● **Drug–drug interactions** These can change the way drugs act in the body or cause side effects you don't expect, and they can involve prescription drugs, OTC drugs, and even vitamins, minerals, and herbs. Very often the effect of one or both of the drugs can be magnified. If you take aspirin and a blood thinner like warfarin (Coumadin) together, for example,

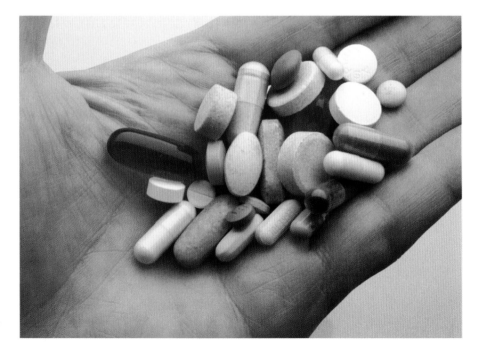

The more medications you take, the greater the chance of interactions or misuse. Even seemingly harmless drugs like aspirin and ibuprofen can pose dangers such as internal bleeding. Make sure your doctor knows about all the drugs, herbs, and vitamins you take.

the combination can thin your blood enough to put you at risk for excessive bleeding. And kava, the popular herbal remedy for stress, could increase the effects of muscle relaxants, sedatives, or antidepressants. In other cases, one drug might prevent another from working properly, such as when an antacid or an iron supplement interferes with the effects of an antibiotic.

- **Drug–food interactions** These occur when a certain food affects the action of a drug. For example, grapefruit juice can enhance the effect of calcium channel blockers and the sleeping pill triazolam because the juice competes for the same enzymes that normally break down these medicines.

- **Drug–disease interactions** These can occur when a drug exacerbates a condition you already have or causes untoward side effects. If you have uncontrolled high blood pressure, for example, you shouldn't take decongestants, which may further elevate your blood pressure.

To help prevent these and other problems, adopt the following safety practices for using drugs. They're all easy to do, and they could keep you from making a serious mistake.

Golden Rules for Safe Drug Use

Read the label. Tackle the fine print of every drug or supplement you take, even if you need a magnifier to do it. Pay particular attention to any cautions about drug interactions and side effects. When you pick up your prescription drug, always check the

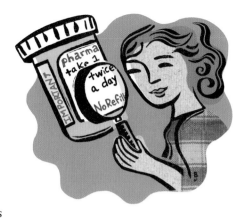

label to make sure it's the right medication. Fatal mistakes do happen.

Avoid overlaps. Many drugs contain the same or similar active ingredients, and you can get too much of that ingredient without realizing it if you take more than one of them. For instance, don't take a blood thinner like warfarin (Coumadin) with aspirin, cimetidine (Tagamet), or vitamin E, which also thin the blood.

Talk with your doctor and pharmacist. Let all your doctors and your pharmacist know which drugs you're taking—that includes OTC drugs and vitamin, mineral, and herbal supplements as well as prescription drugs. (It's a good idea to keep a list of your drugs, with both generic and brand names, in your wallet for easy reference.) Also ask their advice on which OTC drugs are best for you.

Buy all your drugs from one pharmacy. If all your medications are dispensed by the same pharmacist, there's a greater chance that any drug duplications or dangerous interactions will be spotted before a problem occurs.

Don't keep problems to yourself. If you're having side effects or just don't feel right after starting a

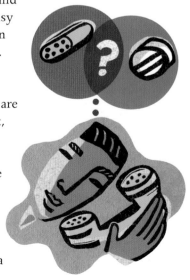

Fast Fact

You might think that older people are the ones most likely to forget to take their medication, but recent research shows that baby boomers are more apt to miss a dose than people over 55. The findings suggest that a busy lifestyle, not age, is the principal culprit.

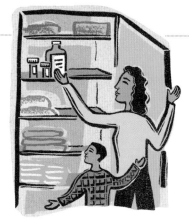

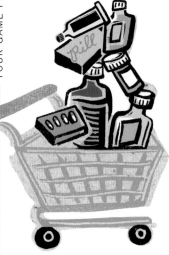

certain drug, don't grin and bear it. Be alert for common symptoms of drug–drug interactions, including nausea or upset stomach, headache, heartburn, and dizziness. If any side effect is causing you more than mild discomfort, call your doctor.

More isn't better. Don't try to supplement your prescription drugs with OTC drugs in an effort to get faster relief. Also, be sure to ask when you can safely stop taking a medication. With OTC drugs, take the smallest effective dose you can. Better yet, see if eating more nutritiously, exercising more, avoiding stress, or making other lifestyle changes will help.

Don't improvise. Follow directions to a "T." If you need to take a drug four times a day, for example, find out whether that really means every six hours—it might not. Don't chew, crush, or break tablets or capsules unless your doctor specifically tells you to. Chewing sustained-release medications could cause them to be absorbed too quickly, resulting in an overdose. Splitting some tablets in half isn't wise either, if they're not meant to be split—for instance, if they're coated to be long-lasting or to protect the stomach. If your doctor recommends splitting pills, ask the pharmacist to do it for you.

Everything in its place. Don't put different drugs in the same container; you can get them mixed up too easily. Keep them in their original containers, even when traveling. Watch where you put the containers, too. Tubes of ointments or creams shouldn't sit right next to your toothpaste, for example. You'll be asking for trouble when you're in a hurry.

Protect others. Never share drugs—they could harm someone they're not meant for. And if you have leftover or expired drugs, flush them down the toilet. Don't just toss them into the wastebasket, because children or pets could be poisoned by them.

Store it right. Keep drugs out of the reach of children, but not in your bathroom medicine cabinet. The bathroom tends to be humid, and drugs should be stored in a cool, dry place, away from direct sunlight. A hall or bedroom cabinet is better.

Avoid the shotgun approach. Some OTC medicines, such as cold remedies, contain as many as five different drugs. To minimize the possibility of side effects and interactions, choose a product with only the ingredients you really need.

Don't economize. Don't take leftover drugs from an old prescription or use drugs that have expired. Out-of-date drugs can be less potent or even toxic.

Never take drugs in the dark. If you keep drugs on your nightstand in case you need to take something during the night, keep a flashlight handy so you can see what you're taking. Don't keep sedatives, narcotics, or tranquilizers by your bed. You could inadvertently repeat a dose if you take it when you're half asleep.

DRUG CAPSULE

Use your pharmacist. One study looked at people over 65 who took five or more medications regularly. Half of them periodically checked their drug regimen with a pharmacist. The control group didn't. Those who did had 25 percent fewer adverse drug reactions than those who didn't.

Be a Smart Online Shopper

In the U.S., people enjoy the convenience of buying drugs online, as well as the ease of shopping for the best prices. But buying from disreputable sources can be risky. In 1999 a 52-year-old Illinois man with episodes of chest pain and a family history of heart disease died after buying an impotence drug from an online source.

The situation is quite different in Canada. Online prescription services from Canadian pharmacies and electronic transmission of prescriptions is not permitted. A limited number of Canadian Web sites offer Internet pharmacy services to customers. These are information-only sites, with consumer information on medications, wellness, and disease management, plus Internet shopping for **nonprescription** drugs. In the United States, there are about 200 Internet pharmacy sites, and some circumvent regulations set by the U.S. Food and Drug Administration by operating offshore. A few supply regulated drugs without a prescription, which poses a serious health risk to consumers. The Canadian Pharmacists Association has the following advice for Canadian consumers and the Internet:

- Do your homework. Check out www.canadian-health-network.ca. to verify that the Internet source of health and medication information you are using is considered reliable.
- Don't let the Internet replace consultation with a pharmacist, doctor, or other health care provider.
- Be cautious about buying medications via the Internet. You may be fooled into thinking a Web site represents a legitimate pharmacy when in fact both the sellers and the products are not legitimate.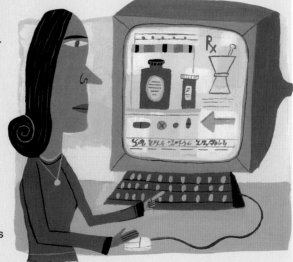
- Make sure that an on-line pharmacy is a licensed pharmacy in good standing in Canada or the U.S. In the U.S., a Web site should have a Verifiable Internet Pharmacy Practice Sites (VIPPS) seal.
- Don't have prescriptions filled by foreign sites even if you are asked to fill out a questionnaire for supposed review by a qualified doctor. Don't trust it.
- Beware of sites that advertise "new cures" for serious disorders.

Common Medicine Mistakes

Even over-the-counter drugs can be dangerous when used improperly. Could you be misusing any of these drugs? Many people do and they don't know it. Make sure you're not making any of these errors.

DRUG	COMMON MISUSES AND PITFALLS TO AVOID
Acetaminophen (such as Tylenol) 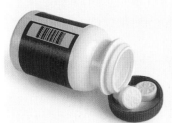	▪ It has few toxic effects if you follow directions, but many people take too much of it. Overdose or misuse can cause serious or fatal kidney or liver damage. Don't take it steadily for more than 10 days. Excessive use can result in rebound headaches when you stop taking it. Keep long-term intake below 4 grams per day. Signs of chronic overdose include bleeding, bruising, sore throat, and malaise. ▪ Check other drugs (such as cold medicines) for the same ingredients to be sure you're not overdosing. ▪ Never drink alcohol while taking it or you'll risk serious liver damage. ▪ If you are too sick to eat, don't take this drug. Taking it while fasting increases the risk of liver problems.
Antacids (such as Rolaids, Tums, Mylanta)	▪ Overuse is common, since people frequently reach for these to cure the ill effects of a poor diet, heartburn, indigestion, smoking, drinking, and stress. Taking too much can cause constipation (possibly leading to intestinal obstruction, especially in elderly people) and kidney damage. ▪ Brands that contain magnesium can cause diarrhea or dehydration. Frequent or protracted use of these can lead to laxative dependence. Products that contain calcium, if taken too often, may cause excessive calcium levels, possibly leading to kidney stones. ▪ Take all antacids 2 to 3 hours before or after your other medications to avoid possible interactions, and don't exceed recommended doses.
Aspirin and nonsteroidal anti-inflammatory drugs (such as Advil, Motrin IB) 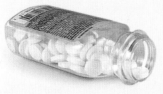	▪ Aspirin may be used too often, or in amounts beyond the recommended dosage. Stomach irritation and stomach bleeding are the biggest risks. Watch for the signs of stomach irritation, including nausea, vomiting, and diarrhea. To minimize stomach irritation, take it with food, milk, or a full glass of water. ▪ Don't lie down for 15 to 30 minutes after taking to avoid irritating the esophagus. ▪ Don't take steadily for more than 10 days. Frequent, excessive use of aspirin for headaches—especially in products that also contain caffeine—can result in rebound headaches when you stop taking it. ▪ Ringing in the ears may signal that you are taking too much. ▪ Don't take daily aspirin for your heart without talking to your doctor first. ▪ Since aspirin increases the risk of bleeding, avoid taking it a week or two before any surgery, including dental surgery.
Cough suppressants and expectorants (such as Benylin DM, Robitussin, Tylenol Cold and Flu)	▪ Some brands contain up to 40 percent alcohol, so avoid drinking alcohol when taking these. ▪ Don't take an expectorant and a cough suppressant at the same time. ▪ Don't take too much for too long. Since some of the prescription cough syrups contain narcotics and can be habit-forming.

DRUG	COMMON MISUSES AND PITFALLS TO AVOID

Laxatives
(such as Correctol, Dulcolax, Senokot, Milk of Magnesia)

■ They're used inappropriately by many older persons who believe they need to have a daily bowel movement (something that's not necessary, as long as stools pass easily).

■ Some people use them inappropriately for weight control, but they're not effective—food is already absorbed before the laxative can work.

■ Discontinue laxatives as soon as normal bowel movements have been reestablished.

■ Don't use them daily for longer than one week without your doctor's advice.

■ Overuse of laxatives can lead to a frustrating constipation-diarrhea cycle. This can hinder your ability to move your bowels and may deplete body fluids and essential electrolytes. It can also affect your absorption of vitamin D and calcium.

■ Avoid constipation by gradually increasing the amount of fiber in your diet through high-fiber foods, drinking at least eight glasses of water a day, and raising your level of physical activity.

■ If you already overuse laxatives, see your doctor. You need medical supervision to stop using them gradually.

■ Do not give children laxatives without your doctor's advice.

Nasal decongestants
(such as Dristan Nasal Spray, Otrivin)

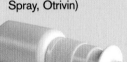

■ Nasal sprays can work so well that some people begin to rely on them all the time. But prolonged use may cause nasal blood vessels to remain swollen, leading to a condition called "rebound congestion." In other words, it can create the problem it's trying to solve.

■ Restrict use to twice a day for no longer than 3 days. Watch for signs of overuse, including inflamed sinuses and nosebleeds.

Sleep aids
(such as Sominex, Nytol, Unisom)

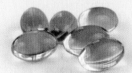

■ People who rely on sleeping pills too often can easily develop a tolerance for them, so that they need to take larger and larger doses of sleep aids to get the same effect.

■ Some older people may have trouble metabolizing the pills, which can remain in their system for up to 96 hours and compromise their alertness.

■ The active ingredient (diphenhydramine) is also found in many OTC cold and allergy preparations. Don't take both at once.

■ If you have liver, kidney, or respiratory problems, enlarged prostate, or glaucoma, consult your doctor before taking any OTC sleep aid.

■ Common side effects of sleep aids include dry mouth, blurred vision, dizziness. Avoid driving and hazardous work until you have learned how the drug affects you. Also, avoid alcohol, which enhances the sedative effect of some sleep aids.

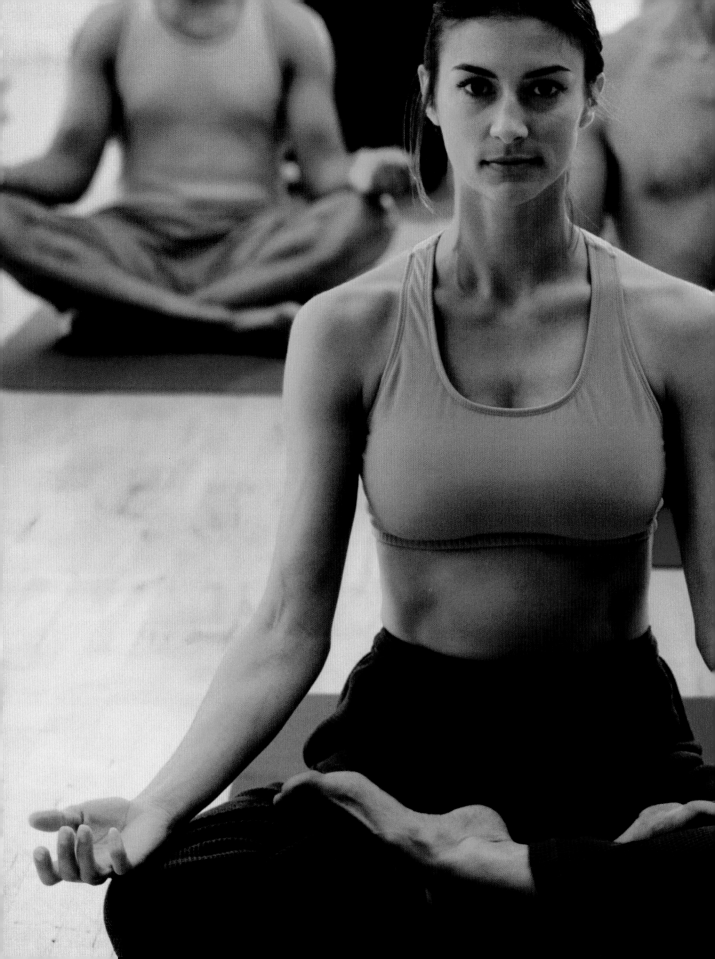

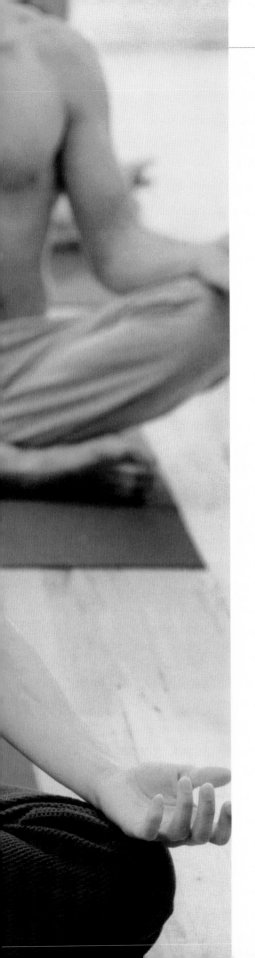

CHAPTER 7

GIVING STRESS THE BOOT

The Health Connection

In the new every-minute-counts millennium, stress is inevitable. But you don't have to let it run your life—or ruin your health.

You know what stress is. It's that teeth-gritting traffic jam when you're late for work. It's your in-laws arriving unexpectedly for a long holiday weekend. It's that shortfall in your bank account this month. In sum, stress is all the aggravations of modern life. But the word *stress* also describes the way your body reacts to these events.

When your heart races, your palms sweat, and your mouth goes dry, that's the stress response. And it's not for nothing: Stress serves a biological purpose. When primitive man spotted a wild beast ready to make a meal of him, his body initiated a chain of events to help him either defend himself or beat a hasty retreat. For instance, his liver converted fats into glucose to supply quick energy. A wave of neurotransmitters, such as serotonin, put his nervous system on alert. Stress hormones surged through his body, raising his heart rate and blood pressure to speed oxygen and nutrients to the brain and major muscles. Hormones called glucocorticoids halted the storage of energy by blocking the transfer of nutrients to fat cells. And his pupils dilated to help him better see his foe—or his escape route.

This "fight or flight" reaction is nature's way of channeling our resources to help us escape immediate danger. The trouble is that work deadlines, money pressures, marriage problems, and a whole host of modern-day difficulties also trigger the stress response—and trigger it more often than nature ever intended, which is bad news for your health.

Paving the Way to Illness

For many years, the link between chronic stress and illnesses like the common cold was the stuff of wives' tales—widely believed but never

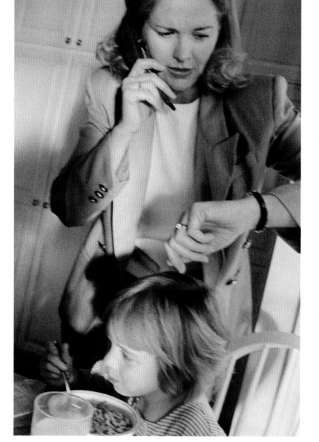

Bane of modern existence, stress isn't a health problem unless it's chronic—and it often is. If stress has become a way of life for you, ask yourself why, then commit to making a change.

Stress: A Double-Edged Sword

The "fight or flight" response can be a blessing in an emergency, but if you trigger it too often, it can undermine your health, increasing your risk of cardiovascular disease, depression, sleep problems, and chronic skin conditions.

REACTION	ADVANTAGE	DISADVANTAGE
You breathe faster.	■ Quick breaths allow more oxygen to enter the bloodstream, providing instant energy.	■ Fast, shallow breathing makes it impossible to relax.
Your heart rate increases.	■ The heart pumps more blood per minute, increasing circulation. This speeds the delivery of energy to the muscles.	■ Increased heart rate over the course of many years can contribute to chest pain, irregular heart rhythms (arrhythmia), and heart disease, as well as increased perspiration or flushing.
Your blood vessels constrict.	■ Blood is redirected to vital organs, such as the heart.	■ Fewer wide-open blood vessels leads to higher blood pressure.
Energy sources such as blood sugar (glucose) and fat are released into the bloodstream.	■ Blood-sugar levels increase, providing more energy.	■ Chronically elevated levels of blood sugar may contribute to adult-onset diabetes. And fat that's released into the bloodstream but isn't used for energy is converted into cholesterol and can contribute to plaque buildup inside your arteries.
Fibrin, a substance that helps the blood clot more easily, is released into the blood.	■ In case of an injury, your body is better able to stanch the bleeding.	■ Blood that clots easily is a risk factor for heart attack and stroke.

proven. But in the past decade or so, the evidence has become so convincing that many scientists and doctors now view stress as a true health hazard. Here are some of the ways in which stress does its damage.

The Immune System. Many studies show that chronic stress weakens the immune system, making us more susceptible to infectious illnesses, including colds and flu. In one study at the University of California, San Diego, researchers found that people under stress had 60 percent fewer active CD8 cells and significantly fewer CD4 cells than other people.

CD8 and CD4 cells are specialized white blood cells that help destroy bacteria, viruses, and cancer cells. The stress hormones epinephrine (adrenaline) and cortisol are most likely to blame.

People under stress also suffer worse symptoms when they do get a cold. In a study at Carnegie Mellon University in Pittsburgh, researchers injected volunteers with the influenza A virus, then quarantined them in a hotel room for seven days. Those under more stress before being injected experienced more intense symptoms, such as greater mucus production.

Fast Fact

Researchers believe that chronic stress may increase your susceptibility to colds by as much as 90 percent.

Stress and the Sexes

Who experiences more stress, men or women? Although men in their forties and fifties are more likely than women to have a heart attack, men don't seem to suffer from more stress—even though stress contributes to heart disease. In fact, a recent international survey of 30,000 people found that women are much more likely than men to be stressed.

The women in the survey reported symptoms including anxiety, depression, insomnia, back pain, and stomachaches. They also described such altered behaviors as a lack of appetite or eating too much (usually sweet or salty foods), exercising too much or not being able to get off the couch, and smoking more or drinking too much.

One reason women experience more stress, some experts believe, is that they tend to have a greater total workload than men since many of them juggle jobs and the lion's share of family responsibilities. Another possibility, according to Alice Domar, Ph.D., director of the Mind/Body Center for Women's Health at Harvard Medical School, is that women feel more stress because they often play the role of nurturer and tend to take care of everyone else first and themselves last (if at all).

So why are women less prone to stress-linked heart disease? Researchers at Duke University found that women's blood vessels constricted less under stress than men's, most likely due to the protective effects of estrogen. Once estrogen starts to decline during menopause, a woman's risk of heart disease rises. Women are also more likely than men to express their feelings and seek support, both of which have been shown to help shield the body from the ill effects of stress.

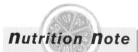

Nutrition Note

The body consumes more vitamin C during times of stress, so when the going gets tough, make sure you get enough. Many experts recommend increasing your intake to 500 mg through food and supplements. Getting more vitamin C may offer an added bonus: In recent animal studies, the vitamin actually reduced levels of stress hormones in the blood.

Heart Disease. Reacting with anger to stressful events only makes a bad situation worse. A groundbreaking 1992 study published in *The New England Journal of Medicine* found that chronic anger contributes to heart disease. Other studies have confirmed this link. Both anger and stress harm your heart by raising your blood pressure. A rapid increase in blood pressure causes tiny injuries to the walls of the coronary arteries. Over time, scar tissue forms and contributes to arteriosclerosis, or hardening of the arteries. Stress also increases your heart rate, and may eventually cause heart-rhythm abnormalities.

Stress makes the blood clot more easily, too—probably in order to stanch bleeding in case of injury. And it raises blood levels of cholesterol, encouraging the buildup of plaque in the blood vessels that feed the heart and making it harder for blood to flow through. All of these factors can lead to a heart attack.

Skin Conditions. Scientists at Tufts University School of Medicine in Boston found that a substance called corticotropin-releasing hormone, or CRH (released by the hypothalamus in the brain in response to stress) may play an important part in chronic skin disorders such as eczema and psoriasis. In the studies, scientists injected CRH into the skin of rats. It triggered a number of allergic skin reactions such as swelling, inflammation, scaling, and itching. When the rats were injected with a drug that blocked the action of CRH, their skin showed no such reactions.

Wound Healing. In a study at Ohio State University, researchers evaluated 36 women based on their reported levels of stress, then produced small blisters on their forearm with the use of a suction device. The women under the most stress healed more slowly than those who were more relaxed. Blood tests revealed that the stressed women produced significantly lower levels of inter-leukin-1 and interleukin-8, compounds that help protect against infection and aid in healing. That's why doctors encourage patients to reduce stress and anxiety levels before undergoing surgery.

The Brain. Some research shows that chronic stress can actually cause a sort of "brain burn"—damage to the part of your brain that controls learning and memory. This may be the result of increased levels of glucocorticoids, stress hormones that can inhibit the function of neurons in the brain's cortex and hippocampus. The effects (slower thinking, trouble handling complex tasks, and either a racing mind or apathy) seem to be more pronounced in older people.

Prolonged stress can even cause memory failure. At Washington University School of Medicine in St. Louis, Missouri, researchers found that exposure to high levels of the stress hormone cortisol over several days can impair "verbal declaration memory," or the ability to remember words, details, and phone numbers. In the four-day study, 51 people were given either a placebo or a dose of cortisol in amounts normally pro-

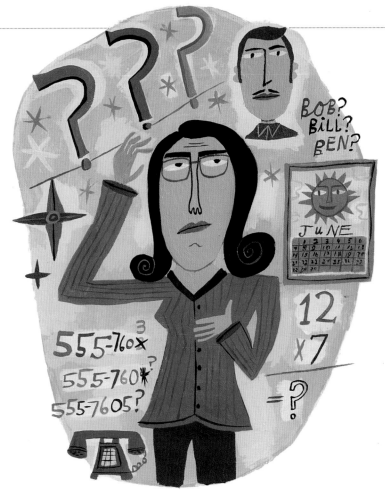

duced by a very stressful event. Of those given the hormone, 93 percent had more difficulty remembering information in a paragraph compared with people given the placebo. Six days after the cortisol doses were stopped, all of the groups performed equally well on memory tests.

A stressful situation can actually heighten your recall. Stress that lasts a few days or more, however, can scramble your memory and interfere with your ability to recollect details such as names and phone numbers.

The Subtle Signs

Listen carefully to your body, since stress can express itself in many ways. Here are a few common examples:

- Unexplained and chronic fatigue
- Anxiety
- Sudden bursts of anger
- Inability to concentrate or remember simple things
- Quick frustration in the face of obstacles or setbacks
- Lack of interest in sex
- Shortness of breath for no reason
- Dry mouth
- Trembling
- Light-headedness
- Irritability
- Sleep problems
- Stomachache or indigestion
- Weight loss or gain

Top 10 Causes of Stress

Over the course of 20 years, researchers at the University of Washington School of Medicine conducted more than 5,000 interviews to establish the top 10 stressors linked to illness or injury. Their results:

1. Death of a spouse
2. Divorce
3. Marital separation
4. Jail term
5. Death of a close family member
6. Personal injury or illness
7. Marriage
8. Involuntary job loss
9. Marital reconciliation
10. Retirement

The Gut. Stress doesn't cause most ulcers, but it may be a contributing factor in many of them. Even lab animals exposed to psychological stress develop ulcers. Stress may also exacerbate irritable bowel syndrome, which causes abdominal pain and diarrhea or constipation.

Weight. Studies at Yale University and the University of Pittsburgh found that high levels of stress may cause you to put on pounds, particularly around the abdomen. During a stressful situation, the liver quickly converts stored fats into readily usable energy (glucose), which then floods into the bloodstream. The more often a person experiences stress, the more the body tries to store fat around the abdomen—near the liver—for anticipated times of crisis. And some people simply eat more when they're under stress.

Good Stress, Bad Stress

Not all stress is negative. Starting a new job, moving to a new home, or awaiting the birth of a grandchild are all happy but nevertheless stressful events. And many athletes probably wouldn't set records if they didn't have competition—and the accompanying surge of adrenaline—powering their muscles. Even negative stress sometimes serves a purpose. Face it, would you fix the roof if you

SELF TEST

How Stressed Are You?

Use this quiz, adapted from information compiled by the U.S. National Mental Health Association, to evaluate the level of stress in your life.

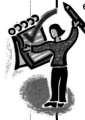

◄ Are you forgetting things more often and finding it difficult to concentrate?

◄ Are you having trouble falling or staying asleep, or are you sleeping too much and still feeling tired?

◄ Do minor problems make you feel really angry or frustrated?

◄ Is it almost impossible for you to stop worrying?

◄ Do you regularly feel nervous and anxious?

◄ Does it seem as if many of the things that annoy you are beyond your control?

◄ Do you often feel inadequate?

◄ Does it seem as if things just never go your way?

◄ Do you get easily upset over things that happen unexpectedly?

◄ Are you unable to cope with everything you have to do?

If your answer to more than one or two of these questions is "yes"—and stays that way over a period of days or weeks—stress is overtaking your life. Read the rest of this chapter for ways to find relief.

weren't worried that it might leak the next time it rains? Would you file your taxes on time without the prospect of a penalty?

What's never good is chronic stress—the daily grind of fear, frustration, and worry that comes from feeling at the mercy of adverse events over which you have no control.

At work, the people who have the least amount of control experience the greatest level of job stress—and the greatest risk of death from cardiovascular disease. According to researchers, stress takes the greatest toll not on top executives but on bus drivers, assembly-line workers, waitresses, and other people with a lot of pressure on the job but not a lot of decision-making authority or power to change their working conditions.

Too much job stress can even shorten your life. Researchers who analyzed 26 years' worth of data found that workers who had little or no decision-making authority throughout their work lives were at increased risk of premature death. In contrast, those who spent more than half their working lives in jobs that allowed them to make decisions were 50 percent less likely than average to die during the study.

Maintaining a sense of control is important even if you're not part of the workforce. Several studies have examined people who live in nursing homes. In one of them, a group of patients was allowed to choose their meals and plan their activities. The other group followed their usual routine dictated by the staff.

Over several weeks, the people in the first group socialized more with others and rated themselves happier

Is It Stress—or Something Else?

Sometimes the symptoms you think are caused by stress may be the result of a serious health problem. For example:
- Intense, squeezing, and prolonged chest pain or a pain that shoots to the left shoulder, arm, or jaw could signal a heart attack. Seek medical help right away, and chew an aspirin, which can help clear the blockage.
- An unwillingness to communicate, socialize, or maintain normal everyday activities may be a sign of clinical depression, which requires professional help and should not be left untreated.

than the people in the second group did. Medical evaluations by doctors who didn't know which patients were in which group confirmed that the people in the first group showed definite health improvements. Most telling of all, 18 months later, there were half as many deaths in the first group as in the second.

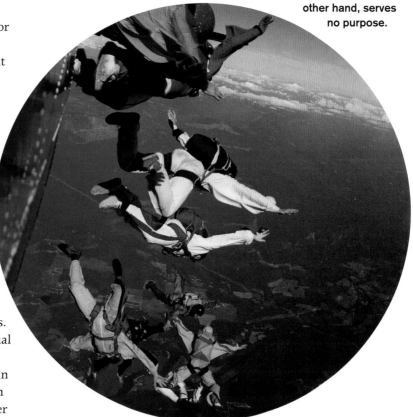

Geronimo!
When you jump out of a plane, your heart rate and blood pressure rise to prepare you for action. Chronic stress, on the other hand, serves no purpose.

Your Anti-Stress Strategy

Like weeds in a garden, stress can take over your life if you don't yank it out by the root.

If you're overly stressed, you probably know it. And while a host of relaxation techniques (see pages 200–203) can help you turn off the stress response, you'll also need to attack stress at the source.

See Molehills, Not Mountains

Does it really matter if your checkbook balances today? Is that spat with your boss truly worth stewing over? One key to stress relief is changing the way you look at things. Consider these questions:

● What's the worst thing that can happen? Is it likely to happen?
● Have you done everything you can about the situation? If so, let it go. If not, taking concrete steps to solve the problem will immediately put your mind more at ease.
● How will the outcome affect your life? Will you remember it a few years from now?
● What would you advise a friend in your situation to do?

Remember, stress-related illness isn't caused by external events but by your reaction to them.

Play Hide...

An obvious approach to avoiding stress is to sidestep the things that cause it, which takes a little planning.

● If traffic jams tie you up in knots, find back roads to your frequent destinations, and time your trips to avoid rush hour.
● Do looming deadlines keep you up at night? Make a contract with yourself to start every project well before you have to complete it. Break up the job into achievable steps and tackle one every day.
● Keep other people's expectations

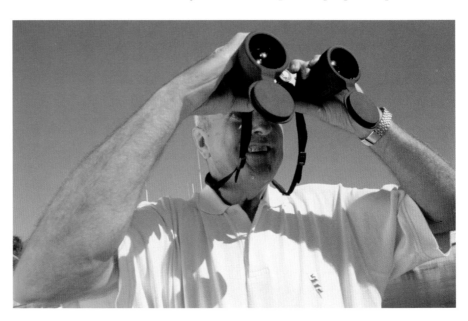

Immerse yourself in a hobby you love and your troubles will seem to shrink. Outdoor activities such as gardening and bird-watching can be especially therapeutic.

in check. Studies show that unclear role expectations or role conflicts are major sources of stress. Insist that the important people in your life tell you what they want from you in unambiguous terms. Then—most important—check their wishes against your own needs and let them know what you can and can't do.

- If certain people you can't avoid always seem to get under your skin, control your interactions with them. See them only when you're relaxed, and tell them directly if there are specific things you don't want to discuss.

...and Seek

At the same time, it's important to seek out activities that provide a refuge from stress. Of course, what you choose depends on what you enjoy. But some hobbies are naturally relaxing. For instance, gardening can be particularly therapeutic since it offers a connection with nature, forces you to slow down, and focuses your attention on other living things instead of yourself (and your problems). Any hobby that absorbs your full concentration can also take you away from your worries, especially activities that require intense focus. For instance, martial arts, racquet sports, golf, and rock climbing all force you to live in the moment.

Take Charge of Your Time

You know the feeling: There's too much to do and not enough time to do it. What's the solution? First, separate what's really urgent from what can wait, and give your full attention

to high-priority responsibilities. Second, delegate whatever tasks you can, and truly let them go instead of continually monitoring their progress. (That goes for housework, too. Avoid the temptation to micromanage your helpers, who probably also happen to be your loved ones. Chores don't have to be done your way; they just have to be done.)

Whatever you do, don't skimp on necessities. No matter how busy you are, you'll be worse off in the long run if you skip meals, curtail exercise, and deprive yourself of sleep, according to Don R. Powell, Ph.D., president of the American Institute for Preventive Medicine.

Some other time-management tips:

- Do your most demanding work when you're most alert, which for most people is around mid-morning or just after a light lunch. Save returning phone calls and other mindless tasks for the afternoon slump, advises Dr. Robert M. Sapolsky, a Stanford University neuroendocrinologist and an expert on stress.
- Let the phone ring. If you have voice mail or an answering machine, let the caller leave a message, then call back when it's most convenient for you.

Nutrition Note

Stressed? Don't reach for junk food. Try these snacks instead:

- Warm milk, yogurt, and tapioca pudding. All supply tryptophan, an amino acid used to manufacture serotonin, a brain chemical associated with relaxation.
- Bread, cereal, and pasta. These feel-good foods induce a feeling of calm by stimulating the release of serotonin.
- Bananas, orange juice, and apricots. These are rich in potassium, which is depleted during periods of intense stress.

DRUG CAPSULE

If specific situations (flying, public speaking, going to the dentist) or short-term pressures (like tax season for an accountant) make your heart pound and your thoughts race, ask your doctor about taking an anti-anxiety medication such as alprazolam, lorazepam, or buspirone. It's safe to take alprazolam or lorazepam for as little as a day or as long as two weeks to relieve anxiety symptoms due to short-term stress. The downside is that both drugs can make you drowsy and sluggish. By comparison, buspirone won't sedate you, but neither will it tame your nerves until you've taken it regularly for about a week, gradually increasing the dose.

- Chop big tasks into bite-size pieces, so they'll be less overwhelming. Chip away at them bit by bit whenever you have a few spare minutes, and they will be done before you know it.
- Just say no. If you really don't have the time to bake for that bake sale or take on that extra project, admit it to yourself first, then find a way to say so.

Tap the Exercise Answer

Exercise is a potent weapon against stress. It helps relieve muscle tension and triggers the release of endorphins, hormones that boost your mood. Plus, it can take your mind off whatever is bothering you. And people who exercise experience milder physical reactions to stress. For instance, studies show that those who exercise before facing stressful situations experience a smaller rise in blood pressure and blood-sugar levels than those who don't. Another bonus: Exercise promotes a longer period of deep sleep, which more fully recharges your body's batteries.

You don't need to be an exercise fanatic to reap benefits. Even a brisk 20- to 30-minute walk or bike ride, three to five times a week, can help (although 30 minutes daily is ideal).

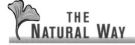

THE NATURAL WAY

Panax ginseng, also called Asian ginseng, is believed to reduce the harmful effects of stress, possibly by balancing the release of stress hormones. It may also enhance the production of endorphins, the body's feel-good hormones. The active ingredient is a compound called ginsenoside, which is extracted from the plant's root. Look for a brand standardized to contain at least 7 percent ginsenosides, and take 100 to 250 mg once or twice a day. Pregnant women, as well as people who take MAO-inhibitors or who have heart-rhythm abnormalities, should not take ginseng.

The trick is to choose an activity you enjoy. Any type of exercise is valuable, but when it comes to stress relief, different varieties have specific advantages.

- Aerobic activities (done at a pace fast enough to work up a sweat, but slow enough to carry on a conversation) help reduce tension, anxiety, and depression.
- Rhythmic exercises (such as bicycling, swimming, running, or rowing) can bring you to a calm state resembling meditation.
- Fast-paced sports (such as tennis, racquetball, or basketball) require intense concentration and take your mind off your worries.
- Solitary sports (such as walking, running, biking, or in-line skating) give you an opportunity to work out any negative, aggressive feelings and calm your mind.
- Team sports provide the benefit of interaction with others.

Practice Optimism

The toll stress takes on your body depends largely on how you cope with adversity. If you tend to withdraw, get discouraged, blame yourself, fly off the handle, or throw back a few stiff drinks, you're letting stress get the best of you. On the other hand, if you tend to look on the bright side, you'll be more immune to life's slings and arrows.

Martin Seligman, a University of Pennsylvania psychologist and author of *Learned Optimism*, has identified attitudes that help people cope successfully with stress. When something bad happens, optimists tell themselves the situation is temporary ("Things will get better soon"). They blame external events,

The Value of Furry Friends

Social support from friends and family affords powerful protection against stress-related illness. But the unconditional affection of a loyal dog or the purr of a friendly feline are helpful, too. In fact, pet owners visit the doctor less often, are less prone to disease, and are more likely to live longer than people who live alone. They also seem to handle stress better.

Researchers at the State University of New York–Buffalo recently studied the stress responses of 48 hard-driven stockbrokers with high blood pressure. The stockbrokers were put through two high-stress situations (being asked to count backward by 17s as fast as they could, then trying, for five minutes, to talk their way out of a hypothetical shoplifting charge). During both tests, their blood pressure soared. Afterward, half the brokers were given dogs or cats to take home.

Six months later, the tests were repeated, with one crucial difference: The pet owners had their animal companions along for company. During the test, their blood pressure readings rose by an average of 8 or 9 points. By contrast, the blood pressure of the people without pets rose an average of almost 20 points. According to study head Karen M. Allen, Ph.D., several of the petless brokers were so impressed by these results that they went out and adopted furry friends of their own.

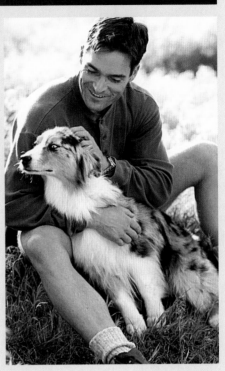

not themselves ("Sometimes these things just happen"). And they view the incident as an isolated event, not part of a larger trend ("This person has a problem with me, but most people don't").

According to psychologists, if you're not a natural optimist, you can learn to be one. When you catch yourself reacting to an event in a destructive way, stop a minute and consider whether there is another point of view, then try to reframe your thoughts. Seeking out the company of optimistic people can also help you cultivate a positive attitude.

For a quick way to stanch the flow of negative thoughts, try this trick: Quickly jot down 5 or 10 things that make you happy in life, and reflect on them. It's a good reality check that helps you refocus on the positive rather than the negative.

If You Need Help

If you feel you're experiencing more stress than you can manage, make an appointment with a counselor or therapist. There is no shame in this; on the contrary, it shows that you're taking control of your situation by getting the help you need.

Ask your doctor or friends for recommendations. Many therapists offer a free get-acquainted session; use it to decide whether you feel comfortable with the person. If you are employed, check your company's benefits plan; some of them offer employee assistance programs that include counseling. For more information, contact the Canadian Mental Health Association (416-484-7750 or www.cmha.ca) or the Canadian Psychological Association (888-472-0657 or www.cpa.ca).

Fast Fact

Research shows that people with strong family ties have milder physical responses to stress.

10 Easy Solutions to Stress

Does stress send you spinning? Don't let it wear you down. Instead, take preemptive action to get it under control—before it controls you. Here are some concrete ways to nip stress in the bud.

1 **Lean on other people.** Studies of both animals and humans show that social contact can help tone down the body's physical response to stress. It can even boost immunity. So cultivate a network of people you can turn to. Share what's bothering you with a friend and ask for some helpful advice. Avoid people who always need something without giving back or who are constantly moody or depressed.

2 **De-clutter your world.** Stop hoarding old magazines, and throw away those old receipts and tax returns you no longer need. Clutter-free surroundings will help prevent the frustration of not being able to find something you need, and give you the reassuring knowledge that everything's in its place.

3 **Eliminate last-minute rushes.** Leave the house 15 minutes early for appointments, set up a system for paying your bills (ask your bank about automatic bill paying), refill your prescriptions a week ahead of time, and stock up on birthday cards whenever you see ones you like. A little advance planning can spare you a lot of headaches.

4 **Keep a journal.** Reflect on your day, your emotions, and your personal goals. Include everything that stresses you, so you can start to recognize patterns and take appropriate action. Writing is also a great way to relax and put things into perspective.

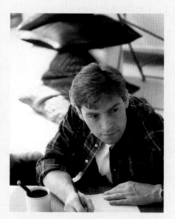

5 **Get organized.** Set aside a place for bills, paperwork, letters. Store items you use most often in accessible places. Spend five minutes straightening your office or main living area at the end of the day. Keep a long-range calendar and a short-range to-do list. Check off items as you finish them.

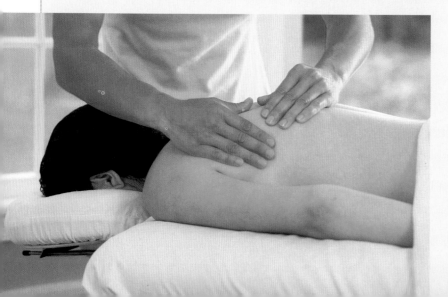

6 **Get a massage.** Massage not only relaxes tense muscles, it decreases the level of stress hormones in the bloodstream and stimulates the release of serotonin, a brain chemical associated with relaxation and a feeling of well-being. Studies show that massage can even lower your heart rate and blood pressure.

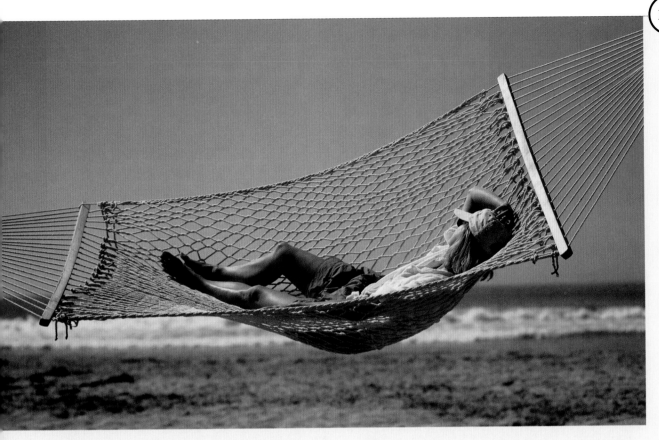

7 Chop your to-do list in half. Most of us set the bar too high. After you've written your to-do list, decide what's most important to you in the long run, then cut the list in half. If you

can't eliminate certain tasks, try to have someone else do them. For instance, hire a neighborhood teenager to do the yard work, or skip cooking and order in.

9 Avoid crowds. Schedule your commute to avoid traffic, go for lunch 15 minutes before the usual rush, make Thursday, not Saturday, your night out, shop for groceries on a weeknight, and order your clothes through the mail.

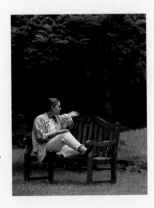

8 Carve time for yourself. Give higher priority to your "relax and renewal" time. Include it in your schedule at least every other day. If you have to cut out an activity to make time for your hobby—or a warm bath—then do it. Or spend some time alone reading or listening to music you love.

10 Laugh a little. When you laugh, you send chemicals called endorphins to your brain that ease pain and enhance your feeling of well-being. Laughter also stimulates the heart, lungs, and muscles and boosts your resistance to infection. If you laugh for 20 seconds, your body gets the same amount of beneficial oxygen—good for stress relief—as it does in three minutes of aerobic exercise. Plus, it's nearly impossible to stay tense while you're laughing. Find cartoons, videos, TV shows, writers, and comics that make you laugh. Share jokes with friends over email.

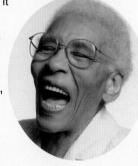

Learning to Relax

Forgotten how to relax? It's not as ridiculous as it sounds. True relaxation can take some effort—but it's worth the work.

Relaxation techniques like progressive muscle relax-ation may help lower blood pressure in people with stress-related hypertension.

Stress—the "fight or flight" reaction—is automatic, turned on in response to danger. The trouble is, unless you literally run away from the problem, there's no outlet for the tension. And that can spell trouble for your health.

You can learn to turn the stress response off by consciously activat-ing what Dr. Herbert Benson, a pioneer in stress research, calls the "relaxation response." Benson was the first to study the physical effects of certain relaxation techniques. He found that by practicing meditation or deep breathing, for instance, you can actually lower your blood pres-sure, slow your breathing, change your brain-wave patterns, reduce your body's oxygen consumption, and even boost some aspects of your immune system.

Any of the following relaxation methods can not only help to relieve anxiety but also foster a sense of well-being and improve your overall health. The more you practice these techniques, the more powerful they become.

Progressive Muscle Relaxation

This technique involves tensing and releasing groups of muscles one at a time to relax your entire body.

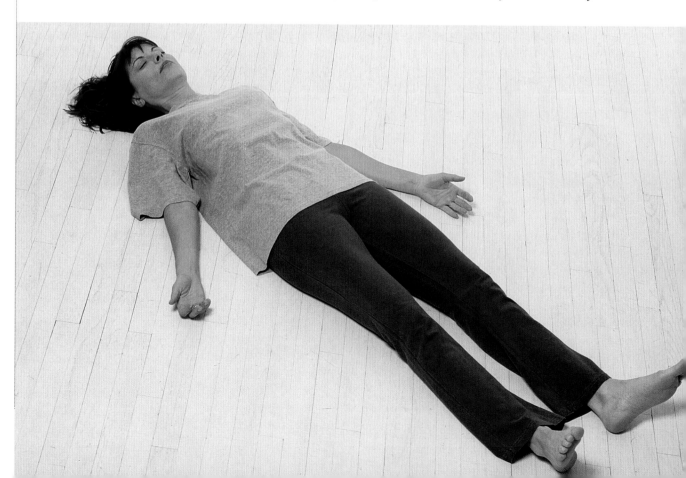

1 Lie on your back on a thick carpet or workout mat.

2 Breathe in deeply, then tense your entire body and hold the tension for several seconds, noticing how it feels. Then let go while exhaling, and notice the difference.

3 Now tense each part of your body one by one, starting with your feet. Point your toes forward, then up. Tense your calf muscles, then relax. Move on to your thighs, then your stomach muscles. Now arch your back slightly, then press it into the floor.

4 Continue tensing individual muscle groups. Make your hands into fists, then let go. Press your arms against the floor, then relax them. Shrug your shoulders, then release. Tense the muscles in your face (wrinkle your brow, clench your teeth, open your mouth wide).

5 When you've finished, lie quietly for a few minutes. Your whole body should feel at rest.

Meditation

There are many different types of meditation. In transcendental meditation, you focus on one thing—usually a word or phrase, also called a *mantra*—in order to clear your mind and achieve a deep state of calmness. Another type of meditation, called mindfulness, involves focusing on your thoughts but not judging or reacting to them.

Here is a basic exercise in transcendental meditation to get you started. Practice this for 20 minutes once or twice a day.

1 Find a quiet place where you won't be distracted or interrupted. Close the door, turn off the phone, and shuffle your pets off to somewhere else. Don't choose a time when you're hungry or have just eaten a big meal.

2 Wearing loose-fitting clothes, sit in a comfortable position.

3 As you take slow, deep breaths, close your eyes and repeat a word or phrase—any one you choose. It could be a neutral word, such as "one" or "om," an inspirational word, such as "peace" or "love," or a religious phrase, such as "The Lord is my shepherd."

Soothing Scents

Researchers have found that essential oils, distilled from plants and flowers, can influence mood and even ease pain. In one New York hospital, a psychologist quelled the anxiety of claustrophobic patients undergoing MRIs (magnetic resonance imaging scans) by pumping the scent of vanilla into the room.

Although some studies have indicated that certain scents, such as lavender, have relaxing properties, any fragrance you like will do the trick. Scents popular for stress relief include ylang-ylang, neroli, sandalwood, eucalyptus, rose, and geranium. Here are a few ways to use them:

● Mix a few drops of essential oil with a carrier oil (such as almond or grapeseed oil) and add it to your bathwater or use it in a massage. (Pregnant women should avoid skin contact with essential oils.)

● Use a diffuser, an electric device that disperses molecules of essential oil into the air. You can even set the diffuser to a timer and awaken to the invigorating scent of citrus oils instead of the buzz of an alarm clock.

● Sprinkle a couple of drops of essential oil on a handkerchief and inhale the scent (people with asthma should avoid inhalations).

Caution: Essential oils can cause skin irritation. Do not apply them directly to your skin unless you dilute them first with a carrier oil. Never take them internally or apply them to sensitive membranes around the eyes, nose, or mouth.

THE NATURAL WAY

To calm your anxiety, consider kava. This popular herb relaxes skeletal muscles without depressing the central nervous system, leaving you calm yet alert. In studies it has been shown to work almost as well at quelling anxiety as tranquilizers and anxiety-reducing medications. Take no more than 250 mg a day. Don't take kava for more than three months without consulting your doctor. Prolonged use increases the chance of side effects such as stomach upset. And don't take kava if you plan to drive, since it may slow your reflexes.

4 When other thoughts enter your mind, simply redirect your attention to your word or phrase. This might be difficult at first, but as you become more adept at meditating, you'll be better able to clear your mind of all distractions.

Deep Breathing

Another way to elicit the relaxation response is to focus on your breathing. During times of stress, we tend to take short, shallow breaths, filling only the upper chest with oxygen. Children, on the other hand, instinctively fill their lungs completely by breathing from their abdomens in what's called deep, or diaphragmatic, breathing.

Deep breathing not only increases your oxygen intake but also helps reduce tension and encourages a state of relaxed alertness. Practice this technique once a day.

1 Lie on your back with your feet slightly apart.

2 Breathe in slowly through your nose. (This filters and warms the air before it enters your lungs.) Keep the tip of your tongue gently touching the roof of your mouth throughout this exercise. If your nose is congested, inhale through your mouth, slightly opened.

3 Count to four as you inhale, imagining the warm air moving deep into your lungs. Make sure that your abdomen—not your chest—expands as your lungs fill with air. Your shoulders shouldn't move.

4 Hold the breath as you count to four again, slowly.

5 Exhale slowly with a whoosh of sound, again to the count of four, imagining any tension moving out

with the air. Contract your stomach muscles to push all the air out of your lungs. Notice your abdomen fall.

6 Pause a second or two, then repeat. As you become more relaxed you may find that you can increase your counts effortlessly, going up to a count of eight.

Visualization

The imagination is a powerful tool. Athletes use it to enhance their performance by "seeing" themselves execute the perfect high jump, triple axle, or jump shot before they actually do it. Along the same lines, if you picture yourself calm and in control, your body will respond in kind. Studies have shown that visualization can lessen anxiety and even ease pain. Here is one simple visualization exercise you can practice daily or whenever you feel stress start to tighten its grip.

1 Take a few deep breaths as described in the deep breathing exercise at left.

2 Now picture a peaceful scene. It might be a meadow, a lake, a mountaintop, the beach, or any place where you feel calm.

3 Immerse yourself in every aspect of the scene. For example, imagine the color of the grass or water, the feel of the warm or cool air on your face, the smell of the salty ocean or pine trees or wildflowers, the chirp of the birds, or the rhythmic crash of the waves. Let these details absorb your full attention for about 5 or 10 minutes. Notice that your breathing is now slower and more regular. When you're ready to disengage, simply allow the image to slowly fade away.

Looking East for Relaxation

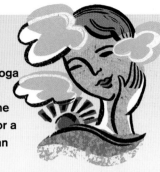

If you feel pulled in a dozen different directions, Eastern practices such as yoga and the others described below can help you find balance. In many of them, defined postures and repetitive movements help focus the mind and relax the body. For maximum benefit, take time to learn the proper technique. Look for a class offered by an experienced teacher. Once you learn the method, you can practice it by yourself at home.

TECHNIQUE	WHAT IS IT?	WHAT CAN IT DO?
Yoga (YO ga)	▪ Means "union." Integrates mind, body, and spirit to foster better health. ▪ Consists of a series of body positions, movements, and stretches. ▪ Most common is the slow-paced Hatha style, which focuses on stretching and breathing exercises. Power yoga, with quick stretching movements that can make you sweat, is also popular.	▪ Strengthen your muscles, improve flexibility, and boost your sense of well-being. ▪ Calm the body. Studies show that doing yoga regularly can reduce your blood pressure, body temperature, and heart rate. Check with your doctor first if you have heart, lung, bone, or muscle problems; people with these health issues may have to limit inverted (upside-down) poses.
Tai chi (tie CHEE)	▪ Developed over 1,000 years ago as a Chinese martial art, it is now practiced in a variety of "schools" or forms. ▪ Often called "moving meditation," it features slow, circular movements and graceful postures combined with deep breathing. ▪ Eases tension in the mind and body.	▪ Strengthen muscles and joints. ▪ Increase circulation and improve balance. ▪ Make you feel tranquil yet alert.
Qigong (chee GONG)	▪ Developed in China as a system of meditation and self-healing exercise. ▪ Based on the Asian concept of chi (chee), or vital life energy. Blocked chi causes illness; stimulating the flow of chi leads to wellness. ▪ Gentle exercises, postures, and breath coordination with visualization.	▪ Promote relaxation. ▪ Boost the immune system. ▪ Increase balance and flexibility.
Reiki (RAY kee)	▪ Developed in Japan in the 1800s from the ancient Buddhist art of healing and relaxation. ▪ A form of healing therapy based on the transfer of chi, or vital life force, from the giver to the receiver. ▪ Resembles massage at times, but some practitioners do it without touching you. You lie on a massage table, fully clothed, while the practitioner places his or her hands in specific positions either on your body or several inches above it.	▪ Restore physical, mental, and emotional health.

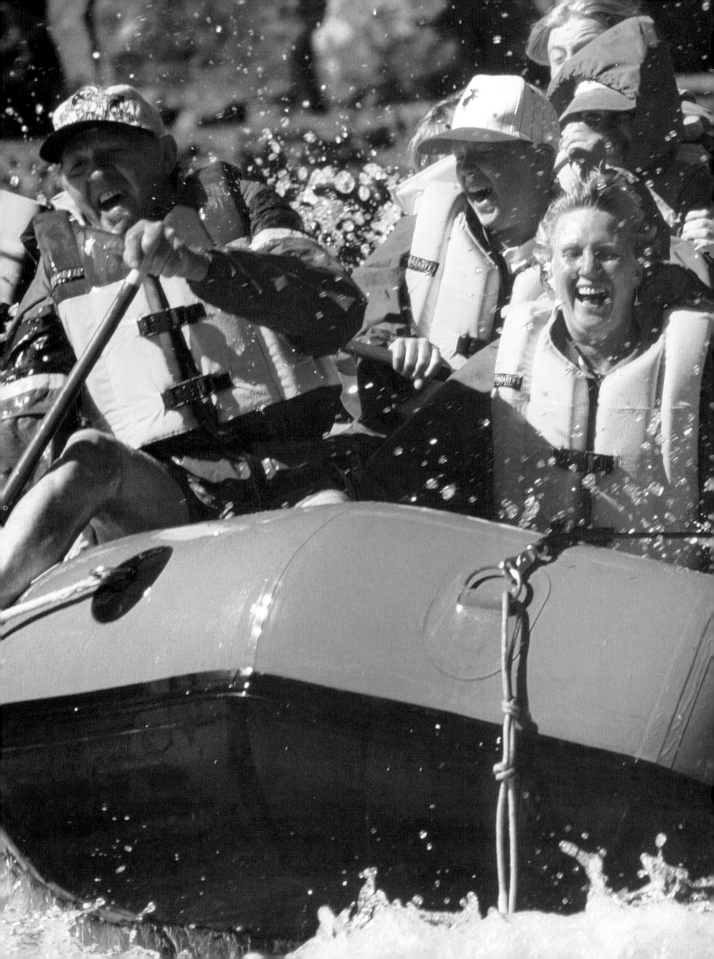

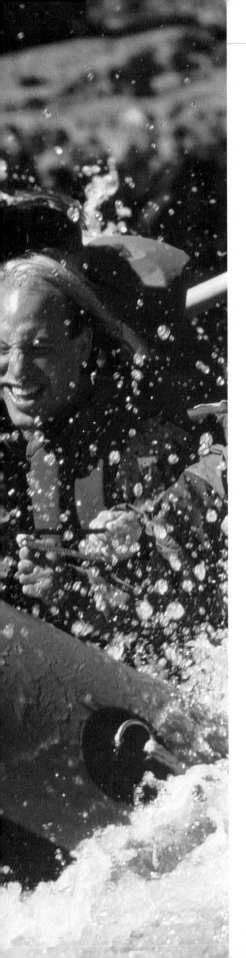

CHAPTER 8

FEELING GOOD

Feeling Good About Yourself

Think your emotional state doesn't affect your health? Think again. The mind and body are joined in marriage, for better or for worse, in sickness and in health.

Scientists are learning more and more every day about the link between your mind and your health. Stress, depression, and anger have all been shown to pave the way to illness and disease. On the other hand, if you feel good about yourself, have a positive outlook, and maintain an active involvement in life, you're more likely to be happy—and healthy.

The Importance of Self-Esteem

Many things—genetics, environment, the food you eat, illness, sleep, even the seasons—influence your emotional state. But at the heart of it is how you regard yourself. If you have a healthy level of self-esteem, you not only cope with life's challenges better than people with low self-esteem, but you're probably more content, confident, and successful. You're probably also healthier. Studies show that positive self-esteem actually helps inoculate people against depression and anxiety, conditions that may pose increased risk of everything from colds to osteoporosis to heart disease.

Most people's sense of worth is rooted in their childhood—in the early approval or disapproval of parents, teachers, and friends. But as we get older, most of us judge ourselves by our sense of how effectively we're managing in the world, especially in the areas of love and work.

Our ability to love and be loved can give our lives a sense of purpose and deep fulfillment. We can also find satisfaction and pride in work-related accomplishments, and the people we meet and work with can reinforce our sense of self and our role in life.

SELF TEST

How's Your Emotional Health?

Measuring your state of mind isn't as simple as tracking your blood pressure. To get a general idea of how you're doing, begin by asking yourself whether you:
◄ are relatively energetic—a self-starter
◄ have a fulfilling, long-lasting relationship with a partner
◄ have satisfying and

secure bonds with friends
◄ are open to new people and new ideas
◄ laugh easily and frequently
◄ seldom feel guilty or regret your decisions
◄ are quick to get over anger
◄ stay in touch with your own feelings
◄ feel depressed only

a few times a year at most
◄ avoid acquaintances and family who are abusive
◄ make decisions spontaneously, without a lot of worrying
◄ have an active, enjoyable sex life
◄ don't abuse alcohol or

other drugs
◄ feel you can go on after a profound emotional upset or loss.
If you answered no to more than one or two of these questions, it may be time to take stock—and take action. Keep reading for tips on boosting your emotional well-being.

Once midlife comes along, however, our self-esteem can take a turn in response to changes in our lives. Marital relationships may change, children may leave home, and we may begin to scale back on work as we approach retirement. Of course, the view in the mirror may not be what it used to be, either.

Bolstering Your Self-Worth

If you find your self-esteem eroding a bit, there are plenty of ways to build it back up again.

- **Reframe your identity.** Redefine what you base your sense of self-worth on. Instead of "sales manager," "stock market analyst," or "mom," start thinking of yourself as "community organizer," "literacy volunteer," "great cook," "gifted gardener," and more.
- **Talk back to your inner critic.** Become conscious of how hard you're being on yourself, and counter a negative attitude with some positive self-talk.
- **Let yourself off the hook.** As the saying goes, it's better to try something and fail than to be successful at not trying anything. Focus on goals that are linked to activities you're really interested in so you'll enjoy a sense of purpose and derive pleasure from the pursuit whether or not you achieve your goal in full.
- **Take time for yourself.** Read the paper, keep a journal, go for a swim. This is especially important for women, who are often so busy nurturing others that they neglect their own needs and interests.
- **Keep your body healthy.** Eat a balanced diet and stay physically active to keep your body in shape, whether it means taking the stairs more or working out with a personal trainer. You'll look better, feel better, and have more energy for new activities.
- **Give yourself kudos.** Remind yourself of your best qualities and make a list. Are you fun to be around, thoughtful, generous? Keep adding to the list (and pull it out whenever you need a boost). Learn to see the positive side of your faults, too. For example, if you gab on the phone too much, remember that you also value your friends and nurture your relationships.

What Midlife Crisis?

A healthy self-image can help you withstand the inevitable stresses in your life, including the very prospect of growing older. For example, it's a great aid during what people commonly—and often dismissively—call a midlife crisis. For some people, this is a time of uncertainty,

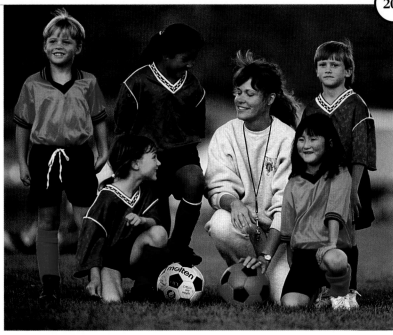

A sense of involvement and purpose is important to your self-esteem.

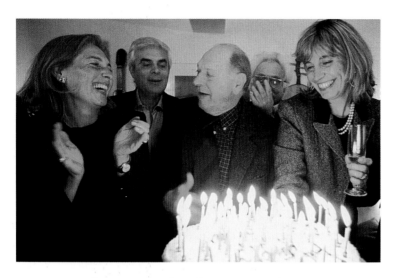

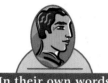

In their own words

Jim Leach, director of communications at Colgate University in Hamilton, New York, recalls how his dad, after retiring from a high-stress engineering job, fulfilled his lifelong dream of becoming a fine woodworker. The skills he'd learned on the job helped him immensely in the design and production of the exceptional vases and boxes he creates. "Now," says Jim, "I've begun to look at ways to extract the parts of my present job that I most enjoy, and I'm trying to figure out how to incorporate them into work I will totally enjoy when I retire."

A milestone birthday can trigger a midlife crisis. Use it to reevaluate your goals and shift your focus to the things that really matter to you.

boredom, anxiety, depression, or even panic. Not everyone experiences it, of course, and for some people, the uncertainty is mild and short-lived. But for an estimated 10 percent of people, the crisis is real.

A midlife crisis usually follows some negative event that challenges your image of your life—a divorce, loss of a job, serious illness, or the death of a loved one. The moment of truth can even be triggered by the simple realization that your children are leaving home or starting their own families.

Whatever activates the crisis, it can flood you with a vague sense of dissatisfaction and prompt you to wonder, Is that all there is? As unsettling as these feelings can be, they offer the potential for change and growth. Viewed in this way, a midlife crisis can be a midlife awakening, an opportunity to reset your goals and appreciate your life in a new way.

To come to terms with yourself and the course your life has taken, you have to step back and take

How to Handle a Midlife Crisis

A midlife crisis isn't necessarily all bad. Here's how to get through it and come out ahead.

● **Give yourself time.** Allow yourself time for reflection and soul-searching. If, in fact, you haven't accomplished what you wanted to in life, now's the time to reevaluate those goals or make changes. For example, if you feel trapped by a job you detest, it may finally be time to make a career move.

● **Don't depend on quick fixes.** You may be impatient for some radical changes (or, yes, even a shiny red sports coupe in your driveway), but remember that, more often than not, change and growth occur as part of a gradual process.

● **Look outside yourself.** Repeat to yourself, as often as necessary, "It's

not all about me." Contribute to the world around you. In doing so, you'll develop a rich capacity for caring that will serve you the rest of your life.

● **Reinvent yourself.** Though you may have based your self-worth on your youth, beauty, or stamina in the past, now's the time to explore other dimensions of yourself. Start by visualizing yourself in different situations and playing new roles—perhaps ones that leverage untapped strengths.

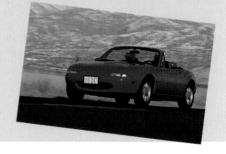

stock. Review your life as it is, with all its triumphs and joys as well as its disappointments and mistakes. Embrace your life without regret, but with gratitude for the lessons you've learned. (See *How to Handle a Midlife Crisis*, previous page.)

A Different Kind of Retirement Planning

One life event that may need some careful navigating is your retirement. This major passage—your long-anticipated reward for years of hard work—can ripple your emotional waters. It can affect your feelings of self-worth, your finances, and even your marriage.

While welcomed by many people, retirement can prompt confusion, anxiety, and depression for others. To avoid these negative feelings, it's important to plan ahead. This means getting your finances in order, finding an avocation that's close to your heart, and establishing personal ties that aren't based exclusively on your professional work. This is especially important for people whose social circle is limited mainly to work-related relationships and who gain their sense of self from their position or profession. These people often find themselves feeling lost after retiring.

Those who are happiest in retirement tend to nurture their relationships and keep themselves busy doing things they enjoy. That might include starting a new business or hobby, or even landing your dream job (for more on this, see page 215). The important thing is not to retire emotionally from life. People who do fare the worst—and are most likely to develop health problems.

For Better or Worse...But Not for Lunch

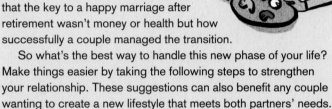

No matter what you do in your retirement, your marriage is going to feel the effects of this transition. You may be surprised to learn that Cornell University researchers found increased depression and marital conflict among newly retired men and women. What's more, a study at Pacific Western University in Los Angeles concluded that the key to a happy marriage after retirement wasn't money or health but how successfully a couple managed the transition.

So what's the best way to handle this new phase of your life? Make things easier by taking the following steps to strengthen your relationship. These suggestions can also benefit any couple wanting to create a new lifestyle that meets both partners' needs. Here's what to do:

- **Be considerate of each other.** Your partner's goals or concerns may differ somewhat from your own. Strive for better understanding. To paraphrase the old saying, try to walk a mile in your partner's moccasins every day.
- **Share household chores** (and don't criticize your partner's housekeeping techniques). Afterward, spend an equivalent amount of time doing things you enjoy.
- **Expand your social network.** Don't rely on your spouse to meet all your social needs. Get involved in activities that provide regular contact with a wide variety of people.

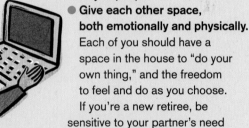

- **Give each other space, both emotionally and physically.** Each of you should have a space in the house to "do your own thing," and the freedom to feel and do as you choose. If you're a new retiree, be sensitive to your partner's need for the time alone he or she may be accustomed to.
- **Chat away.** Increasing the number and variety of things you talk about each day fosters better overall communication. Discuss the news, politics, your cultural and entertainment interests, your vacation plans, and more.
- **Remember you're a team.** Agree that each partner has to buy into a decision before moving ahead. And don't make major decisions quickly. Moving abruptly to that sunny spot in Florida may not be the dream you imagined.
- **Keep a sense of humor.** Being able to laugh at yourself and the predicaments you face is the best tonic.

Staying Connected

It's a fact: People who stay connected socially live longer and remain healthier than those who don't.

Perhaps it's true: People who need people may indeed be the luckiest people in the world. Those who have strong social ties with friends, family members, neighbors, and coworkers enjoy longer, more satisfying, more active lives than those who are socially and emotionally isolated.

The MacArthur Foundation Study of Aging in America and other research studies have confirmed two key facts about social relations:

- **Isolation breeds poor health.** In one study, for example, women who didn't have many opportunities for social contact were found to have higher blood pressure than those who did. Another study revealed that those who had fewer and weaker relationships had two to four times the risk of dying prematurely, regardless of age and other factors.

- **Social support improves health.** For example, a 1999 study conducted at the University of Utah found that older people who have a strong circle of friends have a lower risk of heart disease than those who don't. Support can even help you heal. Women with metastatic breast cancer who were part of a weekly support group lived 18 months longer than those who weren't.

Social interactions can help protect the body from some of the negative physical effects of stress. And people with strong social support have demonstrated less need for pain

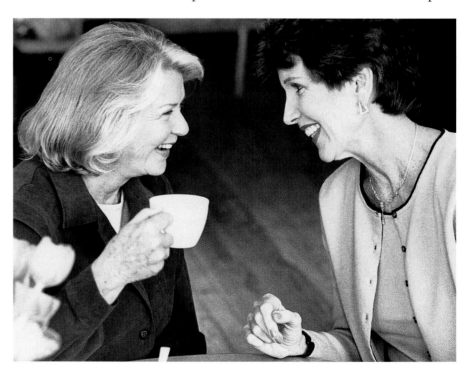

Work harder at maintaining the relationships that make you feel warm and connected, and let go of those that don't.

Ready, Get Net, Go: Finding Old Friends on the Web

The Internet is an excellent resource for finding and reconnecting with long-lost pals, loves, or family members both in North America and around the world. The Web sites below are all free of charge, but others may require a fee to access information.

Start with a general search on a search engine such as Excite (www.excite.com), Yahoo (www.yahoo.com), or Webcrawler (www.webcrawler.com). Simply type the person's name in quotes (to ensure a search for the entire name, not just first or last name). If no matches are found, try one of the more specific search tools below.

Try a people-finder site, such as Anywho (www.anywho.com) and Bigfoot (www.bigfoot.com), which search phone directories (white and yellow pages), e-mail addresses, and toll-free and fax numbers. Missing Friends Network (www.missingfriends.com) searches using the name of a school, hometown, military base, and so on. To learn whether

someone in the U.S. is deceased, use the Social Security Death Index (www.ancestry.com/ssdi/advanced.htm). Populus (www.populus.net) allows you to search by name, city, school, e-mail address, or personal interests. You can find U.S. and Canadian phone numbers, addresses, and maps on WorldPages (www.worldpages.com/ reshome.html). Access the Archives of Canada at www.archives.ca.

Look at Usenet newsgroups, starting with www.usenet-addresses.mit.edu. Newsgroups, much like electronic town halls, allow you to search for a name from messages posted to the Usenet group.

Go to specialty sites using specific info such as military history (www.vac-acc.gc.ca, www.army-buddies.com, www.militaryusa.com/nrrsearch.html), education (www. classmates.com), and fraternity/sorority membership (www.planetalumni.com). For help in organizing a school reunion, go to www.greatreunions.com.

---

medications and faster recovery from illness. They are also more likely to follow medical advice and take good care of themselves. For example, Cornell researchers found that women who were socially connected were more likely to eat lower-fat diets than those who were more isolated.

Making People a Priority

Here are a few of the many ways you can maintain and strengthen established friendships and make new ones, whether you're recently retired, the shyest person on the block, widowed, or simply at a loss for how to meet new people:

- **Initiate casual interactions.** Chat with the clerk when you buy your newspaper, share a joke with the attendant who pumps your gas, or talk to a neighbor you've never spoken to. These interactions help sustain a sense of community.

- **Reawaken dormant relationships.** Catch up with the cousin you haven't talked with in years. Reconcile with long-lost friends. Spend time alone with your brother or sister. These people not only hold your history and link you to your own past, but nourishing these relationships offers opportunities for personal growth.

- **Don't forget to write, phone, or e-mail.** When friends and family move away, stay in touch. The phone and e-mail are the fastest ways to connect, though face-to-face contact is still the best.

- **Leave home.** Maybe you're more comfortable avoiding social situations, but people stop growing when they stop venturing into the unfamiliar. Play cards or golf, take cooking classes, attend religious services, volunteer in a literacy program, or join a gym, investment club, or reading group.

Fast Fact

A study published in the Journal of the American Medical Association *found that people with six or more different types of relationships, including marriage, work colleagues, friendships, and family relationships, were 25 percent less likely to catch a cold than those with fewer social ties.*

Staying in Love with Life

Saying yes to life—engaging your heart, mind, and soul—is the best prescription for staying young at heart.

Make a list of trips you've always wanted to take, then book one.

Aging well isn't just about staying healthy, it's about staying vital, too. Why else do you wish for continued good health if not to prolong your enjoyment of life?

If you tend your happiness, you're also tending your health. Studies have shown that happy people get sick less often and recover more quickly. Optimism has been linked to stronger immune defenses. Happy people, as you might expect, are also more successful at finding a partner than their gloomier counterparts.

Be a Lifelong Learner

Staying mentally active and open to mastering new skills and subjects can add more joy, adventure, and fulfillment to your life, helping to ward off isolation, anxiety, and depression. While you never really outgrow your ability to learn, it can wither if you don't use it enough. Here are some great ways to keep exercising that mental muscle. (See also pages 240-253.)

- **Expand your horizons.** Visit a travel agent and ask about programs such as Routes to Learning (formerly Elderhostel), which organizes educational adventures ranging from day trips to long journeys (613-530-2222). There are opportunities for everything from joining an archaeological dig to museum touring.
- **Bend your mind.** Studying anything new, such as a musical

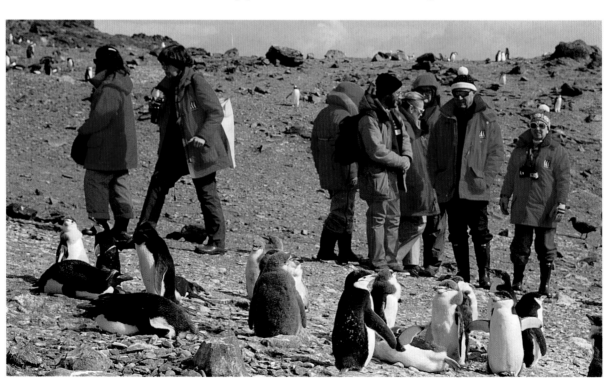

Laugh Your Way to Better Health

Laughter not only feels good, it's good for you, too. Laughing triggers the release of endorphins, feel-good brain chemicals associated with a sense of well-being. It diffuses stress by relaxing the muscles and lowering your heart rate and blood pressure. And it may help you view your situation in a new light.

Humor can also help you heal. Studies at Columbia Presbyterian Hospital suggest that kids who were visited by the hospital's Clown Care Unit healed faster than those who weren't. And researchers at Loma Linda University in California who examined 20 medical students 30 minutes after they viewed a video of a stand-up comedian found that the students' disease-fighting white blood cells shot up 25 percent and their specialized natural killer cells rose by up to 34 percent.

How to inject more levity into your life? Try these tips.

- **Start the day with humor,** be it a cartoon-a-day calendar, a funny Web site, the comics, a radio morning show, or a humorous audiotape played on your commute to work.
- **Make room for whimsy.** Beat a regular path to the comedies at your video store. Even just five minutes of watching a funny film can start to pump your endorphins. Check out a comedy club. Also, take family time to share jokes, tickle each other, and play silly games.
- **Trade jokes in person,** by e-mail, and by fax, and collect cartoons that make you chuckle.
- **If need be, fake it.** Studies show that the physical act of smiling— even if you don't mean it—causes chemical changes in your body that lift your spirits.

> ☐ Subject: Joke
> Date: 28 May 2001
> From: Janice Smith
> To: YOU
>
> How does a crazy person find his way through the forest? Answer: He takes the psychopath.

You have mail!

instrument, prehistoric art, or a foreign language, exercises your ability to think creatively and keeps your mind elastic. Community colleges, adult education centers, and planetariums are great places to expand your educational horizons and maybe find new friends.

- **Be an adult exchange student.** If you're looking for something a bit more unusual, you can always be a foreign exchange student. Room and board is provided by your host family at minimal cost, and you get to study Italian

(or the language of your choice) all day long. For more information, call or write The Talking Traveler, AmeriSpan (800-879-6640), or Languages Abroad (800-219-9924).

Think Positive

When it comes to being happy, a positive attitude helps. Researchers have documented the physical and social benefits of looking at life with a smile. For instance, studies have shown that optimists actually tend to live longer than pessimists.

In their own words

"The skills of optimism do not emerge from the pink Sunday-school world of happy events. They do not consist in learning to say positive things to yourself. What is crucial is what you think when you fail, using the power of 'non-negative thinking.' Changing the destructive things you say to yourself when you experience the setbacks that life deals all of us is the central skill of optimism."

—Martin E.P. Seligman, Ph.D., in Learned Optimism

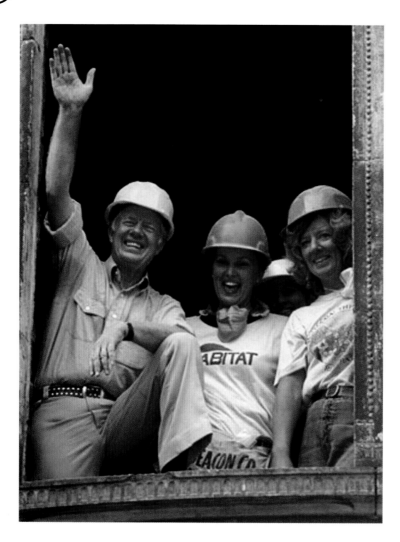

Volunteer organizations such as former U.S. president Jimmy Carter's Habitat for Humanity allow you to help those less fortunate while gaining the social benefits of becoming part of a group.

questions, read up on your condition, and maybe join a support group where you can make yourself and others feel better.

- **Have Thanksgiving every day.** Keep a gratitude journal. Start it with 10 things, both big and small, for which you are grateful (for example, "my partner is in good health"). Keep adding more blessings as they occur to you, and when you're feeling low, curl up with your journal.

- **See with a child's eyes.** Be amazed. Reflect on the wonderment of babies, butterflies, high-tech movies, and so much more.

- **Resolve to stop being unhappy.** You may have to do this in spurts at first to get the hang of it. Try it for a minute, then an hour, then a day, and keep building from there. As Dale Carnegie said, "Act as if you are already happy, and that will tend to make you happy."

Volunteer to Be Happy

Did you know that about 25 percent of men and women over 55 in North America volunteer? As the need for volunteers grows every day, so do the ranks. Be part of this crowd by contacting the Volunteer Opportunities Exchange (www.voe-reb.org), a tool that connects volunteers to organizations, or your local volunteer action center. While gaining plenty of social benefits, you'll also take your mind off your own troubles.

Being involved in volunteer activities could even add years to your

Optimism isn't simply positive thinking—what some psychologists call "passive optimism." Optimism means having a proactive attitude and taking steps to improve the conditions in your life.

Even if you're not a born optimist, you can learn to be one. Start by faking it. Eventually, you might find yourself becoming an optimist just by acting like one. Begin this way:

- **Change your focus.** Instead of seeing problems, try to see challenges. For example, if you are diagnosed with an illness, rather than despairing or relying totally on the doctor's advice, ask plenty of

WARNING

A study by the Mayo Clinic found that, like high cholesterol and obesity, having a pessimistic attitude is a risk factor for early death.

life. According to a study at the University of Michigan's Institute for Social Research, senior citizens who volunteered showed a 67 percent reduced risk of dying during a seven-year period compared with people who did not volunteer.

Embrace Your Beliefs

Studies show that people who attend religious services weekly live an average of eight years longer than those who never do. They are less likely to die of heart disease, have half the risk for depression, require less medication, and are less prone to postsurgical complications.

Some researchers think that believing in a higher power makes it easier to deal with life's difficulties and helps relieve stress—a risk factor for illness. Or it may be that people who have faith generally maintain an optimistic outlook, positively affecting the course of disease.

Spirituality isn't limited to organized religion, of course. It's simply the belief in something larger than yourself. However spirituality enters your life—whether through attending church or temple, praying, meditating, or walking on the beach—studies suggest that it can help you heal.

Rely on Pet Power

Caring for a pet can go a long way toward increasing your sense of fulfillment in life. A furry or feathery friend can help you:

- **Have fun.** There's nothing like a dog or cat to make you laugh and generally entertain you. In one survey of male pet owners, 52 percent confessed to having sung or danced with their dogs.

- **Feel adored.** Pets can be better than friends in boosting your self-esteem. They are never judgmental and always ready to accept and love you.

- **Have someone to talk to.** Pets can help you avoid feeling lonely, which can harm your health. In a study by the American Animal Hospital Association, 57 percent of pet owners claimed that if stranded on a desert island, they'd prefer the company of their pet to anyone else.

What's Your Dream Job?

Experts say a happy retirement depends not on what you retire from but what you retire to. It's a golden opportunity to involve yourself in more meaningful work or activity, a second career, or a lifelong dream. One popular way many retirees are doing this is by landing a part-time dream job, be it fashion model, baseball usher, tour guide, or park ranger.

When sorting out what you'd really like to do, ask yourself these key questions:

1. When you were a kid, what did you want to do? Do you remember why?
2. What have you wanted to do but never had the time for?
3. If you're thinking of doing a particular job:
- Do you have the physical strength and the right temperament for it over the long term?
- How will it help you be happier?
- Are there any fringe benefits to the job (for example, working outdoors, being productive and appreciated, learning new skills)?

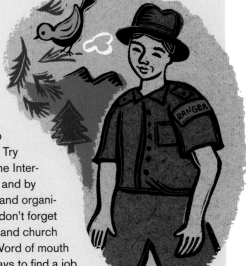

Once you've devised your fantasy job, how do you go about landing it? Try hunting at job fairs, on the Internet, in employment ads, and by networking with people and organizations in the field. And don't forget your friends, neighbors, and church or synagogue groups. Word of mouth is still one of the best ways to find a job.

Managing Your Moods

Worry, anger, and depression are toxic not only to your happiness but also to your immune system and even your heart.

Are you quick to anger? Often anxious or down in the mouth? There's more than your happiness at stake: Scientists have proven that your mood can affect your health.

Beating the Blues

Everyone feels down in the dumps at times. It's perfectly normal and often an appropriate reaction to change. But chronic depression can make you more vulnerable to illness and aggravate such conditions as heart disease and rheumatoid arthritis. Because depression elevates levels of the stress hormone cortisol, which robs bones of calcium, it may also contribute to bone loss, increasing your risk of fractures.

One avenue to staving off depression is maintaining an active social network and staying involved in life. But the fastest way to raise your spirits is to get out and exercise. You'll boost your levels of endorphins, the body's feel-good chemicals. Exercise

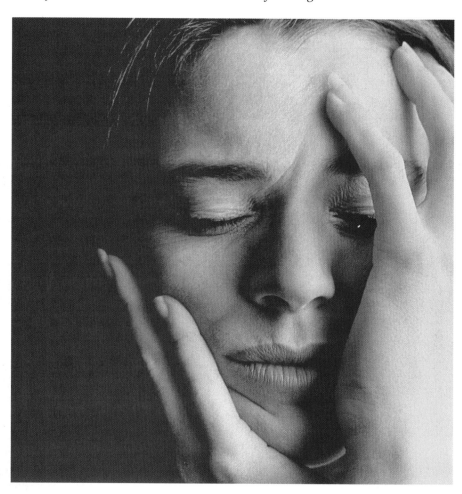

Women are at greater risk for depression than men. People over age 65 are especially susceptible.

can even help prevent depression in the first place. A California study that tracked 1,800 people over 20 years found that those who were physically active at the start of the study were far less likely to report symptoms of depression later on, as were people who took up exercise during the study. People who became sedentary, however, found themselves at higher risk.

Weight lifting is also effective. In one study, people suffering from mild to moderate depression used weight machines three times a week. After 10 weeks, 82 percent no longer showed signs of depression.

If you're interested in natural remedies for the blues, you might consider St. John's wort. This popular herb is prescribed in Germany for depression four times as often as the drug Prozac. In Canada, you can buy it over the counter in drug or health-food stores. (For more information on St. John's wort, turn to page 322.)

If your sad feelings linger for more than two weeks or begin to overwhelm you, talk to your doctor. He may determine that an antidepressant medication is in order. Also seek professional help if you consistently lack energy, feel worthless, take no pleasure in what used to delight you, or experience sleeping problems, significant weight gain or loss, difficulty concentrating or remembering, or persistent thoughts of death or suicide. (See pages 320-323 for more on depression.)

What, Me Worry?

Worrywarts, listen up. A little worrying now and then can be self-protective. Without anxiety you probably wouldn't be compelled to lock your door at night or schedule your regular mammogram. But it's time to lighten up when your apprehensive attitude detracts from your ability to enjoy life.

Too much worrying can lead to a host of problems, such as reduced concentration, poor sleeping habits, and the inability to handle everyday difficulties. What's more, it may also cause physical ills, such as elevated blood pressure.

Before you literally worry yourself sick, try these strategies:

- **See it from a different perspective.** Don't get mired in the details. Talk to yourself about the bigger picture, or imagine what a rational friend would focus on in your situation.
- **Log your worries.** Writing in a worry journal helps create an objective distance between you and your concerns. Jot down your thoughts every day, perhaps first

Fast Fact

Depression isn't "normal" when you get older, but unfortunately it is common. The highest rates for depression in Canada occur among the elderly—ranging from 10 to 15 percent in the community and running as high as 50 percent in nursing homes.

Are You SAD?

If the winter months get you down, you may have what's referred to as seasonal affective disorder (SAD), a mood disorder related to the seasonal ebbing of light. January and February can be particularly difficult, and you may experience low energy, low mood, and weight gain.

If you suffer from SAD, try spending at least an hour a day outdoors, perhaps walking in winter sunlight. If you're unable to get enough daily sunlight, you may be a candidate for at-home phototherapy. This treatment involves sitting in front of an appliance that produces a bright, nonultraviolet light (similar to sunlight) for a few hours each morning. For lasting relief, phototherapy should continue until spring. For more information on SAD, see page 323.

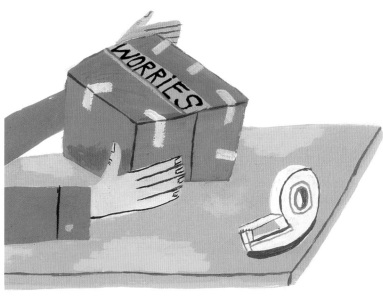

By putting your troubles in temporary storage, you keep them out of sight and out of mind.

thing in the morning before you start your regular routine. Spend about 15 minutes writing and reflecting on what's bothering you.

- **Pack away your worries.** If journal writing isn't for you, create a "worry box" in your mind. Imagine tucking away your anxieties in a small box and closing the lid. Set aside a specific time each day to open the box and examine your worries, but otherwise, resolve to keep it closed.
- **Share your worries with a friend.** Airing your fears helps to lift the burden of worrying and also gives your friends an opportunity to offer comforting thoughts or a dose of reality.
- **Create a personal worry space.** Select a quiet spot in your home where you can focus on your worries without being interrupted. Go there every day for about 10 to 20 minutes. Make sure to maintain a strict time limit, and strive to avoid worrying except when you're in your designated "worry space."
- **Imagine a happily ever after.** See

yourself mastering any difficulty and the problem resolving in the best possible way. Focusing on a happy outcome may even help make it happen. After all, the way we view the future often ends up a self-fulfilling prophecy.

- **Learn how to relax.** Taking a class on stress reduction or meditation can help you slow down those racing thoughts of gloom and doom. Check with your local hospital or community college about programs in your area. Yoga, ballet, and tai chi classes can also help refocus your thoughts.
- **Seek help from a therapist.** If your worries spin out of control continually or if you have exaggerated feelings of distress or apprehension, a therapist or counselor can help you work on ways to regain control.

Taming the Angry Beast

Anger can be a healthy emotion. When you examine and express it constructively, it can lead to personal growth and greater intimacy.

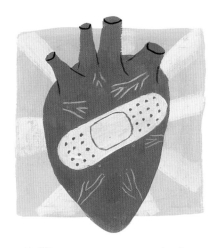

Bottling up your anger can lead to higher levels of homocysteine, a chemical linked to heart disease.

But when you consistently repress it, or when it colors the way you look at life, it can make your life miserable—and possibly lead to serious health problems.

Anger unleashes a flood of artery-damaging stress hormones into your bloodstream, raises your cholesterol levels and heart rate, and suppresses your immune system. Studies repeatedly show links between hostility, repressed anger, and heart disease. A recent study found that both repressing anger and repeated expressions of hostility caused a buildup of homocysteine, a chemical in the blood that's closely associated with heart disease.

Do you recognize hostility in yourself? People who tend to be hostile generally have:

- a cynical mistrust of others (thinking others are too slow, incompetent, stupid, or wrong)
- frequent angry or negative feelings or overreactions to minor events
- aggressive behavior (blowing the horn, yelling, throwing things, and so on).

Researchers have determined that hostile people are more likely to develop life-threatening illness and have a greater chance of premature death than more mild-mannered folks. They are also likely to eat, drink, and smoke more than others.

The issue is not so much anger itself, but the extent to which it permeates your life. The bottom line: If it's chronic, it's dangerous. Does the slightest delay set you off? Do you go berserk in a traffic jam? Do you habitually think others are screwing up? Do you find it hard to forget a slight? These are some of the ways chronic anger can show up. It makes

What to Do with Your Anger

If you are easy to anger and you tend to act out your anger in unproductive ways, put these strategies into practice.

1. Recognize and accept your anger. When you feel angry, be curious about your reaction. Ask yourself:

- What does it do to you physically? (Does it make you clench your jaw? Give you a headache?)
- How do you express it? (Do you become sarcastic? Snap at people? Say hostile, cutting things you later regret?)
- Why did you get so angry? (Was it because your feelings were hurt? Were you frightened? Insulted?)

2. Take responsibility for your anger. Recognize that it's your choice whether or not to become angry. Once you accept responsibility for your feelings, thoughts, and behaviors, you're less likely to react explosively.

3. Talk about your anger. Verbally expressing how you feel is better than acting your anger out and will make you feel more empowered in your personal relationships.

4. Cool off. With time, you may understand what set you off and decide whether action is necessary. If your anger doesn't dissipate or if you find yourself ruminating and getting irritated all over again, try to cool off by:

- counting to 10
- taking deep breaths and focusing on your breathing
- removing yourself physically to a quiet place or going for a walk
- calming yourself by visualizing a serene setting or experience
- meditating
- talking yourself down to a calmer or more positive place
- looking at the event that triggered your anger from another perspective.

5. Learn appropriate ways to express your anger. An anger management program or a therapist can help you learn to defuse your rage. Many times, our inability to deal with anger is tied to unresolved wounds we carry from the past. Discussing your feelings with a professional can help you untangle these emotions.

your life unhappier, of course, but it also alienates the people around you, leaving you isolated.

Learning to acknowledge and express your anger appropriately is the best way to keep it from eating into your life. See *What to Do with Your Anger,* above, for some tips on managing this potentially destructive emotion.

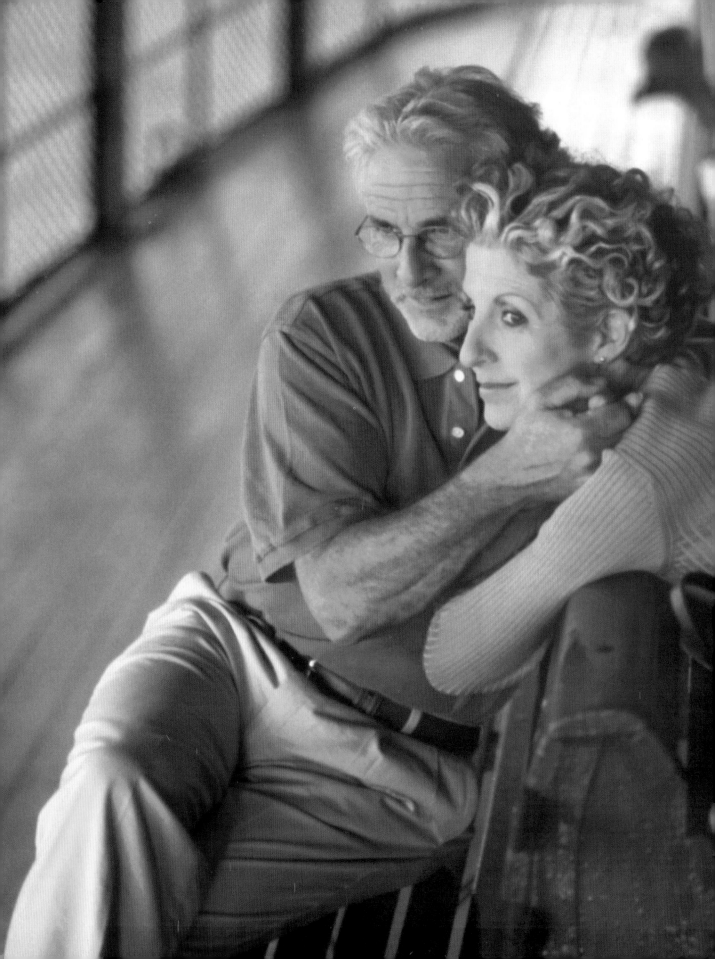

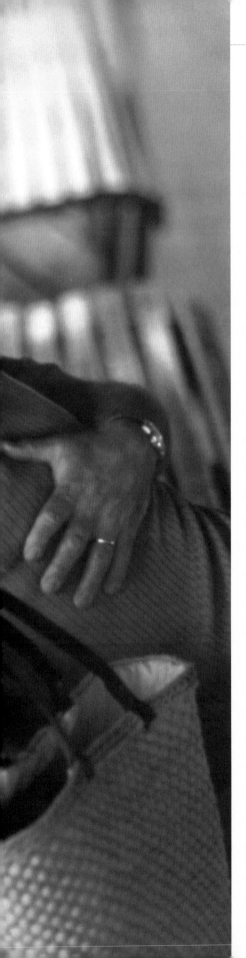

CHAPTER 9

YOUR SEXUAL HEALTH

Better with Age

Judging from the images the popular media put forth, you'd think sex was only for twenty-somethings. Nothing is further from the truth.

If you expect your sex life to dry up over time, you might be in for a surprise. The fact is, many people find that, as the years go by, they enjoy sex more than they ever did before. In a recent telephone survey of men and women age 50 and over, the Association of Reproductive Health Professionals in the U.S. found that two-thirds of those contacted are sexually active and enjoying sex as much as or more than when they were younger. And the 1993 Janus Report on Sexual Behavior, an ambitious study on sex in America, found that men age 51 to 64 had a more active sex life than any other group.

That's good news not only for your relationship but also your health.

Regular sex confers an impressive array of benefits both physical and emotional.

- It's an aerobic exercise that strengthens your heart and lungs.
- It's been shown to boost immune-system function.
- It increases a woman's estrogen production, which can benefit her in a number of ways, such as keeping her hair and skin from drying out and keeping her bones from becoming brittle.
- It may help protect a man from prostate enlargement, since ejaculation empties fluids retained in the prostate gland.
- It's a natural antidepressant because it releases endorphins,

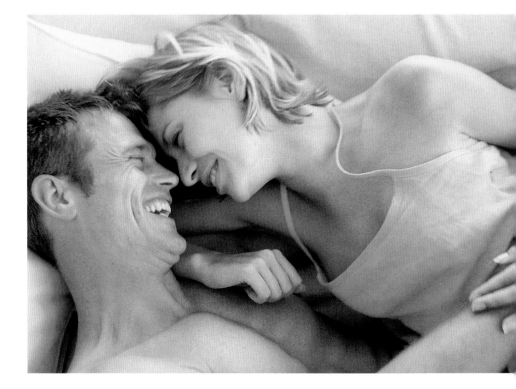

A healthy sexual relationship is key to your partnership and even your health. There are no age limits involved—in fact, many older couples say sex only gets better.

Separating Fact from Fiction

Sex at midlife and beyond is a subject mired in confusion and misinformation. Here are some common myths, and the straight story.

FICTION Beyond a certain age, people have little interest in sex.
FACT There is no age limit on sexuality, but for people age 50 and over, sexual satisfaction depends more on the overall quality of the relationship than it does for younger couples. A National Council on Aging survey in the U.S. reports that among people age 60 and over who have regular intercourse, 74 percent of the men and 70 percent of women find their sex lives more satisfying than when they were in their forties.

FICTION As a man ages, he loses his ability to get an erection.
FACT Aging itself is not a cause of erectile dysfunction. However, diminishing hormone levels do precipitate some changes. A man may need more physical stimulation to become aroused, and his erection may not be quite as firm as when he was younger—but sex is no less pleasurable. While a 25-year-old man might be able to get a second erection as quickly as fifteen minutes after an ejaculation, a 50-year-old man might need several hours.

FICTION Emotional and psychological factors are responsible for a woman's lack of interest in sex at midlife and beyond.
FACT Physical factors can play an even larger role. Hormonal changes at menopause can affect a woman's sexual response. Low estrogen levels can result in vaginal dryness, causing discomfort during sex. And in some women, lower testosterone levels can mean a lack of energy and a weaker sex drive. Other women find their interest in sex increases after menopause, due, in part, to a shift in the ratio of testosterone to estrogen and progesterone.

FICTION A woman loses her ability to have orgasms as she ages.
FACT Many women find increased sexual pleasure after menopause, including more frequent or more intense orgasms.

FICTION Masturbation diminishes your ability to enjoy sex with a partner.
FACT Masturbation can increase sexual pleasure, both with and without a partner. For women, it helps keep vaginal tissues moist and elastic and boosts hormone levels, which fuels sex drive. For men, it helps maintain erectile response.

FICTION A man's inability to get an erection is most likely the result of an emotional problem.
FACT Actually, physical causes—such as circulation problems, prostate disorders, and side effects associated with prescription medications—account for 85 percent of erectile difficulties.

FICTION Couples at midlife and beyond who don't have regular sex have lost interest in sex or in each other.
FACT When older couples don't have regular sex, it's usually because one partner has an illness or disability.

Fast Fact

People who exercise regularly reach orgasm more easily and more often than people who don't.

SimpleSolution

Kegel exercises may increase sexual pleasure and help women achieve orgasm more easily. To do the exercises (developed by a gynecologist to improve bladder control after childbirth), take note of the muscle you use to stop urinary flow, then practice contracting that muscle and gradually releasing it. Work up to 20 contractions three times a day. This exercise can help men, too.

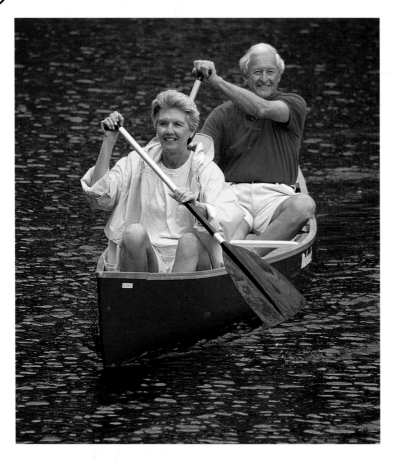

Rediscovering shared interests can add new zest to your relationship both in and out of the bedroom.

brain chemicals that boost mood and reduce the sensation of pain.
- It helps us relax and feel good about ourselves.

When it comes to enjoying an active sex life, your overall health is a more important factor than your age. Common impediments to sexual function, especially for men, are chronic health problems such as high blood pressure, heart disease, and diabetes—and the drugs used to treat them. (What better incentive do you need to eat right and exercise?)

For many women in midlife and beyond, the "partner gap" is a major problem. Researchers have found that only 21 percent of women age 75 and up have a partner, compared with 58 percent of men in the same age bracket.

Change Is in the Air

Of course, sex isn't going to stay exactly the same as you age. But the changes that take place aren't all negative. Once a woman is past menopause and no longer concerned about pregnancy, many couples find it easier to relax and look forward to lovemaking. And partners who are retired or working only part time often have more time and energy for each other, for making love as well as pursuing other shared activities.

By midlife, you know your own body and your partner's intimately, and, hopefully, you've figured out how to communicate what you find pleasurable. It's likely that you've shed any sexual inhibitions, and your sexual confidence and experience probably result in better sex for both of you. Just as important, sex may be more emotionally fulfilling because now it is driven less by hormones and more by the desire to share yourself with someone who loves you. According to the Janus Report, sex after age 65 may take place less often, but respondents reported that it was more gratifying.

Men: Getting in Sync

Starting at midlife, most men notice that getting an erection requires more direct physical stimulation. It also takes longer—which may be a positive change. Since women tend to become aroused more slowly than men, it brings arousal cycles into sync. A slower response also encourages more foreplay, which benefits menopausal or postmenopausal women who may require additional stimulation to achieve sufficient vaginal lubrication.

Recovery time (the time required to achieve another erection after ejaculation, also called the refractory period) increases, but so does the length of time an erection lasts before ejaculation. This can lead to a more leisurely lovemaking style that leaves both partners more satisfied, both physically and emotionally.

Women: Make Yourself Comfortable

During and after menopause, the dramatic decline in estrogen production leads to changes in the body that may make sex uncomfortable, including a loss of elasticity in the vagina and increasing vaginal dryness. An over-the-counter water-based lubricant often solves the problem. If it doesn't, ask your doctor to prescribe a topical estrogen cream that is inserted into the vagina using an applicator, or an estrogen ring, a device about the size of a diaphragm that slips into the vagina and is left in place for three months.

Because your body is changing, what felt pleasurable at one time may no longer feel as nice. For example, since the tissue covering the clitoris shrinks and thins out, direct manual stimulation may feel uncomfortable. Communication is more important now than ever before. Let your partner know what pleases you, and don't be afraid to give pleasure to each other in new ways.

Some menopausal women find that their libido and capacity for arousal and orgasm are diminished. This may be the result of declining testosterone levels (testosterone is the main hormone responsible for sex drive in both men and women). Don't hesitate to discuss the problem with your doctor. If a blood test

confirms that your levels are low, she may prescribe a testosterone supplement. (If you have high cholesterol, you may not be a candidate for testosterone replacement, since this hormone raises cholesterol levels.)

Some women notice that their sex drive actually increases at menopause. That's because estrogen levels decline more dramatically than do levels of testosterone, resulting in a relative increase in testosterone. Women on hormone replacement therapy will not experience this effect, and may actually experience the opposite effect. That's because estrogen affects the proteins that carry testosterone through the bloodstream, making less testosterone available to the body. Your doctor can measure your "free testosterone" to determine if this is a problem.

Returning to Intimacy

It's easy, especially in a long-term relationship, to slip into habits that create emotional distance between you and your partner. Much of your adult life may have been occupied with raising children, cultivating careers, and balancing finances. As these activities plateau, you may find that you don't know how to make the most of the time when you

DRUG CAPSULE

Soon men and women with difficulty achieving an erection or orgasm may be able to remedy the situation with a topical cream that increases blood flow to the genitals. These creams contain alprostadil, a synthetic form of prostaglandin E1, and may be available in the near future.

For women, if lubrication is a problem, your doctor may prescribe a low-dose estrogen cream or vaginal ring to keep vaginal tissues moist and healthy.

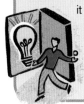

SimpleSolution

Having intercourse regularly helps keep your sex drive in high gear by increasing the production of testosterone in both men and women. In women, it also helps maintain the elasticity of the vagina.

To break out of a rut, break away from the everyday. The "glow" from a special weekend away can linger even after you return.

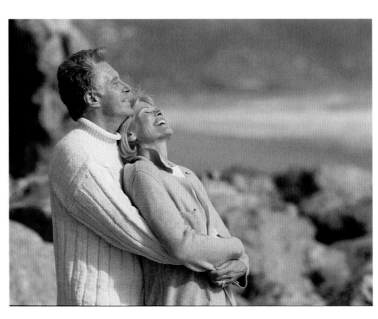

and your partner are alone together. Sex may have become an act rather than an experience, a physical function instead of an emotional connection. Midlife is the ideal opportunity to rediscover each other and the intimacy you once shared.

Of course, intimacy isn't just about sex. It's about sharing yourself with your partner—revealing your hopes and dreams, your worries and fears, your needs and desires. It's about trust, love, and respect. Wild, passionate lovemaking is one way of affirming these feelings. Another way is to snuggle close and enjoy caressing and kissing, even when sex isn't the end result.

Some people find that midlife is a time when long-buried relationship problems surface. For empty nesters and retirees, a change of focus to just the two of you can feel intense. Some relationships buckle under the glare. If your partnership is facing difficulties, consider seeing a marriage counselor to work through your problems. A qualified professional can help you sort out your issues objectively and

> Midlife is the ideal opportunity to rediscover each other and the intimacy you once shared.

develop solutions that meet your needs and your partner's.

Solo Acts

If you are approaching midlife without a partner, you might be thinking about starting a new relationship. For most people, having someone to share life's joys and sorrows is an important dimension of happiness. Just keep in mind that everyone, no matter what their age, is vulnerable to a host of sexually transmitted diseases (STDs), including HIV, the virus that causes AIDS.

Though birth control may no longer be a concern, disease protection is always a priority. Unless you are in a relationship that has been mutually monogamous for several years and both of you are free from STDs, always use latex condoms during sexual intercourse.

Many people, especially women, find themselves without partners later in life. Masturbation is one way to stay connected with your sexuality. In women, it helps keep vaginal tissue healthy. In men, it helps maintain erectile response. Sex toys may enhance your pleasure; mail order and the Internet let you shop from the privacy of your home.

Keeping the Passion in Your Desire

Hormones might be responsible for sex drive, but by nurturing your passion for one another you can be sure to keep desire burning strong. If your sex life has cooled of late, try these tips to help rekindle the flame.

- **Plan your encounters.** Time has a habit of slipping away, becoming filled with activities (even just watching television) you didn't plan. Schedule your amorous adventures so they don't get away from you. Call them dates, if you like. Planning to make love creates anticipation and piques interest. You don't have to go anywhere or do anything special. Set aside an evening, or a morning or an afternoon if your days are free, just for each other.
- **Change your routine.** If you and your partner have been together a long time, chances are you have a fairly established pattern when it comes to making love. The next time you find yourself starting your regular ritual, stop and make a change. It doesn't have to be anything major. Shower together instead of separately, light scented candles, or massage each other with heated body oil. Play music that you heard on your first date. Wear something surprising to bed. Even very small changes can give your love life a new sense of excitement. Or consider a change of venue. For instance, check into a hotel for a romantic getaway.
- **Slow down and enjoy it more.** Even though it's natural for your body to slow down, your brain may still be telling you to move things along at a faster pace. Relax and enjoy the journey. Explore new ways to stimulate your partner outside of intercourse. Take pleasure in both giving and receiving, and let things unfold at their natural pace.
- **Try different positions.** Sometimes health issues make your formerly favorite lovemaking positions uncomfortable or even impossible. If arthritis is a problem, try side-to-side positions, which relieve any need to support yourself or accommodate your partner's weight. Seated positions let you vary the depth of penetration while giving you additional support (especially if you place your back against a wall or the back of a chair). If a man has trouble maintaining an erection, he may want to try lying on top of his partner with his legs outside hers so that she can further stimulate his penis by squeezing her thighs together.
- **Continue your lovemaking over several sessions.** It's great when you have the whole afternoon to indulge in sex, or an evening when you are not tired. But this isn't always the case. Rather than rushing through a "quickie," try breaking off your lovemaking and returning later to pick up where you left off. A man may find that he's enjoyed a lovemaking session giving pleasure to his partner even if he hasn't experienced orgasm himself.
- **Savor the experience.** After lovemaking, delight in the comforts of lying beside each other. Use the time to talk, or simply drift off to sleep together.

Up for some good, clean fun? Put the spark back in lovemaking by changing your routine.

SimpleSolution

A warm bath prior to intercourse can help loosen arthritic joints, making sex more enjoyable. Add a scented bath oil you both enjoy to help set the mood.

Midlife for Women: Managing Menopause

Some women dread "the change" as the end of life as they've known it. Others welcome menopause as the beginning of life as they've dreamed of living it.

Once referred to in whispered tones as "the change of life," menopause does indeed bring about an array of changes. At menopause, a woman's ovaries all but stop producing estrogen. The most obvious result is that she no longer menstruates and is no longer fertile. But there are other implications for long-term health.

At about age 35, a woman's body begins losing calcium. Declining estrogen levels accelerate this loss. During the years leading to menopause, you can lose bone mass at a rate of about 1 percent a year unless you take measures to prevent it. Excessive bone loss results in osteoporosis, a condition in which calcium-depleted bones are weak and susceptible to breaking. Hor-

mone replacement therapy (HRT), calcium and magnesium supplements, and weight-bearing exercise can slow bone loss. Once osteoporosis exists, there are prescription medications that, in combination with exercise and extra calcium intake, can help rebuild bone. (For more on osteoporosis, see page 374.)

The decline in estrogen production also increases your risk for heart disease and stroke. After menopause, a woman's risk of heart attack and stroke rivals that of a man. HRT, regular exercise, and a nutritious diet can help offset these changes.

The Three Stages of Menopause

For women who experience it naturally (not as the result of surgery or other causes), menopause has three distinct stages: perimenopause, menopause, and postmenopause.

1 Perimenopause
Perimenopause, which means "around the end of menstruation," is generally what we think of as the menopause experience. During this time, a woman's ovaries start producing less of the sex hormones estrogen, progesterone, and testosterone. The decline isn't necessarily steady—sometimes hormone levels fluctuate wildly, causing irregular periods. (If you suddenly experience heavy periods, let your doctor know so that she can rule out other causes,

---

What Puts the Hot in Hot Flashes?

Hot flashes, the hallmark of menopause, affect up to 80 percent of women in perimenopause. Like a child playing with a household thermostat, your fluctuating estrogen level confuses your temperature adjustment mechanisms. Your body responds by dilating the blood vessels near the surface of the skin, its usual way of initiating rapid cooling. This may cause flushing or profuse sweating. Because your body isn't really overheated, however, a chill often follows the hot flash. Some menopausal women experience this cycle of what doctors call vasomotor instability only occasionally, or not at all, while for others it is a constant companion. HRT generally eliminates or greatly reduces hot flashes. Without HRT, hot flashes disappear after menopause in most women, when estrogen levels stabilize.

When you have a hot flash, note what you ate or drank beforehand. Potential food triggers include caffeine, alcohol, chocolate, hard cheeses, red wine, tomatoes, chili peppers, and citrus fruits.

such as fibroid tumors and endometrial cancer.) Symptoms such as hot flashes, insomnia, and forgetfulness are at their peak. The tissues of the vagina and urinary tract may become dry and atrophied, possibly making sex uncomfortable and making urinary tract infections more common. During this time it is still possible for a woman to become pregnant.

If you're not sure whether you're in perimenopause, your doctor can order blood tests to measure your hormone levels. Consistently high levels of follicle stimulating hormone (FSH) and low levels of estradiol (the most common form of estrogen), combined with some of the symptoms above, provide compelling evidence.

Women may benefit from beginning hormone replacement therapy (HRT) at this stage. (See page 232 for information on HRT.) Alternatively, your doctor may prescribe low-dose birth control pills as a form of HRT. Advantage: better control of the menstrual cycle. Taking either birth control pills or HRT, however, can make it more difficult to determine when menopause has occurred.

While women can enter natural menopause at any time during their forties or fifties, the average age of menopause in the Western world is 51. Perimenopause begins on average at age 47 and lasts anywhere from 2 to 10 years. Contrary to popular belief, there is no relationship between the age at which a woman started menstruating and the age at which she enters menopause. Chances are, you'll go through menopause at about the same age as your mother and grandmother did. Women who smoke typically enter menopause two to three years earlier than those who don't.

Signs of Menopause

During menopause and the years leading up to it, you may experience some of the following changes. Most are due, directly or indirectly, to fluctuating hormone levels and the decline in estrogen production. Urinary incontinence is caused by a thinning of the vaginal walls and muscles, which support and control the bladder. Many of these changes, such as hot flashes and mood swings, are temporary. Others, such as changes in your skin and vaginal tissue, are permanent unless you undergo estrogen replacement therapy.

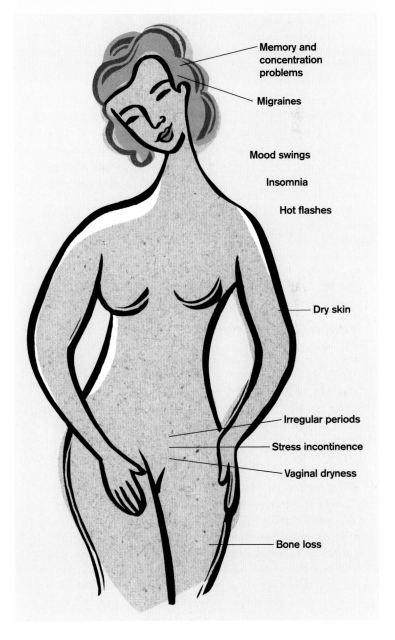

- Memory and concentration problems
- Migraines
- Mood swings
- Insomnia
- Hot flashes
- Dry skin
- Irregular periods
- Stress incontinence
- Vaginal dryness
- Bone loss

SELF TEST

Is It Menopause?

It's not always easy to know whether you're going through peri-menopause, that phase leading up to your last menstrual period. Ask yourself these questions:

◄ **Do you have abnormally heavy periods?** Excessive bleeding is common in women who are nearing menopause, but it may also be caused by uterine fibroids (benign tumors), so check with your doctor.

◄ **Are your periods irregular?** Menstrual irregularity is a hallmark of perimenopause.

◄ **Have you gained weight recently?** Most women put on a little extra weight with the approach of menopause.

◄ **Are you experiencing hot flashes?** These moment- to hour-long episodes of feeling uncomfortably warm, sometimes with skin flushing and perspiration, occur in 45 to 80 percent of perimenopausal women in Western countries. Note, however, that abnormal sensations of heat also occur in hyperthyroidism, a condition that affects some middle-aged women.

◄ **Are you troubled by irritability, poor concentration, mood swings, or forgetfulness?** About two-thirds of perimenopausal women in a recent study reported "sometimes" or "often" experiencing these symptoms. They are especially common among women who have a history of depression.

2 Menopause
In literal terms, menopause is a single, isolated event in a woman's life: her last menstrual period. Of course, you can't know when your last period took place until no others follow, so this is a retrospective determination. Doctors consider that menopause has occurred once you have gone 12 consecutive months without a period.

3 Postmenopause
The period from menopause through the rest of a woman's life is called postmenopause ("after the end of menstruation"). Once upon a time, when living to age 55 was a rarity, this was the beginning of the end. With life expectancy now extending beyond the eighties and even into the nineties, women today may enjoy nearly as many years of life after menopause as before it.

Women continue to face an increased risk of heart disease, stroke, and osteoporosis during postmenopause. For this reason, many doctors recommend HRT following menopause and encourage women to engage in lifestyle behaviors that reduce their risks. These include supplementing with calcium, magnesium, and vitamin D; eating a nutritious, low-fat diet; and getting regular, moderately strenuous exercise. (For more on HRT, see page 232.)

When Menopause Is Early

Menopause arrives early for some women. Here are some common reasons:

● **Surgery.** A woman who has had her ovaries removed, either independently or as part of a total hysterectomy, experiences immediate menopause. Other types of abdominal surgery can interrupt the flow of blood to the ovaries, causing follicles to die.

● **Premature ovarian failure.** Women who enter menopause while they're in their thirties or even twenties may have illnesses that cause their ovaries to stop functioning well ahead of schedule. A thorough medical evaluation is appropriate.

● **Polycystic ovary syndrome (PCOS).** This medical condition interferes with ovulation, causing inflammation and scarring that damages and destroys follicles.

● **Autoimmune disorders.** These include insulin-dependent diabetes, hypothyroidism, rheumatoid arthritis, and lupus.

● **Cancer treatments.** Chemotherapy and radiation therapy often trigger early menopause. Women taking tamoxifen to reduce their risk of breast cancer may also enter menopause early.

Menopause and Your Brain

Your ovaries and uterus aren't the only organs in transition as you go through menopause. Because of declining estrogen levels, your brain experiences a number of chemical changes that can alter the way you think and feel.

Early evidence suggests that decreased estrogen levels may alter how the brain encodes and retrieves data. Researchers using magnetic resonance imaging (MRI) have discovered, for instance, that menopausal women who don't take estrogen may experience less activation of the left brain during the encoding of information. Perhaps that's why some women reportedly have trouble with rational or analytical "left-brained" thought processes such as those involved in balancing a checkbook or making decisions. Marian Van Eyk McCain, in *Transformation Through Menopause,* calls this effect "cottonhead." If indeed it exists, it seems to be temporary. And studies show that estrogen replacement may reverse it.

Scientists are only beginning to understand the complex effects of estrogen on the brain. In animals, the hormone has been shown to stimulate the growth of dendrites, hairlike projections that facilitate communication between neurons (brain cells). It also seems to boost levels of the neurotransmitter acetylcholine. And it appears to help protect neurons in certain areas of the brain—especially the hippocampus, a region critical to learning and memory—from damage that leads to cell death. The possibility that estrogen may delay or possibly even prevent the onset of Alzheimer's disease is currently being investigated. So far, studies have yielded mixed results.

The Memory Connection

Can't remember where you left the car keys or why you walked into the kitchen? Some women notice temporary lapses in short-term memory as they approach menopause, and it's possible that shifting estrogen levels may be partly to blame.

Researchers have discovered that areas in the brain involved in memory are estrogen-sensitive. And women taking estrogen show more activity in brain areas associated with memory. Some studies have shown that women taking estrogen performed better on memory tests than those not taking the hormone. But other studies have failed to confirm these results. Regardless, the majority of women may not experience any memory problems as they go through menopause.

Menopause and Mood

What about mood swings? Some women experience them, probably the result of fluctuating hormone levels. But, contrary to popular belief, women do not suffer an increased risk of depression during this period. In fact, research shows that menopausal women actually have a lower incidence of depression than younger women.

Estrogen seems to affect how thoughts are processed. Lower levels, combined with changes associated with aging, may mean less analytical ("left-brained") thinking and more creative ("right-brained") thinking.

HRT and Other Options

HRT—or maybe a natural alternative? It's a personal decision to make after you've reviewed the pros and cons and discussed your long-term health risks with your doctor.

Hormone replacement therapy, or HRT, replaces the estrogen (and if you still have your uterus, the progesterone) that your body no longer produces. Though a number of hormones play a role in menopause, it's estrogen that causes the unpleasant symptoms many women experience. HRT greatly reduces or eliminates many of these discomforts in most women. It may also lower the risk for long-term health problems such as osteoporosis and heart disease, though studies have yet to identify the direct correlation, and the benefits stop if you stop taking it.

While HRT is not for everyone, your doctor might suggest it if:

- Frequent hot flashes interfere with your sleep or interrupt your regular daily activities.
- You are at increased risk for osteoporosis (see page 375).
- Vaginal dryness and tissue changes make sex uncomfortable.
- You are troubled by other menopausal symptoms, such as mood swings, irritability, urinary incontinence, or frequent urinary tract infections.

HRT generally is not appropriate for women with a history of:

- Cancer of the breast or endometrium (uterine lining), in yourself or in immediate family members such as your mother or sisters.
- Blood clots or a clotting disorder.
- Liver problems.

The decision to undergo HRT is a highly personal one, made with your doctor after exploring your options and considering your health status and medical history. After careful consideration, you and your doctor may decide that the benefits of HRT significantly outweigh the risks.

The Benefits

In the short term, HRT provides dramatic relief from the discomforts of menopause, especially hot flashes, vaginal dryness and irritation, and mood swings. Most doctors also believe HRT offers protection against osteoporosis and heart disease, though some studies show conflicting results. Harvard University's ongoing Nurses' Health Study and the National Institutes of Health's Women's Health Initiative are two of the most comprehensive studies of the effects of HRT on women who are primarily in good health. These and other studies provide strong and consistent evidence that estrogen replacement, in combination with calcium, slows and often stops bone loss, significantly lowering the risk of osteoporosis.

Findings are less conclusive regarding estrogen's role in protecting against heart disease. While there seems to be a relationship between estrogen and heart disease, researchers don't fully understand it. Heart disease is uncommon in women under age 50 who are menstruating, but it

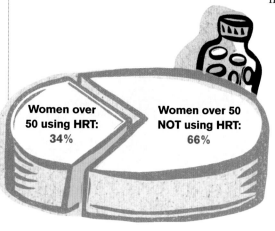

Women over 50 using HRT: 34%

Women over 50 NOT using HRT: 66%

is the leading killer of women over age 50. The difference is thought to be estrogen, which appears to lower blood cholesterol levels.

Women undergoing HRT have a lower incidence of heart disease, but whether or not HRT is the reason has yet to be determined. (Perhaps women on HRT simply take better care of their health in general.) Scientists were surprised by early findings of the Women's Health Initiative, which indicated that women on HRT actually experience a small increase in heart attacks, strokes, and blood clots in the lungs. Final results are not expected until at least 2005. One thing is clear: Estrogen does not seem to provide heart benefits for women who already have heart disease.

Other ongoing studies are looking at estrogen's role in lowering the risk for Alzheimer's disease and Parkinson's disease.

DRUG CAPSULE

Evidence from small studies suggests that antidepressants such as Paxil and Prozac may help relieve hot flashes.

HRT Options

There are several ways to undergo HRT. You may use one form of HRT, such as taking estrogen and progestin in pill form, or a combination of forms, such as an estrogen patch and progestin pills. The regimen depends on your symptoms, your health risk factors, and personal preferences.

FORM OF HRT	COMMENTS
Estrogen pills alone	▥ Appropriate only for women who have had their uterus removed.
Cyclic therapy: estrogen pills, with progestin added for the second 10 to 14 days of the month	▥ Mimics the menstrual cycle. Possible side effects: breast tenderness, bloating, and some bleeding when progestin is stopped.
Combined continuous therapy: estrogen and progestin taken daily	▥ Lower dose of progestin (because it is taken more often) may minimize breast tenderness. May cause irregular bleeding.
The patch: available with estrogen alone (you also need to take progestin in pill form) or as a combo patch that releases both estrogen and progestin	▥ Placed on the lower trunk and changed every three or four days. Lower dose, so fewer side effects. Patches are better than pills if you are at risk for gallstones (see page 338). Appears to protect bones and minimize hot flashes and vaginal dryness as effectively as oral estrogen does. The adhesive may cause skin irritation; if it does, try a different brand.
Gels	▥ Similar to the patch but without skin reactions.
Estrogen vaginal creams	▥ Helpful only for vaginal dryness and atrophy and to reduce the risk of urinary tract infections. Some estrogen may enter the bloodstream, so depending on the dose, you may need to take progestin pills to offset an increased risk of endometrial cancer.
Natural estrogens (estriol, estradiol, estrone): available in cream or pill form	▥ Some people believe these are safer than synthetic estrogen because they are weaker, but hard scientific evidence of their efficacy is scant. Researchers don't know whether natural estrogens alone, without progestin, may increase the risk of uterine cancer.
"Natural" progesterone: available in cream or pill form (not approved for sale in Canada)	▥ Natural progesterone is less likely to cause the side effects, such as breast tenderness and bloating, that synthetic progesterone can cause. No data exists on its effects on the endometrium or bones.

The Risks

The main drawback to HRT is its link to certain kinds of breast cancer. Estrogen seems to fuel growth in breast cancer cells. Health experts disagree on whether the estrogen used in HRT has the same effect as the estrogen your body produces. Most doctors do agree, however, that women who've had breast cancer or have a strong family history of the disease should forgo HRT. Long-term estrogen replacement (more than 10 years) can raise your breast cancer risk by as much as 30 percent. Short-term HRT (up to 5 years) is not associated with increased risk.

This 30 percent increase should be put in context. Among women age 60 to 65 who don't take HRT, 3 in 1,000 develop breast cancer. Among those in the same age group who take estrogen alone for 5 years, 4 in 1,000 develop breast cancer. This is still a very small risk, one that must be measured against the cardiovascular benefits of HRT. Remember that heart disease kills about 11 times more women each year than breast cancer.

Until recently, researchers believed that adding progestin to estrogen treatment counteracted the increase in breast cancer risk. But surprising research published in 2000 indicated that, in thin women, the combined therapy may actually elevate risk further. Adding progestin still is important because it helps guard against endometrial cancer.

The confusion doesn't end there. Some studies suggest that estrogen replacement increases the risk of blood clots. Others show no increase or even a reduced risk. Most doctors recommend against HRT if you have a personal or family history of blood clots or clotting disorders.

Clearly, researchers are still sorting out the effects of HRT, so it's important to discuss your options with your doctor and reevaluate your decision as new information becomes available. Meanwhile, be sure to perform monthly breast self-exams and schedule regular mammograms.

The Now-and-Later Approach

Some women go on HRT as they go through menopause because their symptoms are bothersome, then stop for a decade or so if they're at low risk for osteoporosis and heart disease. At age 60 or so, they might reconsider HRT for its protection against these diseases.

Some opt instead to take the drug raloxifene (Evista), a selective estrogen replacement modulator (SERM) that seems to confer many of estrogen's long-term health benefits without the increased breast cancer risk. However, raloxifene is a new drug, and no long-term data exist. Also, it may increase hot flashes. If osteoporosis is your main concern, your doctor might prescribe a nonhormonal drug called alendronate (Fosamax) to enhance bone density.

Adjusting to HRT

In the beginning, HRT may cause side effects such as breast tenderness, weight gain, and uterine bleeding, most of which disappear within six months to a year. If they still trouble you, your doctor can adjust the dose, type, or schedule of your medication. Estrogen seems to increase migraines in some women, though in others it lessens their frequency and severity.

DRUG CAPSULE

If you don't want to take HRT, you may want to try an estrogen cream or vaginal ring for vaginal dryness and for protection against urinary tract infections. Estrogen in this form does not guard against heart disease, osteoporosis, or hot flashes, however.

Natural Alternatives for Menopause Relief

ALTERNATIVE	HOW IT HELPS	COMMENTS
Soy	■ Soy contains isoflavones, plant compounds that act like a weak form of estrogen and may ease mild menopausal symptoms. They also appear to lower cholesterol and reduce bone loss. Aim to get 30 to 50 mg isoflavones from food daily. Different soy foods contain different amounts, so check the label. Roasted soy beans, tofu, and soy milk are three ways to eat soy. (For tips on adding more soy to your diet, see page 50.)	■ Studies have yielded mixed results on whether or not soy works. The only way to know for sure is to try it yourself. Scientists don't know whether very high doses might increase the risk of breast cancer, just as estrogen does. Isoflavone supplements are not recommended at this time.
Flaxseed	■ Flaxseeds are another source of plant estrogens. Grind some in a spice grinder and add 1 to 2 tablespoons to cereal and other foods.	
Black Cohosh	■ This traditional Native North American remedy contains plant hormones, and it has been shown to be helpful in relieving symptoms such as hot flashes, bloating, depression, insomnia, and vaginal dryness. Take 40 mg of dried rhizome and root a day, or look for a standardized extract containing 1 percent 27-deoxyaceteine and take 8 mg a day.	■ Don't take if you are having heavy periods, since it may increase menstrual flow. Don't confuse black cohosh root with blue cohosh, a potentially dangerous herb.
Chasteberry	■ Also known as chaste tree berry and vitex, this herb is widely used in Europe for the relief of menopausal symptoms. It helps restore progesterone levels, which plummet during menopause. Take 30 to 40 mg once a day.	
Vitamin E	■ Some women find that high doses help relieve hot flashes, night sweats, and vaginal dryness. Try taking 400 IU once or twice a day. Vitamin E may also protect against heart disease, although studies have yielded conflicting results.	■ Check with your doctor before taking more than 400 IU vitamin E a day. Higher doses are contraindicated for people with diabetes and certain other medical conditions.
St. John's Wort	■ This herb may combat mild depression and insomnia. Try taking 200 to 300 mg of standardized extract containing 0.3 percent hypericin three times a day.	■ This herb can take four weeks to become effective. Do not take it along with other antidepressants (see warnings on page 105).
Acupuncture	■ A Swedish study reports that acupuncture helps ease insomnia and hot flashes. Some women agree.	
Exercise	■ Studies show that one to three hours of exercise a week can significantly reduce hot flashes. Weight-bearing exercise such as walking and weight lifting help prevent osteoporosis, and aerobic exercise helps guard against heart disease.	

Midlife for Men: A Change of Pace

Slowing down?
Don't worry.
A leisurely pace
can lead to more
creativity, which
can take love-
making to a
whole new level.

There's no such thing as "male menopause," since menopause means the end of menstruation, and men don't menstruate. But that doesn't mean men's bodies don't change at midlife.

One of the biggest changes is the decline in available, or "free," testosterone. The body continues to produce nearly the same amount of testosterone, but in older men, a protein may lock onto the hormone, reducing the amount available to the body. Testosterone levels peak when a man is in his late teens and early twenties. At age 50, you have about 75 percent of the free testosterone you had at age 25. By age 75, you have half. For most men, this is still more than enough to maintain enjoyable sexual function, though response and recovery times are slower.

Other changes occur that can impede your ability to get an erection. Your blood vessels lose elasticity, so they don't respond as quickly to demands for increased blood flow. Blood vessels can also become clogged with fatty deposits that limit the amount of blood that can pass through them (another excellent reason to stick with a low-fat diet).

Many of the changes take place so gradually they seem to sneak up on you. One night you start making love and it dawns on you that while your mind is ready, your body seems to be waiting for a special invitation. Actually, your body may be inviting you to take your time and build sexual tension more gradually. Consider it a chance to find alternate routes to a familiar destination—and enjoy the scenery along the way.

Testosterone Peaks and Valleys

Men experience a gradual decline in available testosterone from about age 45 to age 70, when a marked drop occurs. That doesn't mean your sex life has to stall. The best predictor of an active sex life after age 60 is an active sex life in your younger years.

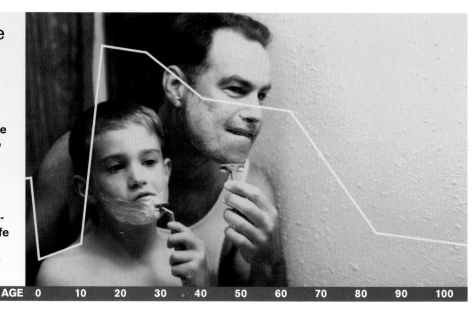

| AGE | 0 | 10 | 20 | 30 | 40 | 50 | 60 | 70 | 80 | 90 | 100 |

Erectile Problems

For some men, the problem isn't that their erections aren't what they used to be, it's that they find it difficult to get or maintain an erection at all. Until recently, many doctors considered erectile dysfunction to be more in the mind than in the body. But now doctors know that physical problems cause 85 percent of erectile difficulties. Common culprits include arteriosclerosis (hardening of the arteries, which restricts blood flow to the penis), diabetes (which can damage blood vessels and nerves involved in erections), and high blood pressure—or the drugs used to treat these problems. Spinal cord injuries, strokes, surgery or injury to the pelvic area, and groin injuries that damage the penis or testicles can also interfere with erectile response.

Emotional factors can complicate the situation. It's natural to feel distressed when you want to perform and your body refuses. Unfortunately, stress just makes matters worse. So try to relax, and, most important, keep the lines of communication open between you and your partner.

The Viagra Factor

When these little blue pills hit the market in the U.S. in 1998, millions of men couldn't wait to give them a try. In fact, doctors wrote more than 16 million prescriptions for them in their first two years on the market.

For once, the hype was accurate. Sildenafil citrate, better known by its brand name, Viagra, improves erectile function for 80 percent of the men who use it. It works by suppressing an enzyme produced in the penis that breaks down nitric oxide, which is required for an erection. Viagra requires between 30 and 60 minutes to take effect, and physical stimulation is still required to get an erection, which can last 45 minutes to an hour.

Viagra is not perfect. Like any drug, it has side effects, which can include headaches, diarrhea, flushing, and tinted vision. Men who take heart medication that contains nitrates are not candidates for Viagra, since the drug combination can cause a sudden and dangerous—even fatal—drop in blood pressure. Viagra has not been shown to improve erections in men who are not impotent.

Another impotence drug, apomorphine (Uprima), may soon be approved in the U.S. by the FDA. It works by increasing the levels of the brain chemical dopamine in an area of the brain thought to be important to erections. Since its mechanism is different from that of Viagra, this drug may prove to be beneficial for men who have found Viagra ineffective. And unlike Viagra, it's safe for men who take nitrate drugs.

Uprima comes in a tablet that's placed under the tongue and is absorbed into the bloodstream. It produces an erection within minutes. But this drug, like any other, has side effects. They include nausea, vomiting, and dangerously low blood pressure that can lead to fainting.

Other Treatments for Erectile Problems

One of the newest and most promising treatments for erectile dysfunction is a drug called alprostadil. It's a synthetic form of prostaglandin E1, a hormone that causes the smooth muscle tissue in the penis to relax,

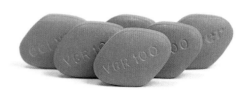

Due to Viagra's instant success, pharmaceutical companies are in a heated race to develop a Viagra-like remedy for female sexual dysfunction.

Fast Fact

An estimated 3 million Canadian men are affected by erectile dysfunction.

Sex and Heart Attacks

For most people, even those who have had heart attacks or coronary artery bypass surgery, sex that culminates in orgasm places no more stress on your heart than climbing a flight or two of stairs without resting. Statistics show that fewer than 1 percent of heart attack deaths occur during or following sex, and those often involve extramarital sex and alcohol consumption. Heart specialists believe it's a combination of stress (fear of getting caught) and elevated blood pressure (from the alcohol) that puts the fatal strain on the heart, not the act of sex. If you've recently had a heart attack, follow your doctor's advice. Most people can resume sexual activity in 12 to 16 weeks.

allowing the increased blood flow that causes an erection. You can inject alprostadil directly into the muscles of the penis with a very fine needle, or use a disposable applicator to insert it, like a suppository, into the urethral opening. Erections occur within 15 minutes. The drug should not be used more than three times a week. Other treatment options include suction devices, implanted pumps, and surgery to repair damaged blood vessels.

Testosterone: Worth a Try?

If hormone replacement therapy works for women, can it help men? A number of studies have looked at testosterone replacement therapy (TRT) as a way to offset the natural decline in blood levels of available testosterone that occurs in a man's body as he ages. Although the decline doesn't interfere with normal sexual functioning in most men, it can cause a slower sexual response and contribute to diminished sex drive, lack of energy, and even hot

New on the market is a clear gel that delivers a measured dose of testosterone through the skin.

flashes similar to those women experience during menopause.

Doctors may prescribe testosterone injections or skin patches for the small percentage of men who experience a severe decline in the hormone. But replacement therapy should be approached with caution because it may aggravate benign prostatic hypertrophy, or enlarged prostate (see *Protecting Your Prostate,* next page). There is also some suspicion that TRT may increase the risk of prostate cancer, although long-term studies are needed before doctors can be sure. If you take TRT, your doctor should monitor you closely for signs of the disease.

Natural Approaches

There are also several nondrug options that are worth a try.

● **Go for ginkgo biloba.** It may offer a natural remedy for men with mild erectile difficulties. The herb appears to improve circulation by relaxing blood vessels, helping more blood reach the penis. If you are taking aspirin or prescription blood thinners (such as

DRUG CAPSULE

More than 200 medications can cause erectile difficulties. The main culprits are the drugs used to treat high blood pressure, heart disease, depression, allergies, and gastric distress. Changing the drug, dosage, or timing of your medication can help, so talk with your doctor.

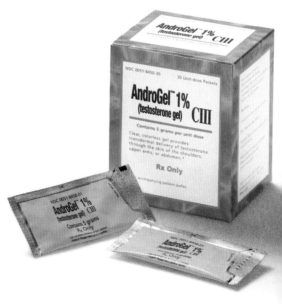

Coumadin), be aware that ginkgo can increase their effects, so check with your doctor before taking it.

- **Get enough zinc.** Adequate intake of this mineral is important to the production of testosterone. Foods rich in zinc include yogurt, fortified cereals, wheat germ, nuts and seeds, shellfish, and poultry.

- **Try losing weight.** According to a recent study, men with a 42-inch waistline were nearly twice as likely to have erectile dysfunction as those with a 32-inch waist.

- **Give up cigarettes.** Smoking damages blood vessels, including the tiny capillaries in your penis. This can make it difficult to achieve and maintain an erection.

Protecting Your Prostate

Nestled deep in your pelvis at the base of your bladder is a chestnut-size gland called the prostate. It is vital for proper bladder operation and control of urine flow, but its primary role is to make semen and then propel it through the penis.

For reasons no one fully understands, the prostate begins to enlarge as you enter your fifties and sixties. As it gets bigger, it presses against the urethra, the tube that transports urine out of the bladder. The bladder wall compensates by pressing out harder, creating an urge to urinate more frequently, even when there is very little urine stored. The condition, called benign prostatic hypertrophy or hyperplasia (BPH), is often left untreated if it's not causing symptoms. BPH does not lead to prostate cancer and does not interfere with sexual function.

Some men, however, do experience symptoms, which can include a

The herb saw palmetto has proven remarkably effective against symptoms of prostate enlargement.

sudden, urgent need to urinate, especially at night; a weak urine stream; or difficulty starting to urinate. Over time, bladder strain can cause bladder or kidney damage, bladder stones, and incontinence.

Several medications are available to treat BPH. However, some of them inhibit testosterone production, which can diminish sexual desire and interfere with erections. Your doctor can adjust your medication if you experience these side effects.

A popular natural alternative is the herb saw palmetto, which has been shown to significantly relieve symptoms of mild to moderate BPH, although it won't shrink the prostate. Take 160 mg of the herb twice a day between meals. Saw palmetto can be taken safely on a long-term basis. Other natural approaches include flaxseeds or flaxseed oil, which help prevent the swelling of the prostate, and pumpkin seeds, rich in zinc, a mineral shown to reduce the size of the gland and help relieve symptoms. Avoid decongestants and spicy or acidic foods, which may make symptoms worse.

If you think you have BPH, see a doctor to rule out prostatitis (inflammation of the prostate), a more serious condition often caused by an infection and accompanied by low back pain, burning during urination, fever, joint and muscle aches, and pain within the pelvis or scrotum.

Fast Fact

Nine out of ten men who live into their seventies and beyond can expect to develop some type of prostate problem.

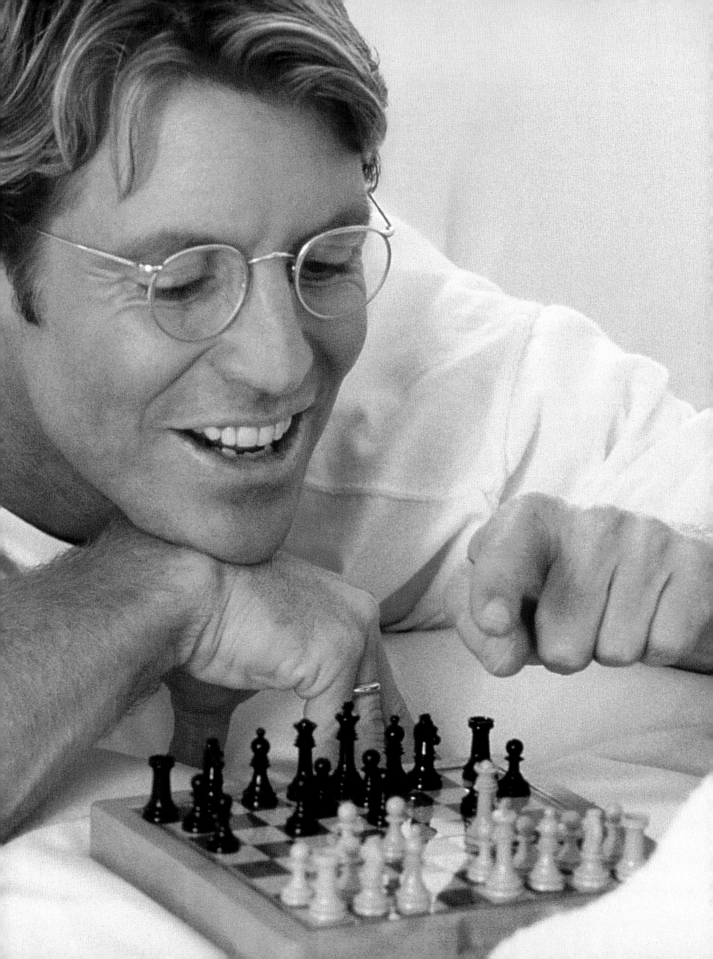

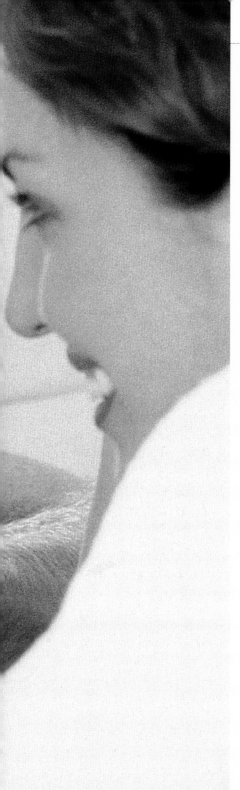

CHAPTER 10

MAINTAINING YOUR MEMORY

YOUR GAME PLAN FOR GOOD HEALTH

The Brain Drain Myth

The truth is, mental decline in old age is greatly exaggerated—and there's no age limit to learning new things.

Worried that your failing memory may be a sign of aging—or worse?

Relax. You don't have to panic every time you forget a name or misplace your keys. Yes, some mental processes do slow down a bit in the course of normal aging. But changes in memory are generally mild and rarely impair your ability to function well on a day-to-day basis. What's more, lifestyle and attitude can go a long way toward preserving memory. And it's never too late—or too early—to start building your defenses. Consider these findings, culled from the MacArthur Foundation Study on Aging in America:

● **Learning makes a difference.** The better educated you are—and the more you continue to keep learning new things—the greater the likelihood you'll maintain high cognitive functioning. Scientists aren't exactly sure why. Perhaps

it's because education early in life has a positive effect on brain circuitry, or simply because educated people are more likely to pursue intellectual hobbies that challenge the brain. One thing is certain: Aging doesn't diminish your ability to make new mental connections, absorb new information, and acquire new skills. Need proof? Just think of all the technology that older people have mastered that didn't even exist a few years ago, such as the automatic teller machine (ATM) and now the Internet.

● **Physical fitness is one road to brain power.** If you want to keep a sharp mental edge, you need to stay physically fit and maintain good lung function. Exercise supplies the brain with oxygen. It may also boost levels of a chemical substance called nerve growth factor that promotes the growth of new brain cells—something scientists long thought impossible.

● **A stimulated brain doesn't deteriorate.** You're much more likely to stay mentally sharp if you believe in your ability to solve problems, meet challenges, and influence events—and put yourself to the test every day. Many people find their job is their prime source of mental stimulation, providing opportunities to take initiative, form judgments, and make decisions. That's one reason why people who go straight from a fulfilling career to an easy chair may experience a sharp decline in

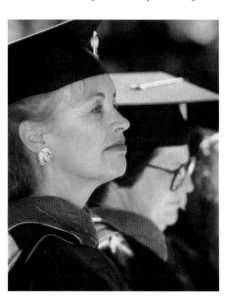

Flex your mental muscle: Continuing your education—either formally or informally—helps keep your faculties in top form.

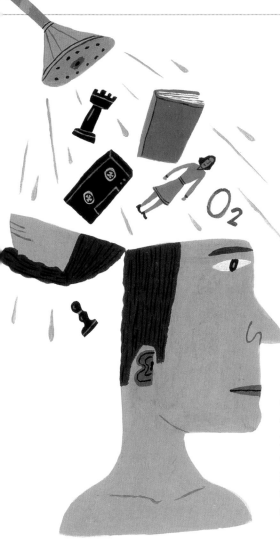

A shower of stimulation feeds the brain, forcing its neural pathways to continue to grow. So take up the chess challenge or crack open a classic.

random words from a long list could recall 15 after completing some memory training. In another study, people who seemed to be losing their ability to decipher directions or move logically from point A to point B improved significantly—and permanently—after taking just five "how-to" sessions. In fact, they did better than young people who hadn't received any training.

Forget All Those Memory Myths

The MacArthur Foundation studies have overturned much of the standard thinking on how aging affects memory and brain power. Many of the findings have provided jumping-off points for further research.

Myth 1:
Memory simply gets worse as you get older.
Not necessarily. Age-related cognitive changes may be fewer and less

cognitive function. On the other hand, if you're retiring from a job that centered on monotonous, repetitive tasks, retirement can be a time of tremendous mental growth. The key is to maintain a can-do attitude and pack your days with activities that demand initiative, flexibility, and problem-solving ability. It doesn't matter whether you're getting paid for the work. Plunge into mind-challenging volunteer activities, or become a student again.

● **You can train your brain.** Memory-building exercises really work. In one study, older people who initially struggled to recall 5

You're Not Too Old to Learn

Some mental processes do slow down a bit in the course of normal aging. About a third of older people have some difficulty with retrieval—the ability to spontaneously recall the names of people, places, and things (that "tip of the tongue" phenomenon)—an area where memory training can make a real difference. But in terms of learning new skills and information, older people are at no disadvantage. Research conducted by the Dana Alliance for Brain Initiatives in the U.S. showed that aging does not affect the amount of material you can absorb in a given period. And once you've learned it, you'll probably retain it as well as a younger person.

Information Superhighway

Neurons—nerve cells in the brain—send, receive, and store the signals that add up to information. They are connected by hairlike filaments called dendrites, which receive and process information from adjacent neurons. The information passes across gaps called synapses. If synapses aren't activated regularly, dendrites atrophy, reducing the capacity to learn and recall information from memory.

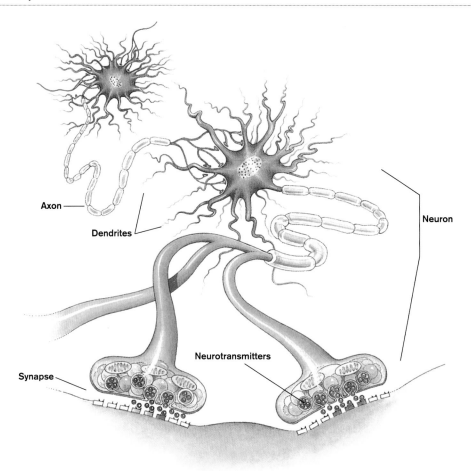

Axon

Dendrites

Neuron

Neurotransmitters

Synapse

SimpleSolution

To stay in mental shape, keep working. A Japanese study of 80-year-olds found that employment enhanced mental agility.

Those who worked a normal day had sharper minds than their contemporaries who had retired at 60. And brain function was improved even among employees who worked just one hour a day.

pronounced than previously thought. Recent research shows that older adults can perform as well as younger people on most mental tasks. One MacArthur investigation followed a large group of individuals for 28 years to track changes in mental fitness, including their ability to:

- use words and numbers accurately
- see relationships between different shapes
- draw appropriate conclusions from a given set of facts.

In the oldest group, ages 74 to 81, at least half of the participants showed no signs of mental decline in these functional areas. This finding is supported by a 1995 study of 65,000 older men and women, in which scientists at England's Manchester University reported that IQ slips by at most 5 percent between the ages of 50 and 80.

Myth 2:
Brain cells flake away at the rate of 50,000 a day, explaining age-related mental decline.

Scientists believe that brain mass shrinks about 10 percent during your lifetime, but this doesn't necessarily lead to diminished brain power. It seems that the complexity and strength of the brain's circuitry is more significant than brain size.

Researchers now believe that most mental decline is a result not of shrinking nerve cells (called neurons) but reduced density in the dendrites, hairlike filaments that branch out from the ends of neurons and receive and process information from adjacent neurons. Dendrites develop throughout life, whenever we acquire new knowledge or learn new skills. Information passes to dendrites across connections called synapses. If those synapses aren't activated regularly, dendrites can atrophy and connections between neurons can weaken, reducing the brain's ability to learn and retrieve information from memory.

If you get proper nutrition, exercise, and mental stimulation—and don't have Alzheimer's disease—dendrites in the aging human brain can actually grow longer and denser. This enhanced network of connections enables brain cells to connect in multiple ways, enriching thought processes and helping to compensate for cellular shrinkage. The increasingly elaborate interconnections between brain cells—the wisdom of age—may help you:

- better understand the long-term consequences of decisions
- know when and where to get more information before arriving at a decision
- be more sensitive to religious and cultural issues
- realize that issues are complex and that no course of action is necessarily perfect.

Myth 3:
Once you lose it, it's gone.
Scientists long believed brain cell loss or damage was permanent, but new studies refute the notion that we're born with all the neurons we'll ever have. Scientist Fred Gage and colleagues at the Salk Institute have found compelling evidence of neurogenesis, the birth of neurons, in the adult human brain. Researchers

Dendrites develop throughout life, whenever we acquire new knowledge or learn new skills.

aren't certain how or even whether these newborn cells function in learning and memory processes, but it seems possible.

Similar investigations into the brain's capacity to regrow or heal itself are ongoing in labs around the country. Researchers at the Massachusetts Institute of Technology reconfigured the brains of newborn ferrets so their eyes were connected to regions of the brain where hearing normally develops. The result? The ferrets went on to develop fully functioning visual pathways in auditory brain tissue. The implication is that functional hearing, sight, and touch—and perhaps language and emotions—are not completely isolated in specialized regions of the brain, or at least those regions are not set in stone at birth.

Researchers are also racing to test a new technology for brain repair: the harvesting and manipulation of stem cells, immature cells that can be grown in culture dishes in the lab and then grafted into living tissue. Once these cells are introduced into the brain, chemical signals may cause them to develop into specialized brain cells and then form appropriate connections with other neurons. If this process is successful, it may eventually be possible to restore function to injured brains. At Harvard Medical School, stem cell implants into the brains of seemingly senile or stroke-impaired rats and primates hint at good recovery.

Fast Fact

Research at the University of Kentucky shows that only about 5 percent of memory impairments are due to brain disorders such as Alzheimer's. Stress, depression, poor health, improper nutrition, and a lack of exercise are far more prevalent—and preventable—causes.

YOUR GAME PLAN FOR GOOD HEALTH

Maximizing Your Memory

Can't recall the name of someone you just met? Learn the tricks the experts use and keep your memory sharp at any age.

What is memory anyway, and how does it work? The process by which the brain first acquires information, then stores it and retrieves it when needed, is an amazing yet mysterious phenomenon. But thanks to advanced technology, including positron emission tomography (PET) and functional magnetic resonance imaging (MRI), researchers have begun to map brain function—our brain wiring—giving us a much better idea of how memories are created.

Thought in Action

Memories are laid down as sequences of electrical activity that connect brain cells, or neurons, in various parts of the brain. These electrical pathways link all your senses and connect your sensory input to your physical and emotional responses, storing it all into memory.

When you recall something, you don't retrieve a single piece of data from a neatly organized file located in one specific area of your brain— it's much more complex than that. Think of the word "hammer" and your mind instantly recalls the name of this tool, its appearance, its weight and texture, its function, the sound it makes when hitting a nail—each piece of data drawn from a different region of your brain. In recalling your third-grade teacher, you assemble, in just a split second, the various aspects of her appearance, her personality, and perhaps the sound of her voice, and project that multilayered image on the screen we refer to as our "mind's eye."

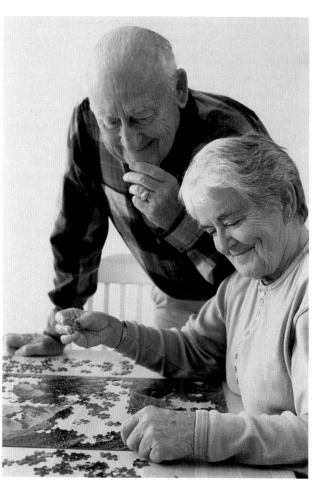

Research backs it up: Older people can hone analytical and spatial skills by solving puzzles and playing complex games.

The Short and Long of It

A memory begins the moment you take in information through your eyes, ears, nose, skin, or taste buds. Sensory impressions are fleeting, however, lasting only a few seconds, unless you consciously decide to remember the information and "encode" it either visually or verbally. Encoded information is first held in short-term memory, but only for about 30 seconds to a few minutes, because capacity there is limited. As new information enters your short-term memory, it bumps out the oldest information that was there.

There are no set rules governing what the mind moves to long-term memory and what it "cleans out." Something that garners special interest or attention is a good candidate for long-term storage, especially if two are more senses are involved and the information is somehow associated with an existing memory.

There is virtually no limit to how much we can store in long-term memory, and the information there is never lost (although it may not always be easily accessed).

Making Memories Stick

Follow these cues to help turn your moment-by-moment experience into memory:

- **Focus on one thing at a time.** Face it: You can't remember every fact that comes your way. Decide what's really important to remember and pay close attention when this new information is presented.
- **Be an active listener.** Hearing is not the same thing as listening. Some people find it useful to jot down notes or "play back" the gist of what they've just heard, as in "Let me see if I understand you correctly. You want me to . . ."
- **Eliminate distractions.** When you were younger, it may have been easy to study with the television on or the radio blaring. Now that you're older, you probably have to eliminate distractions for best mental performance. Some people find they need total quiet in order to concentrate.
- **When you're laying down memory, use as many senses as you can.** Years ago many elementary students easily memorized a long list of prepositions by learning to sing them to a familiar tune. They were processing input along several tracks at once: cognitive, visual, auditory, and motor. Fifty years later that memory is still there.
- **Practice, practice, practice.** Repeated exposure strengthens the brain's electrical pathways and greatly improves recall. Remember how many hours you spent memorizing multiplication tables? Give new learning the time it needs.
- **Put new information in context.** It's much easier to remember something meaningful than something abstract or random. For best retention, associate new learning with something you already know. The more linkages you develop around a piece of information, the greater the likelihood that one of them will jog your memory.
- **Sleep on it.** Adequate sleep is important in two ways. First, your mind works much more effectively when you're not tired. Second, preliminary research at Harvard Medical School indicates that most people need six to eight hours of

sleep—at least two cycles of deep sleep per night—for their brain to go through the chemical changes needed to integrate new skills or facts into long-term memory.

- **Reduce stress.** Stress, whether in the form of anxiety or depression, can be a major impediment to memory, interfering with concentration and weakening the motivation to learn.

- **Address sensory impairments.** You can't remember information you don't take in. For some older people, memory problems start with sensory deficits. If you have vision or hearing problems, talk to your doctor.

- **Become a creature of habit.** Make things easy on yourself. Pick one spot to leave your eyeglasses, keys, and wallet. And park your car in the same general area whenever you go to the mall.

- **Drink plenty of water.** Be sure you're getting a minimum of eight cups a day, more if you drink caffeinated beverages. Dehydration can cause numerous problems, including an electrolyte imbalance that can affect your brain.

- **Make smart lifestyle choices.** You can enhance memory function by following the advice you've read throughout this book: Eat nutritiously, make time for aerobic exercise at least three days a week, limit alcohol consumption, and avoid smoking.

Tips from the Memory Experts

Ever wonder how memory trainers manage to rattle off hundreds of names and long number sequences? They've mastered the use of mnemonic techniques, tricks, and shortcuts that help us capture information and store it in memory. Most of these tricks work by consciously increasing the amount of mental processing around any single piece of data. Ironically, although many of the standard memory enhancement techniques are age-old, they are supported by the latest findings on how the brain processes new input.

The principal techniques are association, visualization, imagination, and organization. See how they come into play in these everyday memory challenges.

Name that face. Names are everyone's number one memory bugaboo. The next time you meet a new person, scan his face and pick out a single feature—perhaps freckles, a dazzling smile, or a receding hairline. Now make a conscious link between that feature and the person's name. Say you meet a man named Tom Shipley. Notice that his blue eyes are the color of the ocean, and imagine him as the captain of a ship, with a tomcat as his first mate. The more ridiculous the image, the better, because exaggeration can make a visualization even more memorable. The key is to make a strong association between the name and the visual image so calling forth one will trigger the other. Strengthen that memory track by repeating the name several times during the conversation. You might also try picturing what the name looks like in print.

Finders, keepers. Association and visualization can also help you avoid misplacing your reading glasses or losing your parking stub. To fix some piece of information in your memory, associate it with a visual image or at least one additional sensory cue. For instance, when you put your glasses on the bathroom counter, notice how the lenses pick up the reflection of the lights over the vanity. As you tuck that parking stub into your raincoat pocket, note how the yellow ticket contrasts with the olive cloth and feel the stiff outline of the ticket against the soft fabric of the pocket lining. To remind yourself to buy lemons at the store, imagine their tartness on your tongue as you add them to your mental shopping list.

Sentence the subject. Take the first letter of the words you want to remember and construct a new word or sentence. Remember how your piano teacher taught you the notes in the G clef? *Every good boy does fine.* Use the same technique to commit a short shopping list to memory: milk, eggs, lemons, lettuce, oranges, walnuts. *Male eagles look lively over Winnipeg.* You can also try to spell out a word or two from the first letters of your shopping items. This list, for example, spells out *mellow*.

Chunk it. Long number sequences—credit card numbers, Social Insurance Numbers—are organized into subsets to make them easier to remember. Most telephone numbers consist of just seven digits (broken into two or three subsets) because that's all that short-term memory can handle at one time. The same technique can be applied to words. Say Thursday's to-do list has these random jottings: eggs, pick up clothes at cleaners, newspaper, bread, buy a nightgown, fill up car, drugstore, catsup. Here's one way to chunk the information for memory efficiency:

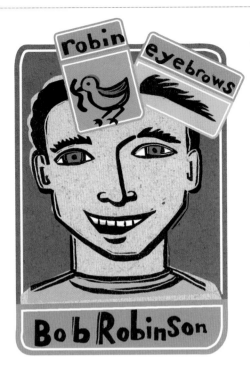

To remember a name, think of a visual image based on the name and link it to a prominent feature on the person's face. For instance, to remember Bob Robinson, picture a robin bobbing between the man's bushy eyebrows.

Foods	Places	Ns
eggs	drugstore	newspaper
bread	gas station	nightgown
catsup	cleaners	

Chain it. Think serially, making up a mini-story that strings together the items you want to remember. The sillier and more outrageous the story, the better. You might memorize Thursday's to-do list this way: *As I drive into the gas station I almost hit a man leaving the drugstore. He gets mad and throws eggs and catsup at my car. As he runs off, he knocks down a woman leaving the cleaners, carrying her nightgown. The incident is written up in the newspapers.*

Be a reporter. Have something important to remember? Pretend you're a reporter and write a story lead that zeroes in on the who, what, where, when, and why of the information. Exaggerating some aspects of the story will make the information even easier to remember.

Exercising Your Mind

Want to keep
your brain fast
and nimble?
It takes two kinds
of exercise—
aerobic and
neurobic.

You probably already know it from observation, and researchers have confirmed it in study after study: Older people who stay physically active and fully engaged in stimulating pursuits are mentally sharper than those who live out their sunset years in a recliner in front of the TV. And staying physically active and mentally challenged is the best way to boost your brainpower at any age.

Keep It Flowing

Aerobic exercise is one key to maximizing brain fitness. Researchers, citing animal studies, suggest that physical exercise may actually increase the number of neurons in the brain. Moreover, the cardiovascular conditioning gained from regular aerobic activity helps prevent hardening of the arteries, which may have brain benefits. According to the American Medical Association, people in poor cardiovascular health are three times as likely to suffer a decline in cognitive function as the healthy elderly.

Keep It Growing

There's another kind of exercise that can enhance mental fitness. Coined "neurobics" by Lawrence Katz and Manning Rubin in their book *Keep Your Brain Alive*, it's a type of mental exercise that strengthens the brain's natural affinity for learning new things. In his work at Duke University, neurobiologist Katz observed that many of the brain's neural pathways are vastly underused. They need extra stimulation to reach their potential. Recent research has revealed that when you combine your senses in novel and unexpected ways, your brain produces a chemical called neurotrophin, a kind of fertilizer that strengthens brain circuits by almost doubling the size and complexity of your dendrites.

Neurobics encourages you to accomplish ordinary tasks in new ways, by using all five of your senses, not just your overloaded visual and auditory channels. It teaches you to break away from brain-deadening routines and seek offbeat experiences that stir up activity in nerve pathways you don't normally use. It's a great way to stay ready to master new learning challenges.

Fast Fact

Experiments show that animals who are housed in environments enriched with many social activities, toys, and areas to explore develop heavier brains than animals who live in small, drab, unstimulating environments. They also learn better and develop more connections between neurons.

Mental Muscle

One study found that older people who stay mentally alert frequently:

- play complex games, such as chess, Scrabble, or bridge
- read, often at a local library
- keep abreast of current events
- talk regularly with others
- solve crossword puzzles
- use estimating skills and solve math problems in their head
- learn new skills
- help with their children's businesses or care for grandchildren
- write, paint, play a musical instrument, or engage in other creative hobbies.

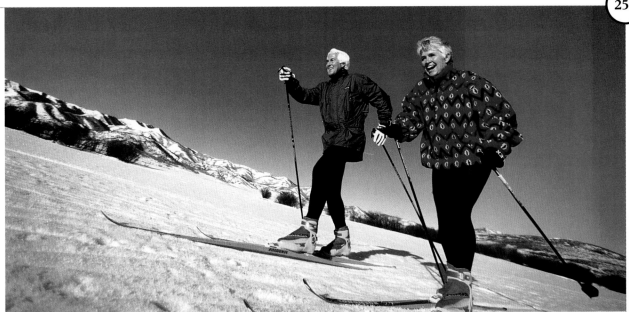

Try a neurobic exercise right now: Cross the room with your eyes closed. In doing so, you're challenging your brain to perform a task that is interesting and potentially frustrating. Besides activating your spatial memory, you'll be forcing your senses of touch, smell, and hearing to perform in unaccustomed ways. Your brain will absorb all kinds of fresh sensory input and create new linkages between neurons. Even something as simple as brushing your teeth with your nondominant hand or getting dressed with your eyes closed helps build neural circuitry.

Maintain good mental function with daily physical activity that boosts blood circulation and keeps oxygen and key nutrients flowing to the brain.

A Neurobic a Day

Neurobic conditioning is easy. Just use at least two of your senses in unexpected ways throughout the day. While it seems simple, doing things in new ways actually triggers complex activity in the brain and, over time, packs a real punch in terms of enhanced mental fitness. Here's a week's worth of activities to start you off.

SUNDAY	MONDAY	TUESDAY	WEDNESDAY	THURSDAY	FRIDAY	SATURDAY
See things differently. Challenge your spatial sense by wearing an eye patch or a Post-it note over one lens of your eyeglasses.	**Reroute yourself.** Take a new route on your daily commute to work or shopping. If you drive, open the windows and let all the sights, sounds, and smells rush in.	**Could you repeat that?** At dinner, have the family eat the entire meal without speaking aloud, communicating with only gestures and facial expressions.	**Be a backseat driver.** Challenge your visual and spatial sense and change your perspective by riding in the backseat instead of driving.	**Nose around.** Place a strong-scented substance, like pine oil, in a cup and ask someone to hide it in your home. Find the cup with your eyes closed, using smell and touch and your spatial memory.	**Stack 'em up.** Fill a cup with an assortment of coins and, without looking, use your sense of touch to sort them into stacks of the same denomination.	**Park yourself.** Sit on a park bench with your eyes closed. Listen to the sounds and smell the aromas around you, and piece together a picture of the scene. Then make up a story about it.

Brain Games

Want to exercise different parts of your brain? Here's a grab bag of memory games, mental challenges, and puzzles to try. You'll find the answers at the bottom of page 257.

1 Test Your Digit Span

On a piece of paper, make a vertical list of the letters A through O. Now, starting with line A in the exercise below, look at each line of numbers, then turn the page and write them down from memory on your sheet. Continue until you can no longer remember the sequence correctly. Most people can memorize seven digits without too much trouble. But you can increase your capacity by visualizing the shapes of the numbers as you say them aloud several times, jotting them down as you memorize them, chunking them into groups of three or four, associating them with part of a number sequence you already know (like an address or birth date), or recognizing a pattern in the numbers—for example, even numbers followed by odd numbers, numbers in ascending or descending order of value, and so on.

A 9537
B 04429
C 719503
D 4932187
E 60443659
F 138274992
G 2848688808
H 73656243317
I 934637830507
J 7564132958503
K 24179553573060
L 621487346596832
M 8574068300583237
N 79948328574639102
O 649301948672883755

2 The Three Hats

There are three black hats and two white hats in a box. Three men (we will call them A, B, and C) are blindfolded. Each of them reaches into the box and places one of the hats on his own head. No man can see which color hat he has chosen. The men are then positioned in such a way that A can see B's and C's hats, B can see only C's hat, and C cannot see any of the hats.

When A is asked if he knows which color hat he is wearing, he says no. When B is asked the same question, he says no. When C is asked, he says yes, and he is correct.

What color is C's hat, and how does he know?

Adapted from brain-teaser.com

3 Connect the Dots

Using only 4 lines, connect all nine dots without lifting your pencil.

4 So That's It!

In your cellar are three light switches in the OFF position. Each switch controls a lightbulb on the floor above. How can you determine which switch controls each bulb? You may operate any of the switches, but you may go upstairs only once to inspect the bulbs.

Adapted from brain-teaser.com

5 Memory Master

Here's a fun way to get your synapses firing. Ask a friend to arrange the contents of your junk drawer on a tabletop, and cover the items with a cloth. When the cloth is removed, you have 60 seconds to memorize the items. When the cloth is replaced, jot down as many as you can remember. Take turns, substituting new items and rearranging the display. Try increasing your recall by using some of the memory enhancement techniques introduced on pages 247 and 248: Associate the items with something else, chunk them in categories, chain them to make a story, and so on.

6 Word Wizard

Come up with as many words as possible using the letters found in the following words. Increase the challenge by competing against a partner or working within a time limit.

mercenary   *cryogenics*

7 Picture This

Use all the following elements to make three different pictures. There are no right answers, but you can increase your options by varying the size and orientation of the elements.

2 rectangles ▢▢   2 triangles △△

2 periods ●●   2 commas ❞

8 Ls L L L L L L L L

8 Lend an Ear

Which U.S. states are represented here?

My sore eye

In tennis shoes

My wise cousin

No decoder

Let's lose Anna

Have a mini-soda

An arid zone

9 Go Figure

In 1990, a person is 15. In 1995 that same person is 10. How is that possible?

10 Practically Speaking

Place a button in an empty wine bottle, and cork it. How can you remove the button without removing the cork or breaking the bottle?

11 Tic Tac Toe

Place 6 Xs in the puzzle without placing 3 in a row.

12 Name That Number

Study the following sentences to discover the embedded telephone and Social Insurance Numbers and the technique used to encode them.

Telephone numbers

Monkeys are fun to watch as they
swing from branches.
Kittens usually like to take naps
in the warm sunshine.

Social Insurance Numbers

A big animal is here sitting on our front step.
Giraffes have long necks to reach
the highest branches.

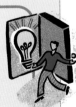

SimpleSolution

Looking for more memory games and puzzles? There's an ever-expanding assortment in bookstores and on the Internet. Two of the best online sites are brain-teaser.com and logic.com.

Guarding Your Brain Health

Worried about your memory? Take heart: No more than 10 percent of all people age 65 and up get Alzheimer's disease.

Everyone forgets things from time to time, and we've seen that normal aging is associated with some slowdown in thought processing and memory formation. But people who have ongoing problems storing and retrieving memories are said to have a memory disorder.

Impaired memory can range from mild to severe and is often the result of a disease or injury that affects the brain. Severe cases can be due to dementia, a state of generalized, progressive mental deterioration—not just forgetfulness, but diminished language, visual, and spatial skills, as well as deficits in judgment and problem-solving ability. Alzheimer's disease is the most common form of dementia. (For more on Alzheimer's disease, see pages 296-299.)

Another common cause of memory loss among the elderly may surprise you. It's depression. Scientists using the latest brain-scanning technology have noted that persistent melancholy thoughts actually cause the brain metabolism to switch off in the thinking part of the brain and switch on in the emotional part of the brain. Fortunately, there are several effective interventions, and it's usually possible to reverse depression-induced memory loss. (Read about depression and its treatments on pages 320-323.)

Time for a Checkup?

If memory lapses are beginning to affect the quality of your life, talk to your doctor. Diagnosis may involve a review of your medical history, a physical and neurological exam, standard laboratory tests, cognitive assessments, and possibly a computerized tomography (CT) scan or magnetic resonance imaging (MRI) to

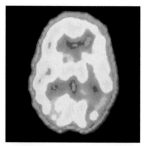

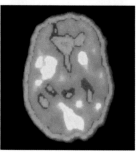

Depression can hamper cognitive function. A scan of a normal brain is shown at top. On bottom, depression has decreased activity in the prefrontal cortex.

Not Quite Alzheimer's

Researchers have identified a new category of memory loss: mild cognitive impairment, or MCI. People with MCI are not disoriented or confused, like those with Alzheimer's disease, nor do they have trouble with language, abstract thinking, or their attention skills. However, their mental and functional abilities decline faster than those of the average person their age, and they may have difficulty recalling facts, keeping appointments, and remembering to pay bills.

People with MCI apparently have a small hippocampus, an area of the brain closely tied to learning and memory. Having MCI seems to increase the risk of developing Alzheimer's.

Currently, the National Institutes of Health in the U.S. is funding research on whether a combination of vitamin E and the drug donepezil (Aricept) might slow the progression from mild cognitive impairment to Alzheimer's. Trials are also under way to determine the effectiveness of the COX-2 inhibitor drug rofecoxib (Vioxx), currently used to treat arthritis.

Food for Thought

One of the best ways to preserve your brain and nervous system is to give them a steady supply of essential nutrients. Poor eating habits, combined with poor food absorption, can contribute to cognitive problems. Here's the latest advice:

RECOMMENDATION	WHY IT'S IMPORTANT
Stick to a low-fat diet to control cholesterol.	■ A diet high in fatty red meats and whole-fat dairy foods can boost cholesterol levels, clogging arteries and reducing oxygen flow to the brain.
Consume low-fat dairy products and lean meats.	■ These are good sources of carnitine, an amino acid essential to proper brain and nerve function.
Increase your intake of whole grains and legumes.	■ Beans and whole-grain breads and cereals contain lecithin, which the brain uses to make acetylcholine, an important neurotransmitter.
Eat foods rich in vitamins C and E and supplement your diet.	■ These antioxidants can protect the brain from damage by neutralizing free radicals and helping reduce protein-plaque deposits associated with mental decline. Vitamin C food sources include broccoli, citrus fruits, leafy greens, strawberries, and tomatoes. Boost vitamin E with almonds, vegetable oil, nuts, seeds, and whole-wheat flour. Also consider taking supplements.
Eat foods rich in B-complex vitamins or cereal fortified with them.	■ Recent research suggests that even moderate shortfalls in vitamin B_{12} and folic acid can contribute to mental decline, and possibly the onset of Alzheimer's disease, by elevating blood levels of homocysteine (an amino acid). Fortified breakfast cereals, wheat germ, nuts and seeds, and vegetable oil are good food sources.

pinpoint or rule out these other common contributors to memory loss:

- poor nutrition, especially deficiencies in B vitamins
- endocrine disorders
- side effects of common medications (see page 256)
- vision or hearing problems
- anxiety or stress
- dehydration
- alcohol use
- isolation and inactivity
- sleep problems
- grief.

Although there are currently few drug treatments for memory problems beyond these treatable causes, researchers expect to develop some within the next decade. In the meantime, it pays to know what you can do to help prevent memory problems in the first place.

DRUG CAPSULE

Studies indicate lower rates of Alzheimer's disease among arthritis patients and others who regularly take non-steroidal anti-inflammatory drugs (NSAIDs) such as aspirin, ibuprofen, and naproxen. Acetaminophen has no effect on inflammation and hasn't shown any effect on Alzheimer's risk. Consult your doctor before starting long-term use of NSAIDs.

Memory-Zapping Meds

Many drugs and drug combinations can affect cognition and memory. Sometimes you can avoid the problem by having your doctor substitute another medication or reducing the dosage. Here are the most common offenders.

TYPE OF DRUG	EXAMPLES
H2 blockers of stomach acid	■ Famotidine (Pepcid)
Antidepressants	■ Amoxapine (Asendin) ■ Amitriptyline (Elavil)
Antipsychotic drugs	■ Haloperidol (Haldol) ■ Thioridazine (Mellaril)
Antiviral drugs	■ Amantadine (Symmetrel)
Blood pressure drugs	■ Methyldopa (Aldomet) ■ Propranolol (Inderal)
Sedatives	■ Flurazepam (Dalmane) ■ Diazepam (Valium)

WARNING

Recent studies link high blood pressure with impaired mental ability. High blood pressure exacts a toll on your arteries and capillaries, reducing blood flow and oxygen to the brain. If left untreated over 10 years, chronic hypertension can lower your memory by 2 to 3 points on a 100-point scale.

An Estrogen Link?

Estrogen seems to play a key role in memory function by mopping up free radicals (unstable oxygen molecules), supporting nerve cell repair, reducing cellular inflammation, and boosting levels of acetylcholine, an important neurotransmitter.

Researchers associate the higher frequency of Alzheimer's disease in women with the drop in estrogen that comes with menopause. A 1996 study of more than 1,000 women showed that using estrogen for up to a year reduced Alzheimer's risk by a remarkable 60 percent. The risk fell even further when women stayed on the hormone for longer periods. More recent studies have shown risk reductions in the 30 to 50 percent range. And some—but not all—studies of postmenopausal women on hormone replacement therapy (HRT) link higher estrogen levels with improved memory.

The results, though impressive, are not clear cut. One recent study of postmenopausal women in the early stages of Alzheimer's disease showed no change in their rate of cognitive decline as a result of HRT. And other researchers have noted that it can be difficult to differentiate the effects of estrogen therapy from other factors. For instance, women who undergo HRT tend to be better educated and, for reasons unknown, higher levels of education are associated with lower Alzheimer's risk.

Estrogen replacement therapy is not without risks (see pages 232-234 for more information), and no one should initiate it solely for the potential brain benefits. Discuss the pros and cons with your doctor.

Get with Ginkgo

Used for thousands of years in Asian cultures to boost energy and mental alertness, ginkgo biloba is an antioxi-

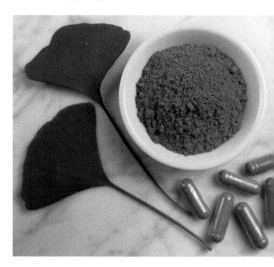

The herb ginkgo biloba helps improve the flow of blood, and therefore oxygen and nutrients, to the brain.

dant herb with blood-thinning properties. It is thought to increase blood flow to the brain (as well as the heart and extremities). Studies at the National Institutes of Health in the U.S. are looking at the herb's role in supporting cognitive function, perhaps by increasing the production of adenosine triphosphate (ATP), a chemical that figures prominently in brain metabolism. Ginkgo may not boost memory in healthy people, but it may help older people with nar-

rowed arteries, who have diminished blood flow to the brain.

Choose a product standardized to deliver 24 percent flavoglycosides and 6 percent terpenes. Ginkgo can increase the effects of blood thinners such as aspirin and Coumadin, so check with your doctor before taking it. Besides ginkgo, you might also want to include ginger, ginseng, and rosemary in your diet. All are antioxidants thought to stimulate blood flow to the brain.

Brain Games Answer Key

Below are the anwers to the puzzles on pages 252-253. (Questions 1 and 5 don't require answers.)

2 Man A must not see two white hats on B and C, or he would know that his own hat must be black. So A's answer establishes that B and/or C must be wearing a black hat. If B saw that C was wearing a white hat, he would know his own was black. But when B cannot tell which color he is wearing, C knows that he must be wearing a black hat, and he answers correctly.

3

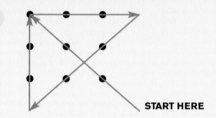

START HERE

4 Turn on switch 1 for five minutes, then turn it off. Turn on switch 2, and immediately inspect the bulbs. The hot bulb is controlled by switch 1. The lit bulb is controlled by switch 2. The bulb that's cold and unlit is controlled by switch 3.

6 Here are some possibilities:
mercenary—many, meany, mean, meaner, mane, careen, career, year, near, nearer, rear, ream, reamer, cream, creamer, nary, marry, merry, carry
cryogenics—yogi, scion, scone, scenic, cog, coy, cry, crying, gone, ego, nice, cone, nose, rice, gory, cringe, sing, singe, yes

7

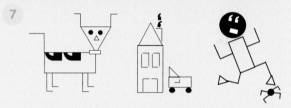

8 Missouri, Tennessee, Wisconsin, North Dakota, Louisiana, Minnesota, and Arizona. Devise your own phrases that sound like the syllables in the names of each of the other states.

9 The person lived in the B.C. era.

10 Push the cork into the bottle and then shake out the button.

11

X	X	
X		X
	X	X

12 **Telephone numbers** 733-252-4548; 774-244-2347
Social Insurance Numbers 136-246-235; 844-525-378
The number of letters in each word corresponds to the number in the sequence. For example, "quiet" has 5 letters, "a" has 1 letter, and so on.

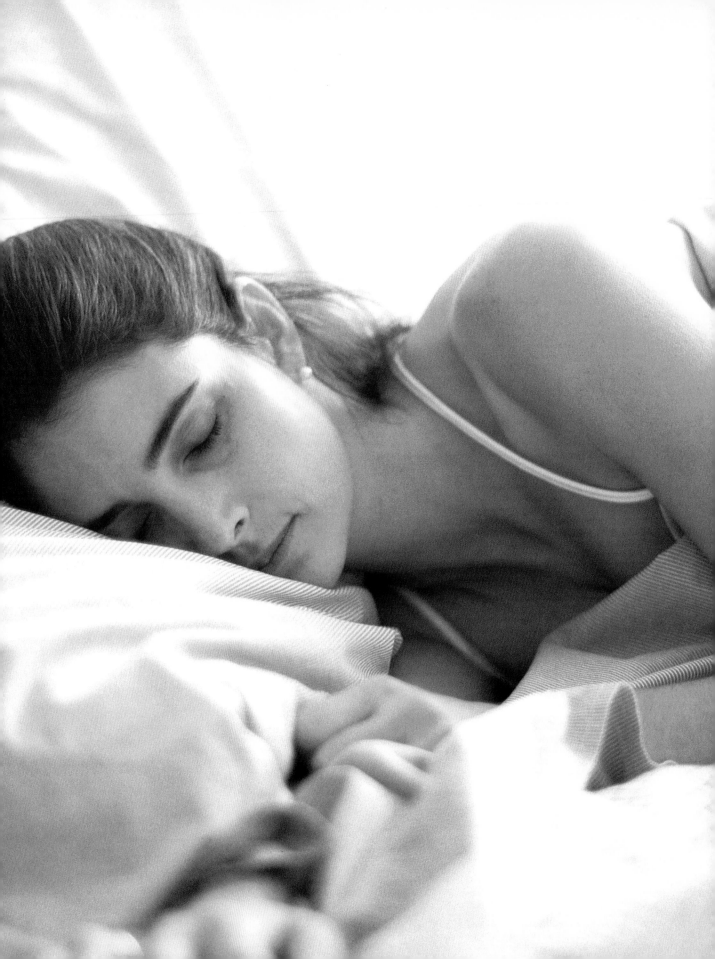

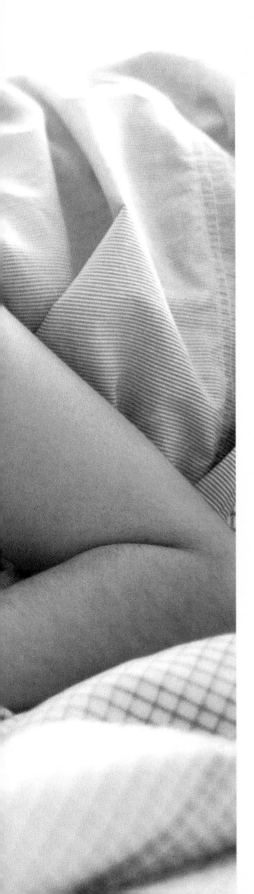

CHAPTER 11

GETTING ENOUGH SLEEP

What's Keeping You Up at Night?

Tossing and turning? Waking up too early? Sleep problems can be more than harmless annoyances: They can jeopardize our health.

Most people assume that after a night of sleep they will wake up feeling well rested and ready to go. A good night's sleep is a real blessing—and it's critical for our physical and mental health. For instance, scientists recently discovered that people who sleep at least six hours (including two periods each of deep sleep and REM sleep) have better memory formation than those who sleep less.

Yet many people skimp on sleep in order to save time. And as we age, deep, restful sleep can be harder to come by. Some 40 percent of people over age 60 complain that their sleep isn't what it used to be. And they're not imagining things. With age, sleep often becomes fitful and light. People over age 60 may wake up more than 20 times a night—twice as often as younger people. Such unproductive sleep does more than make you feel tired and grumpy the next day; it can impair your cognitive function and harm your health (see *The Dangers of Sleep Deprivation,* below).

How Much Sleep Do You Need?

Although your sleeping patterns may change, you probably still need as much sleep as you did when you were younger. Most adults, whether

The Dangers of Sleep Deprivation

Sleep is critical to the proper functioning of your brain and body. Deep sleep restores the physical body, and experts believe that dream sleep restores the mind, perhaps by clearing out irrelevant information. As research shows, losing even one night of sleep can lead to:

- **Weakened immunity.** Many studies have shown that sleep deprivation can interfere with immune-system function. A trial at the University of California, San Diego, for example, found that missing four hours of sleep on one night resulted in significantly decreased activity of T-cells, a type of disease-fighting white-blood cell. After a night of regular sleep, T-cell activity returned to normal.
- **Increased stress hormones.** In a University of Chicago study, lack of sleep was linked to increased production of the stress hormone cortisol, which over time is thought to raise the risk of memory impairment and age-related insulin resistance.

- **Less efficient glucose metabolism.** In the same study, sleep-deprived participants showed a 30 percent decrease in their ability to both secrete and respond to insulin, a condition that resembles an early stage of diabetes. The upshot? Sleep deprivation might exacerbate or hasten the onset of type 2 diabetes.
- **Impaired cognitive functioning.** In various studies, researchers have demonstrated that lack of sleep can interfere with memory, concentration, learning, logical reasoning, and mathematical calculation.
- **Increased risk of car accidents.** The National Highway Traffic Safety Administration in the U.S. estimates that drowsiness is the leading factor in some 100,000 auto accidents every year. In one study, researchers found that people who were sleepy during the day had twice as many car accidents as those who weren't sleepy.

What Happens During Sleep

While we're asleep, our brains follow a sequence of activities that occur in cycles. Each cycle contains five phases of sleep, known as non-REM (rapid-eye movement) stages 1, 2, 3, and 4, plus REM sleep. The stages progress from stage 1 to REM, then the cycle repeats, for an average total of four or five cycles per night. Between ages 50 and 60, you begin to spend more time in stages 1 and 2 sleep and less time in deep sleep. In older people with insomnia (particularly women), stage 4 sleep can be absent. Poor stage 4 sleep is believed to be a factor in chronically painful conditions such as fibromyalgia.

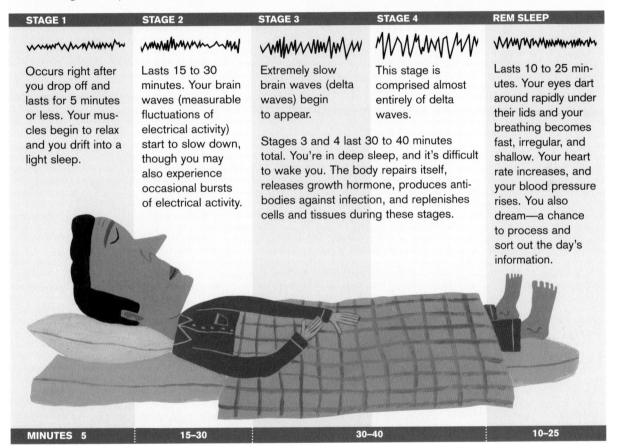

STAGE 1	STAGE 2	STAGE 3	STAGE 4	REM SLEEP
Occurs right after you drop off and lasts for 5 minutes or less. Your muscles begin to relax and you drift into a light sleep.	Lasts 15 to 30 minutes. Your brain waves (measurable fluctuations of electrical activity) start to slow down, though you may also experience occasional bursts of electrical activity.	Extremely slow brain waves (delta waves) begin to appear. Stages 3 and 4 last 30 to 40 minutes total. You're in deep sleep, and it's difficult to wake you. The body repairs itself, releases growth hormone, produces antibodies against infection, and replenishes cells and tissues during these stages.	This stage is comprised almost entirely of delta waves.	Lasts 10 to 25 minutes. Your eyes dart around rapidly under their lids and your breathing becomes fast, irregular, and shallow. Your heart rate increases, and your blood pressure rises. You also dream—a chance to process and sort out the day's information.
MINUTES 5	15–30	30–40		10–25

they're 25 or 75, need seven to eight hours of shut-eye each night. According to a survey by the National Sleep Foundation in the U.S., only one-third of adults say they get eight hours a night during the week. As many as one-third of those polled reported sleeping less than six hours. Women age 30 to 60 seem to be the most sleep-deprived group.

True, some people might get by with a mere five hours of slumber, while others might need ten. The actual number of hours slept may be less important than the consistency of your sleep pattern. If you're waking up refreshed after seven hours or even less and you don't need an alarm to wake you, you don't need to be concerned. But if your sleeping pattern is off, or if you're putting in the time required for a good night's rest but just can't seem to get much sleep, start looking for suspects.

YOUR GAME PLAN FOR GOOD HEALTH

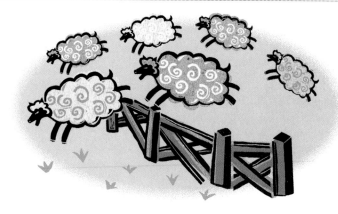

If you wake up at night and can't get back to sleep, don't count sheep. Get out of bed and do a relaxing activity until you feel sleepy again.

Counting Endless Sheep

Perhaps you are among the estimated 40 percent of adults who experience insomnia, the most common sleep disorder in Canada. It can involve difficulty in falling asleep, waking up and having a hard time getting back to sleep, or awakening too early. If it lasts only a few days, it's called transient insomnia; if it lasts a few weeks, it's called short-term insomnia. The problem is chronic if it happens most nights of the week and lasts a month or more.

The most common form of insomnia is learned insomnia, in which a few sleepless nights lead to anxiety about being unable to get to sleep, making it even harder to do so.

However long it lasts, insomnia is not a disease in itself but a symptom of another problem, or several problems, whether physical, emotional, or behavioral. Common culprits include the following:

- **Stress.** Many experts consider this to be the leading cause of short-term sleep disturbances. Common triggers include job-related pressures, marriage troubles, or a serious illness or death in the family. Usually the insomnia disappears when the stressful situation passes. If stress hormones are still pumping in your body by the time you're ready for bed, they'll inhibit the production of melatonin, a hormone that helps induce sleep. High levels of stress hormones can also block the restorative effects of growth hormone, which aids in the manufacture of new cells.

- **Alcohol and caffeine.** Too much caffeine or alcohol, especially when it's consumed too close to bedtime, can ruin a good night's sleep. Caffeine, a stimulant, can make it difficult to fall asleep.

Cat Naps: Naughty or Nice?

The body's natural rhythms have two peak times for sleeping, nighttime and midafternoon. Even if you're not chronically sleep deprived, that post-lunch urge to nap can sometimes be overpowering. Should you succumb? The answer is yes—if it doesn't interfere with your nighttime sleeping. Brief naps improve productivity, creativity, and problem-solving skills, and they may reduce accidents at work. Studies show that people have more active brains after a nap, so they pay closer attention to detail and are better able to make critical decisions.

The optimal nap length is 20 to 30 minutes. If you sleep longer, you'll pass into deeper, slow-brain-wave sleep that will make it hard for you to awaken and leave you feeling groggy for about half an hour afterward. Napping for more than an hour will probably interfere with your sleep that night. A longer nap may also diminish the total amount of sleep you need at night, making you wake up earlier than usual, or making it difficult to stay asleep.

Its effects can last for up to 10 hours after you consume it, especially in older people, whose metabolism is slower. And although alcohol is a sedative and may help you doze off more quickly, it can disrupt sleep later, when the effect wears off.

- **Pain and chronic medical conditions.** Some people don't sleep well because a medical condition is making them uncomfortable. The pain of arthritis, heartburn, a sore back, or a headache can wake you up and make it hard for you to get back to sleep. In a random sampling of adults in the U.S., one-fourth reported having pain that disrupted their sleep 10 or more nights per month. Chronic conditions such as fibromyalgia, Parkinson's disease, and diabetes can also make it difficult to fall asleep or cause you to awaken during the night.

- **The ups and downs of female hormones.** At the beginning and end of the menstrual cycle, low progesterone levels can make it difficult to sleep. If you think your hormones are contributing to your sleep problems, try keeping a sleep diary for a month. It can help you determine when in your cycle you should avoid caffeine, alcohol, and other things that could make the problem worse. During menopause, hot flashes caused by fluctuating levels of estrogen can cause restless nights. Estrogen replacement therapy often helps.

- **Medications.** Certain medications, such as corticosteroids and some drugs used to treat high blood pressure, asthma, and depression can interfere with sleep. So can thyroid drugs if the dose is too high. Some common over-the-counter (OTC) drugs, decongestants for example, contain stimulants, such as pseudoephedrine, and some aspirin formulas contain caffeine. If you're having trouble sleeping, review your medications with your doctor.

- **Depression.** Sleep laboratory researchers have observed sleep abnormalities in people with depression, including reduced periods of slow-brain-wave sleep and an early onset of the first episode of REM sleep. Research has shown that as many as 90 percent of people with depression have sleep disturbances. These can range from early waking to excessive sleeping. Antidepressants can help.

OTC Sleep Solutions

Transient and short-term insomnia are extremely common and, by definition, short-lived. Figuring out the root of the problem can help clear it up. It may be as simple as skipping that afternoon cup of coffee or keeping a more regular sleep schedule by making sure to go to bed and get up at the same time every day.

If stress is the cause, consider learning a relaxation technique, such as deep breathing or meditation (see pages 200-203). One study found that people who practiced relaxation techniques and smart sleep habits

(see pages 200-203)

Fast Fact

Migraines that occur during the night or early in the morning may be caused by lack of sleep. In one study, 65 percent of migraine sufferers who were treated for sleep problems reported that their headaches went away.

Light or interrupted sleep is a problem for many older people. One solution: exercise. It increases the duration of deep sleep, from which you are less likely to awaken.

Can Melatonin Get You to Sleep?

Melatonin is a natural hormone produced by the brain's pineal gland. During the day, our blood levels of melatonin are fairly low, but come bedtime, this gland revs up production, releasing more of the hormone into the blood. Though it doesn't make you fall asleep directly, melatonin may initiate changes in your body that set you up for sleep. Levels peak by around 2 A.M. and gradually fall back to normal daytime levels around 7 or 8 A.M.

It was once thought that our melatonin production tapered off as we got older, but a recent Harvard study found no difference in melatonin levels in the young and old. People just seem to produce varying levels of it.

Melatonin supplements might help you fall asleep faster, but they won't necessarily help you stay asleep. Some evidence shows that 1 or 2 mg a day may help some people, but possibly only those with a melatonin deficiency. And since there are no clinical trials on melatonin, doctors aren't sure of its long-term effects. If you want to try it, proceed with caution and don't exceed 1 or 2 mg, since more than that can actually disturb your sleep. Melatonin has not been approved for sale in Canada; however, it may be imported for a three-month supply.

WARNING

Daytime sleepiness is associated with heart disease among people age 65 and older. A study in the Journal of the American Geriatrics Society *found that men and women who reported feeling sleepy during the day were more likely to have heart disease.*

(see *Easy Ways to Catch More ZZZs*, page 268, for tips) reduced by 75 percent the amount of time it took to fall asleep at night—from 76 minutes to 19 minutes.

Many people turn to OTC sleep aids, such as Nytol, Sleep-Eez, and Sominex, for relief from a sleepless night. In fact, people buy more non-prescription sleeping pills than any other type of drug. Most experts agree, however, that the drugs are not a very effective solution to insomnia. If you often have trouble sleeping, your best bet is to improve your sleep habits. OTC drugs can be helpful, however, in breaking the cycle of occasional short-term insomnia.

These drugs aren't addictive, but they can leave you feeling drowsy the next day. Older people are particularly susceptible to next-day drowsiness from medication because their metabolism is generally slower,

so drugs stay in their system longer. Alcohol and other depressants exaggerate the drowsiness.

Antihistamines are the main active ingredient in most of these medications.

If minor pain is the only thing keeping you awake, try taking non-prescription pain-relieving brands such as Tylenol, Advil, or Motrin IB, which won't cause daytime tiredness. If you have angina, heart arrhythmia, breathing problems, chronic bronchitis, glaucoma, or difficulty urinating due to an enlarged prostate gland, check with your doctor before taking OTC sleeping pills.

Heavy-Duty Help

If your insomnia persists, see your doctor. She may need to adjust your current medications, treat you for stress or depression, or refer you to a sleep disorder clinic. There are hundreds of these clinics around the country, most of them associated with universities or hospitals. If you go to one, you will be examined and then monitored overnight, while you sleep, for any underlying conditions, such as sleep apnea (see *Dangerous Snoring: Sleep Apnea*, page 265) or periodic limb movements disorder (see page 267), that might be interfering with your sleep.

About half of patients who visit a doctor for sleep problems come home with a prescription for sleep medication. But remember that even prescription medications treat only the symptom, not the cause, and many can also cause next-day drowsiness.

The drugs can also cause rebound insomnia—making the sleeplessness return with a vengeance—when you stop taking them. The longer you

If you often have trouble sleeping, your best bet is to improve your sleep habits. OTC drugs can be helpful, however, in breaking the cycle of occasional short-term insomnia.

take them, the greater your chances of experiencing rebound insomnia or withdrawal. In any case, you shouldn't use sleep aids daily or for longer than three to six months. Taking a pill once every two or three days as needed will break the cycle of sleeplessness and reduce your chances of drug dependency.

The most commonly prescribed anti-insomnia drugs are benzodiazepines, hypnotics that inhibit the excitability of nerve cells called neurons. Well-known benzodiazepines include Dalmane, Restoril, and Halcion.

Unlike these drugs, the recently introduced drug zaleplon (brand name Starnoc) is not a benzodiazepine and causes no drowsiness the next day, provided you take it at least four hours before wake-up time. A study showed that it can be taken safely for up to a year without causing withdrawal symptoms when you stop.

Benzodiazepines are potentially dangerous if taken with alcohol, and they can cause side effects when taken with the ulcer medication Tagamet. Long-acting benzodiazepines (Valium, Dalmane, Librium) can remain in the body for days in older persons and should be avoided if possible. Halcion, though metabolized quickly, has been associated with short-term memory impairment and confusion.

Antidepressant medications such as Paxil are commonly prescribed for insomnia caused by depression. These drugs pose less risk of dependency than standard anti-insomnia medications.

Dangerous Snoring: Sleep Apnea

If you snore heavily, you may have obstructive sleep apnea, a disorder that affects more than 3 percent of the Canadian population, and often goes unrecognized. If you have it, you literally stop breathing for brief periods of time. A potentially serious and even life-threatening condition, sleep apnea is most common among overweight men, although women also are affected. According to the National Sleep Foundation in the U.S., 28 percent of men over age 65 and 24 percent of women over age 65 suffer from the condition.

Obstructive sleep apnea occurs when the tongue or the soft palate in the back of the throat relaxes during sleep and blocks the flow

A new sleeping pill, zaleplon (Starnoc), leaves your system in a few hours and causes no aftereffects. It can even be taken after you've gone to bed if you have trouble falling asleep.

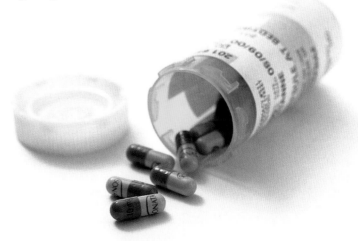

of oxygen through the airways. You may stop breathing perhaps 20 to hundreds of times each night for 10 seconds or longer each time. Usually you wake up during these lapses, but you won't remember doing so. You may also snore loudly and gasp suddenly for air, a signal that your brain is jump-starting your breathing. When the night's over, you'll probably wake up exhausted.

The health danger comes from the higher carbon dioxide and lower oxygen levels that result when you don't breathe regularly. These changes increase your chances of developing high blood pressure, stroke, heart attack, heart failure, diabetes, and kidney failure.

In a less common condition called central sleep apnea, the airway tissues are normal but the brain's respiratory center malfunctions. The cause is typically vascular or degenerative brain disease.

It's important to see a doctor if you suspect you have sleep apnea to avoid further health complications—and car accidents. In a study that compared adults with sleep apnea with people who were legally drunk, those with apnea scored worse than those who were drunk on a test measuring reaction time.

What to Do for Apnea

Sleep apnea ranges from mild to severe, and how you treat it depends on the severity of your symptoms and whether the apnea is obstructive or central. If you are experiencing mild apnea, or even just heavy snoring, try sleeping on your side instead of your back to help prevent your soft palate and tongue from relaxing into the back of your throat.

If your neck size is greater than 17 inches, or if you have more than one chin, losing weight may be the answer. You probably have fatty deposits on the inside of your neck that constrict your airway and contribute to your snoring problem. Obstructive sleep apnea usually improves with weight loss and, in some cases, completely disappears.

If apnea is a problem, avoid alcohol and sleeping pills, which relax your muscles and make the problem worse. Smoking is also detrimental because it can make your throat swell, narrowing your air passages. Finally, consider trying nasal breathing strips, available at your drugstore. You can tape these strips over the bridge of your nose to keep your nostrils open while you sleep.

If your sleep apnea is severe, a doctor can fit you with a soft plastic mask you wear while sleeping. Called a CPAP device (which stands for continuous positive airway pressure), the mask allows you to inhale pressurized room air, which keeps your air passages open.

To keep yourself from rolling onto your back in the middle of the night— a habit that encourages snoring—sew pockets into the back of your pajama top and stuff them with tennis balls, or roll up some socks and tape them to the back of your sleepwear.

If these approaches don't help, you may need surgery to increase the diameter of your breathing passages. This might involve removing adenoids, tonsils, or other tissue growths, although success rates are only about 65 percent. Laser surgery is another option and usually requires three or four outpatient sessions.

One of the newest treatments for apnea uses radiofrequency energy to reduce the volume of the tongue. During a 45-minute outpatient procedure, a physician attaches an electrode to the base of the tongue. It transmits low levels of radiofrequency energy, which shrinks the tongue. A 1999 study showed that patients who had this treatment experienced a 50 percent reduction in sleep interruptions.

Running Undercover: Restless Legs

Another medical condition that can disturb your sleep is restless legs syndrome (RLS), which affects more than 5 percent of Canadian adults and is more common in people middle-aged and older. RLS causes achy, crampy legs that feel as if you need to stretch them. Ironically, you experience it when you're resting, not when you're using your legs.

Doctors aren't sure exactly what causes the syndrome, but it may be associated with vitamin or iron deficiencies, anemia, thyroid disease, peripheral nerve disorders, excessive caffeine intake, and certain chronic diseases such as diabetes or rheumatoid arthritis.

Many people—an estimated 45 percent of those over 65—may have a similar malady called periodic limb movements disorder (PLMD), in

---

Is Your Snoring Suspicious?

How do you tell the difference between plain snoring and sleep apnea? If your snoring is moderate and steady, you most likely don't have a problem. Loud, gasping noises that awaken you or your partner are more suspicious.

Your doctor can make a preliminary diagnosis by asking you some simple questions. You can get confirmation of the diagnosis by undergoing a test called polysomnography at a sleep disorder center, where you'll be monitored while you sleep. One of the things that will be measured is your blood pressure, which is typically very low during sleep. If your blood pressure rises during the night, you probably have serious apnea.

Stanford University has recently developed what seems to be a highly accurate test to help doctors spot sleep apnea in five minutes. By considering various markers such as weight, height, neck circumference, and dental overbite, a doctor can determine whether your airway is likely to be blocked during sleep. Still in trials, the test is not used widely yet, but it promises to be a useful diagnostic tool for both doctors and dentists.

---

which the legs or arms kick every 20 to 40 seconds throughout the night, but only during sleep. If you have RLS, movement is continuous and occurs whenever you're at rest. Treatment is the same for both conditions.

If your leg movements are keeping you up, try massaging your legs or getting out of bed and walking around. Soaking your legs in cool water or using a heating pad may help. Avoid caffeine, alcohol, and nicotine and try to find techniques to reduce stress, because all these may aggravate the condition. Over-the-counter pain relievers—including acetaminophen or ibuprofen—can provide some relief.

If you can't manage the problem on your own, see your doctor. Prescription drugs including controlled-release levodopa/carbidopa, amantadine, pergolide, and bromocriptine (all are also used to treat Parkinson's tremors), and benzodiazepines (hypnotics) can help.

In their own words

"By any measuring stick, the deaths, illness, and damage due to sleep deprivation and sleep disorders represent a substantial problem for American society."
—*from* Wake Up America: A National Sleep Alert, *a report of the National Commission on Sleep Disorders Research*

Easy Ways to Catch More ZZZs

Say good night to sleep problems. Here are 10 effective strategies for getting a better night's sleep that don't require a trip to the drugstore.

If you've had one or two bad nights lately, you can probably solve the problem by taking some of the measures below. These strategies may require you to change your sleeping habits, but the effort is well worth it in the long run.

1 Make your bedroom a haven for sleep. Your room should be quiet and sufficiently dark, because darkness prompts the pineal gland to produce melatonin, the hormone that induces sleep. Heavy drapes can help keep the light out, and a fan or white-noise machine can help drown out any annoying sounds.

Cool temperatures help you sleep, so set your thermostat appropriately. For better air circulation, open a window or use a fan. If the air in the room is too dry, buy a humidifier.

2 Become a creature of habit. A nighttime routine can be very effective in letting your body know when it's time to sleep. Go through whatever rituals help you get mentally prepared for sleep. (Read a few pages of your novel, spend 5 to 10 minutes on personal grooming, meditate, stretch.) It's also critical to go to bed and get up at the same time every day—even on weekends.

3 Reserve your bed just for sleeping and sex. Avoid working, paying bills, reading, or watching television in bed. If you associate your bed only with sleep, you'll be more likely to fall asleep when you get under the covers for the night.

4 Tame your tummy. Going to bed either hungry or too full can disrupt your sleep. Don't have a big meal too close to bedtime or the digestion process might keep you awake. Also, if you lie down after stuffing yourself you can end up with gastric reflux—stomach acid backing up into the esophagus. If you're hungry, have a snack rich in carbohydrates, which trigger the release of the brain chemical serotonin, associated with relaxation. Try a graham cracker or bowl of cereal. Pair it with some milk or a slice of turkey, both rich in the amino acid tryptophan, which also induces sleep.

5 Watch the caffeine. Too much caffeine throughout the day, even if it's not consumed right before bedtime, can contribute to fitful slumber. Once you hit 50, your metabolism slows, so caffeine may stay in your system longer—up to 10 hours. Limit yourself to two cups of tea, coffee, or cola, taken at least 6 hours before bedtime. If that doesn't work, try cutting out caffeine altogether.

6 Tap the exercise answer. It's a simple fact: If you're physically tired at the end of the day, you'll sleep better. In a study from Stanford University School of Medicine, a group of 50- to 76-year-olds who had complained of sleep problems began moderate exercise for about half an hour four times a week. Compared with a similar group of people who didn't exercise, the more active group slept an average of one hour

SimpleSolution

Wearing socks to bed may not look sexy, but it could help you get a date with the sandman. A study reported in the journal *Nature* found that participants whose hands and feet were toastier fell asleep faster. Why? Warming your extremities increases blood flow to those areas, rerouting it from your internal organs and lowering your core body temperature—a prerequisite for nodding off.

more each night, took less time to fall asleep, spent less time napping, and reported an overall improvement in sleep quality. Outdoor exercise is especially helpful. By exposing yourself to sunlight (particularly in the afternoon), you help prevent midday sleepiness and reinforce your body's circadian rhythms (your 24-hour body clock). Exercise at least three hours before bedtime.

7 **Soak it up.** Take a warm bath an hour or two before bed. Your body temperature will slowly drop after you get out of the tub, making you feel tired. Don't bathe right before bed, however, because it can briefly stimulate you enough to make it hard to fall asleep.

8 **Drift off naturally.** Investigate the benefits of chamomile, valerian, kava, passionflower, skullcap, catnip, or hops. These herbs can be taken in tea and other forms. A cup of chamomile tea before bedtime may be all you need to relax. If you're trying valerian, the suggested dose for the concentrated form is equal to two to three grams of the root a day. But don't combine valerian with alcohol or mood-regulating drugs. If you're using kava, try a dose of between 60 and 120 mg before bedtime.

9 **Don't toss and turn.** If 30 minutes go by and you haven't fallen asleep, don't lie in bed feeling frustrated. Get up and do something relaxing, like listening to soothing music or flipping through a magazine. Or make yourself a cup of warm milk.

10 **Buy the right bed.** A bed that's too soft can cause poor sleep postures (which can also lead to muscle stiffness and back problems). If you're leaving a divot in the mattress when you get up, it's too soft. Replace your mattress if it's more than 10 years old, and buy one that's as firm as you can tolerate but still comfortable.

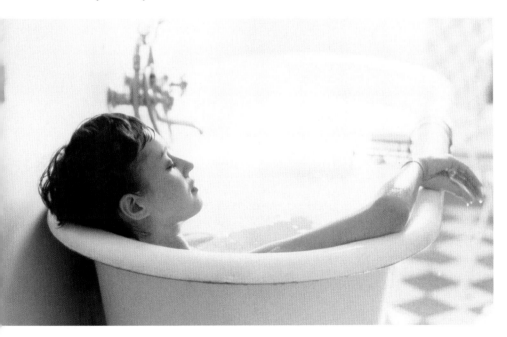

Adding soothing essential oils like rose, lavender, or marjoram to your bathwater can make a prebedtime soak even more relaxing. Mix the oil in a carrier oil, such as vegetable oil, before adding.

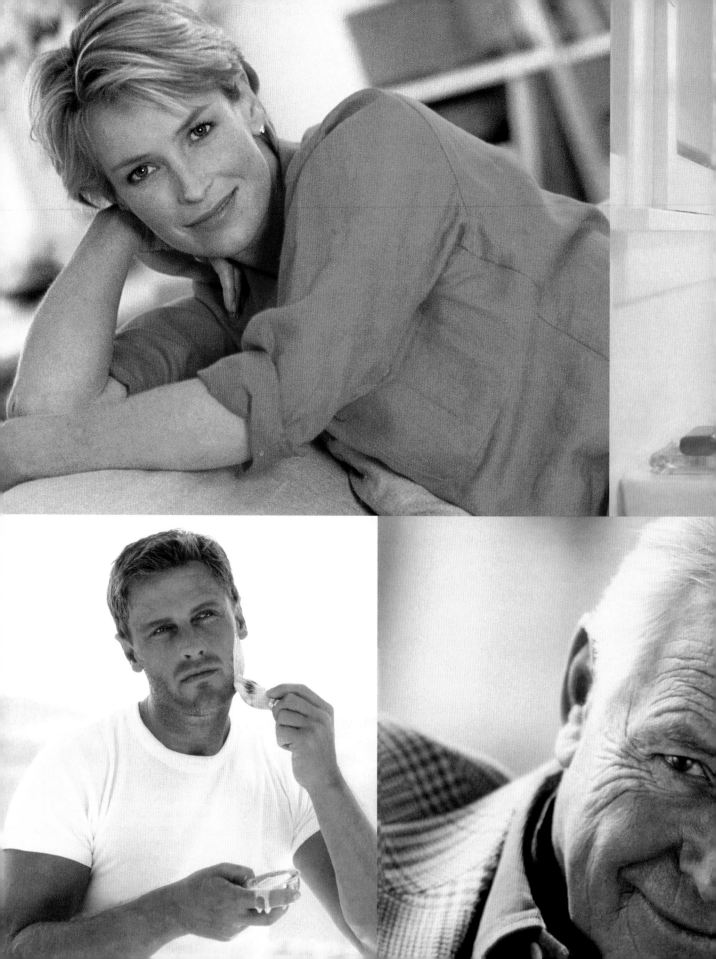

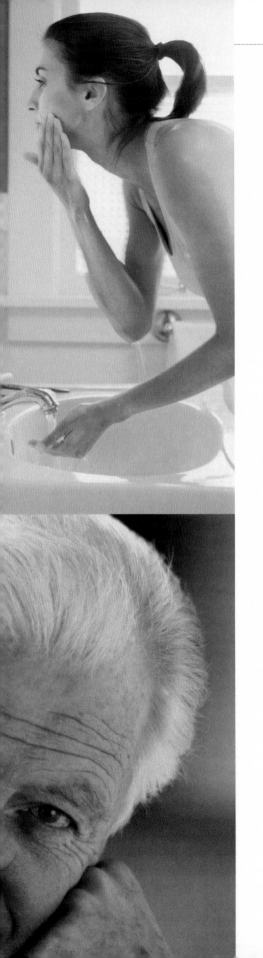

CHAPTER 12

LOOKING GREAT

Putting Your Best Skin Forward

Does your skin look older than it should? It's not too late to put the brakes on the aging process—and maybe even reclaim that youthful bloom.

If you want to look your best—and who doesn't—what should you think about first? Your skin. Skin that's healthy looking (with or without wrinkles) radiates a youthful glow no matter what your age. On the other hand, skin that shows the telltale signs of a poor diet, a nicotine habit, or too much time in the sun can add years to your appearance.

Why Does Your Skin Look Older?

You may think you're seeing the same old face every morning, but you're not. Your skin's top layer, the epidermis, replaces itself about every 27 days through washing and friction. Your new exterior is created below, in the much thicker second layer, the dermis. In this layer are collagen, the ropelike protein fibers that support the skin, and elastin, protein fibers that provide elasticity. There is also a protective cushion of fat, which creates the pleasing contours that fill out and shape your face and body.

As your skin ages, collagen and elastin break down, and your subcutaneous fat shrinks, making the bony areas of your face more prominent. The skin becomes thinner, making tiny blood vessels and any uneven coloration easier to see. With time and gravity, this thinner, less elastic skin begins to sag. Repeated smiling and frowning also leave their marks.

Basic Skin TLC

No amount of creams, lotions, or cosmetic procedures can do as much for your skin as a nutritious diet and

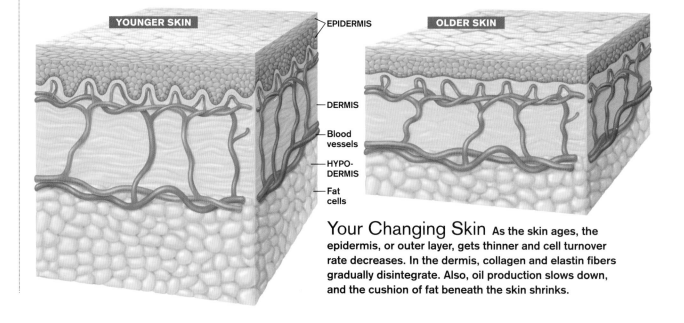

YOUNGER SKIN   EPIDERMIS

DERMIS

Blood vessels

HYPO-DERMIS

Fat cells

OLDER SKIN

Your Changing Skin As the skin ages, the epidermis, or outer layer, gets thinner and cell turnover rate decreases. In the dermis, collagen and elastin fibers gradually disintegrate. Also, oil production slows down, and the cushion of fat beneath the skin shrinks.

The sun is to blame for up to 90 percent of wrinkles, not to mention the dreaded leathery look.

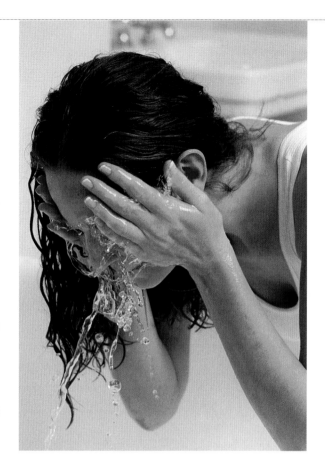

exercise. For radiant, youthful-looking skin, you need a regular supply of all the basic nutrients, including protein, fat, vitamins, minerals, and plenty of water. The antioxidant vitamins (such as E, C, and A) are especially important since they help counter the effects of free radicals, those unstable oxygen molecules that are thought to accelerate aging by causing cell and tissue damage.

Exercise is also important because it pumps more oxygen-rich blood through your body, which speeds the elimination of toxins and expedites the growth of new cells. Your skin needs about 7 percent of the oxygen you take in. If you exercise less as you get older, you will take in less oxygen—and your skin will show it.

Avoiding the Skin Wreckers

Taking care of your skin also means avoiding the things that can ruin its appearance.

- **Too much sun.** The sun is to blame for up to 90 percent of wrinkles, not to mention the dreaded leathery look. Ultraviolet rays break down the underlying structure of skin and damage cell membranes and DNA. They also boost the production of enzymes that break down collagen. Though wearing sunscreen won't reverse existing damage, it can help prevent further wrinkling and also protect

against skin cancer. See *Screening Yourself from the Sun,* page 275, for sunscreen tips.

- **Smoking.** As if you needed another reason to quit, smoking is a curse to your skin. It constricts blood vessels, decreasing blood flow and depriving skin of some of the oxygen it needs. It also introduces toxins and steps up free-radical damage to a super-charged pace. For help in quitting, see pages 166-173.

- **Too much alcohol.** Because alcoholic beverages dehydrate the body, overindulgence can leave your skin looking drier and older. For better overall health, limit your intake to no more than one drink a day if you're a woman, two if you're a man, and offset the dehydration by drinking plenty of water throughout the day.

Gentle cycle: If your skin is very dry, washing your face once a day may be enough.

SimpleSolution

Skin too dry? Take shorter showers, and adjust the tap to luke-warm. Most women shower for about 12 minutes—twice as long as necessary. Prolonged exposure to hot water strips skin of oil and replaces it with water, which leaves skin drier as it evaporates.

SimpleSolution

To keep skin from drying out, use a humidifier to put moisture back in the air that air-conditioning and winter heating take out.

● **Too little sleep.** They don't call it beauty sleep for nothing: During sleep, the body regenerates collagen and keratin (a protein in the skin's top layer). Lack of sleep can dull the complexion and make those dark circles under your eyes worse. Raising the head of your bed by putting blocks under the legs may help reduce under-eye puffiness by allowing fluid that collects there to drain away.

● **Too much stress.** Skin breakouts are common when you're under stress, and even without them, your skin can look pale or ruddy and drawn. Relaxation techniques—and vacations, of course—can do a world of good. Treat yourself to a face or body massage. It will not only help you relax, but also improve blood and lymph circulation, accelerate the elimination of toxins, and speed the delivery of oxygen and nutrients to your skin.

Simple Skin Care

Caring for your skin doesn't have to involve a lot of expensive products or even much effort. In fact, many people do more harm than good to their skin by using harsh soaps and

Good Skin Food

You are what you eat, as they say, and nothing shows it more quickly than your skin. For that radiant glow, make sure you get enough of the following:

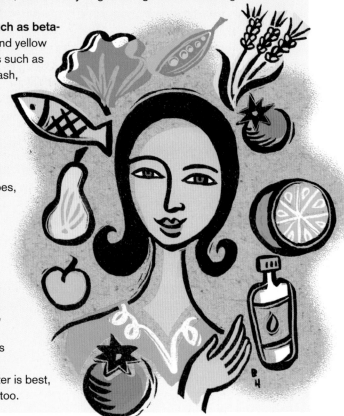

● **For carotenoids (such as beta-carotene):** orange and yellow fruits and vegetables such as apricots, yellow squash, sweet potatoes
● **For B vitamins:** liver, sardines, eggs, whole-grain cereals
● **For vitamin C:** citrus fruits, strawberries, tomatoes, green vegetables
● **For vitamin E:** vegetable oil, green leafy vegetables, whole-grain cereals, wheat germ
● **For essential fatty acids:** salmon, trout, mackerel, tuna, supplements such as evening primrose oil
● **For water:** Plain water is best, but fruit juices help, too.

abrasive masks and washing too often. For most people, here's the only daily routine you need.

1 Cleanse Wash your face once or twice a day with a mild, nonfoaming soap (such as Dove) or cleansing lotion (such as Trifan). Use your hands, not a washcloth, which can be rough on the skin and may also harbor bacteria. Steer clear of buffing pads and face scrubs, which strip skin of its protective layer and boost oil production, encouraging breakouts. If your skin is oily, wash twice a day with a mild pH-balanced liquid cleanser that's astringent enough to lift grease.

2 Tone If you use an astringent or clarifying lotion after cleansing, choose one that's vinegar-based (to soften the skin and relieve itchiness) over one that contains alcohol, which is drying.

3 Moisturize Apply moisturizer after showering, while skin is still damp. Moisturizers don't actually add moisture to the skin, they simply help lock in the moisture that's already there. If your skin is dry, choose an oil-based product. If your skin is oily, look for a water-based lotion. There's no need to choose an expensive brand; price is not an accurate gauge of effectiveness. Apply any product gently around the eyes since skin there is thinner and more likely to wrinkle as a result of repeated tugging.

If your skin is sensitive or prone to redness or chapping, use an over-the-counter anti-itch moisturizing lotion, such as Sarna-P, or keep skin soft with a mild, nonirritating product such as Aveeno lotion.

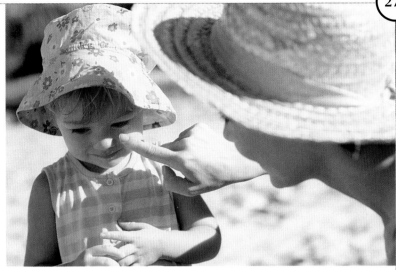

Screening Yourself from the Sun

Sunscreen is your ticket to young-looking skin. Be sure to use it—and use it properly.

Don't skimp on sunscreen—most people apply too little. Use it daily, regardless of season or weather, and reapply it often for best protection.

- **Wear sunscreen daily,** rain or shine, summer or winter. Don't assume fog, mist, or clouds will shade you, since 80 percent of the sun's rays penetrate them. And don't rely solely on protection from a beach umbrella or wide-brimmed hat, since 85 percent of rays bounce off sand, water, snow, and concrete. Also use sunscreen if you sit near a window at the office or home, since UVA rays penetrate glass.
- **Choose a broad spectrum sunscreen** to guard against the longer UVA rays associated with aging and the shorter UVB rays that cause most skin cancer. Opt for a product with a sun-protection factor, or SPF, of 15 or greater, meaning it will take 15 times as long for your skin to burn. Non-greasy formulas are available for people with oily skin.
- **Slather it on.** Dermatologists recommend using about an ounce of

WARNING

Don't take your face to just anyone. Choose a physician who is accredited by the Royal College of Physicians and Surgeons (the body that accredits specialists in Canada.) For help finding a specialist in dermatology in your area, contact

- *Canadian Dermatology Association in Ottawa, at 613-730-6262. They will provide you with a list of dermatologists to choose from.*
- *The Canadian Society for Aesthetic (Cosmetic) Plastic Surgery at 1-800-263-4429, www.csaps.ca. This web site contains information about procedures and locating a specialist in your city.*

product on your face, ears, and neck—much more than most people use. Apply it about 30 minutes before going outside to give the skin time to absorb it, and reapply every two to three hours.

- **Hands-down protection.** The skin on your hands is thin, which is one reason the hands are among the first areas to show signs of sun damage. To prevent age spots and wrinkles, don't skip your mitts when you apply sunscreen.
- **Pay lip service.** To guard your lips from the sun, use a lip balm or lipstick that contains sunscreen. Squamous cell skin cancer is most aggressive when it strikes the lips.
- **Run for cover at noon.** When possible, stay out of the sun from 10 A.M. to 3 P.M., when the sun's rays are at their strongest.

Wrinkle Relief

Even if you're careful in the sun, some wrinkles are inevitable with age. But you don't have to accept them without a fight. While you probably can't erase your wrinkles completely, there's plenty you can do to make them less noticeable.

- **Tretinoin.** Originally used to treat acne, tretinoin sloughs away dead skin cells, allowing new cells to rise to the surface. It also boosts production of collagen, the spongy tissue beneath the skin's surface. Tretinoin topical preparations (such as Retin-A and Renova) can soften wrinkles, reduce blotchiness, and even reverse signs of sun damage. It may also make the skin look firmer.

  You'll need a doctor's prescription for either Retin-A or Renova,

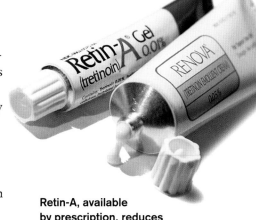

Retin-A, available by prescription, reduces the appearance of fine lines, wrinkles, and age spots. Renova contains the same active ingredient combined with an emollient, and may be gentler on sun-damaged skin.

a product that combines retinoic acid with an emollient so it's less drying than Retin-A. With consistent use, you'll see results within months. Even with just a pea-size drop, the skin usually tingles and turns red and may even peel in the first few weeks of treatment. Excessive amounts can cause small capillary rupture over time. Because these products make your skin more sensitive to the sun, use them only at night, and be sure to wear sunscreen during the day.

- **Don't count on retinol.** This ingredient is found in many over-the-counter skin-care products. It's often listed on the label as vitamin A or retinol palmitate. Despite what the label may say, there are no human studies that support any anti-aging claims.
- **For a gentler approach, try AHAs.** Alpha hydroxy acids, or AHAs, also referred to as glycolic acids, are fruit acids that slough off dead skin and speed up cell renewal. Various products contain different concentrations of AHAs. Products sold over the counter have

concentrations of less than 10 percent. When using these, be patient; it can take up to six months for them to soften fine lines. Some products contain higher concentrations, which may actually thicken the skin's dermis, as tretinoin preparations do. Like tretinoin products, these may be strong enough to cause irritation.

AHAs increase the skin's sensitivity to sunlight, so it's important to wear sunscreen. Don't use AHAs around the delicate tissues of the eyes unless the cream is specially formulated for that area. Stick to one product at a time (don't combine tretinoin preparations and AHAs). And don't go overboard; a dime-size amount is enough for the whole face.

● **Look to estrogen.** While no one should take estrogen purely for the fringe benefits, it's true that women undergoing hormone replacement therapy are less likely to have wrinkles. One reason is that estrogen counteracts the slowdown of oil-producing glands that normally comes with age. And according to one study, women who took estrogen for a year increased their skin's thickness by 12 percent.

Tackling Liver Spots

Despite their name, liver spots, also called age spots, have nothing to do with the liver and little to do with age, although they tend to appear in people over age 55. These small, dark patches that develop on the face and hands are the result of cumulative sun exposure.

If you want to minimize liver spots, bleaching creams can be effective with extended use. Products range from mild over-the-counter brands (it may take about six months of use to see a difference) to much stronger prescription creams. No matter which you try, also use a sunscreen or the spots won't budge.

Tretinoin preparations can improve the quality of damaged skin in general and may lighten spots. Or the spots may be frozen off with liquid nitrogen. A chemical peel or laser resurfacing (see pages 280-281) may also help. See your dermatologist.

Don't confuse age spots with hyperpigmentation, an unusual darkening of the skin that can be a sign of an adrenal insufficiency or a side effect of certain medications. If your age spots are larger than a quarter, irregularly colored from light to medium brown, or as dark as black coffee, alert your doctor.

Over-the-counter anti-wrinkle products may or may not be strong enough to soften fine lines, and you'll have to use them for long periods to see any change. The ones available through a dermatologist are much stronger and more effective.

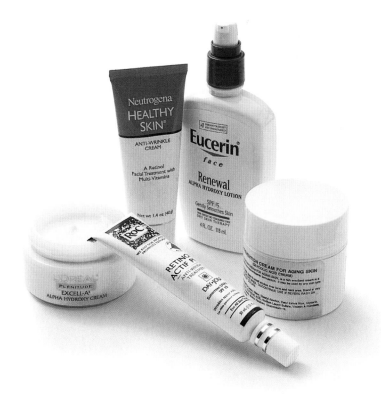

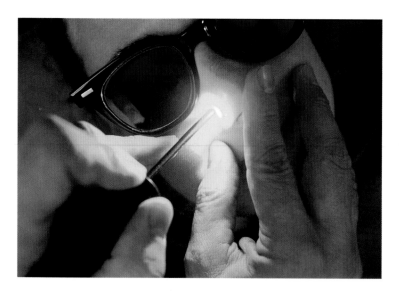

Laser treatment can be effective in eliminating broken capillaries around the nose and cheeks.

Fast Fact

Having 50 to 100 or more moles doubles your risk of skin cancer. If you've had four irregular moles larger than the diameter of a pencil eraser, your risk jumps 28-fold.

Itsy Bitsy Spider Veins

Spider veins, those hair-thin networks of bluish-purple veins and red capillaries that form near the skin's surface, are of little consequence medically. (Unlike spider veins, varicose veins bulge toward the surface of the skin on the legs and may throb or itch.) But if you find them unsightly, you can banish them with help from your dermatologist.

Sclerotherapy is the most widely used treatment for spider veins on the legs and thighs. After numbing the area, a saline (saltwater) solution is injected in the veins. The solution inflames the lining of the veins and makes them collapse, and the veins are ultimately reabsorbed into the body. There's little adverse reaction to the saline, though more than one treatment is usually necessary.

Laser procedures also can be effective. The energy of a specific wavelength of light heats and collapses these small blood vessels without affecting surrounding tissue. A typical laser session might run $100 to $150. More than one session may be required.

To prevent more spider veins from forming, break the habit of crossing your legs. Avoid standing for long periods and limit high-impact activities such as running.

Ugh! Cellulite

You've seen it. You loathe it: that dimpled skin (the orange-peel effect) that can develop around a woman's kneecaps, thighs, and buttocks. Cellulite is simply fat under the skin. The fat becomes dimpled when adhesions of fibrous connective tissue under the skin pull it down, pushing up the fat on either side, much like a tufted quilt. No one knows exactly what causes this to occur, although age, gender, and heredity seem to play a role, affecting the strength of the connective fibers and the thickness of the skin. (Women tend to have thinner skin than men, so fat pockets are more visible.)

Is there a cure? Some creams supposedly reduce the appearance of cellulite, but there is no reliable evidence that these products work, and most experts agree they don't. Liposuction removes fat, but it can damage the fine network of capillaries, lymph vessels, and collagen fibers, setting the stage for the return of cellulite. Skin with cellulite may actually look worse after treatment.

While there are no miracle cures for cellulite, exercise helps, especially strength training. Losing weight may also help, although there are plenty of thin women with cellulite, so there's no guarantee. In the meantime, drink plenty of water to hydrate your cells, and consider applying a self-tanning lotion to make your thighs—and the rest of you—appear slimmer.

Seeing Red

Rosacea is a condition marked by mild flushing and facial redness, along with pimples and tiny red streaks from dilated blood vessels. The cause is unknown. Rosacea is harmless, but can it be unsightly. In men, rosacea usually centers on the nose, often making it appear bulbous. Onset is usually at age 35 to 50.

Your dermatologist can prescribe an antibiotic, either in ointment or pill form, that will control rosacea, but the condition may return after you stop taking the medication.

To help prevent rosacea from returning, avoid direct sunlight and beauty products that contain fragrances, alcohol, witch hazel, menthol, and oils of peppermint and eucalyptus, all of which may aggravate the condition. Limit your intake of foods and beverages that cause blood vessels to dilate, including alcohol, spicy foods, caffeine, and hot drinks. Reducing stress can also help.

Here are a few natural approaches that are worth a try.

- Counter inflammation with omega-3 fatty acids, found in oily fish (such as mackerel and salmon), flaxseed oil, and evening primrose oil. Try taking 1,000 mg of evening primrose oil three times a day or 1 tablespoon of flaxseed oil a day.

- Be sure to get enough vitamin A, which supports healthy skin. Check your multivitamin and make sure that it contains 5,000 IU. If you're already getting enough of the vitamin and rosacea persists, taking a separate supplement of 15,000 IU a day may help minimize flare-ups.

- Also be sure to get enough of the B vitamins; a deficiency is common in people with rosacea.

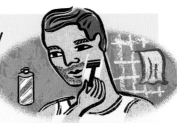

For Men Only

Men have their own skin-care issues and may not want to shop around for answers. Here are some solutions geared for you:

PROBLEM	SOLUTION
A cabinet full of products	■ Use an all-in-one cleansing gel. If it contains an alpha hydroxy acid, it can remove dead skin cells and heal razor bumps and ingrown hairs. Also look for a multifunctional shower product—a scalp-face-body wash that contains clay to absorb excess oils.
Razor burn	■ Prevent it by softening your beard with a preshave softener. Shave in the shower or after your shower, and follow up with an aftershave balm for protection.
Blackheads	■ Start with a cleanser with alpha hydroxy acid to remove dead surface cells that may plug pores, and finish with a "scrub" or "scruffing" lotion that uses abrasive particles to unblock pores and prevent blemishes and ingrown hairs. You can also switch to a moisturizer for oily skin—it may contain antibacterial ingredients and salicylic acid, both of which discourage blemishes.

Playing Skin Tag

Healthy skin may develop skin tags—small, soft, flesh-colored flaps that usually appear on the neck, armpits, or groin. Skin tags are easily removed by a doctor by freezing them with liquid nitrogen.

Seborrheic keratoses are harmless dark or flesh-colored pebbly nodules that may appear anywhere on the skin but usually on the face, temples, or torso. They are more common in older people. A doctor can remove them by freezing them off with liquid nitrogen or cutting them out with a scalpel under local anesthesia.

Fast Fixes

What if you want to take a more aggressive approach to younger-looking skin? A quick nonsurgical cosmetic procedure might work for you. Once the exclusive domain of the rich and famous, these procedures (sometimes called "nooners" because they can be done in a lunch hour) are now more common among ordinary folk. In the U.S. alone, almost 5 million such procedures were performed in 1999, up a whopping 66 percent from the previous year according to the American Society for Aesthetic Plastic Surgery. Most popular

PROCEDURE	WHAT IT IS	PROS
Botox injections	■ Botox is a paralyzing poison that's safe when used in minute doses. Injected into eyebrow furrows, crow's feet, and forehead and neck creases, it binds to the nerve endings of muscles to inactivate them. Once the muscle is immobilized, lines on the skin surface smooth out.	■ Removes the tired, angry look. Shots take less than three minutes and leave no scars, stitches, or hospital bills. Only a topical anesthetic is used, enough to counter the sting of the shots. Swelling lasts a half hour or less, though it takes two days to two weeks to see results.
Microdermabrasion	■ Known as the "power peel," this procedure involves a device that moves a fine spray of aluminum oxide particles over the face, neck, chest, and hands to sand away lines and lighten brown spots and other skin imperfections.	■ This skin-smoother and brightener is noninvasive. It involves no laser and no recovery time. Improvement is gradual, generally taking 6 to 10 treatments before change is visible. Results are permanent.
Chemical peel	■ An acid solution is swabbed onto the skin to remove the entire epidermis, or outer layer, and perhaps some of the dermis, or inner layer, too. The depth of the peel depends on the strength of the acid, which is generally about 20 times stronger than most AHAs. It's typically left on for two minutes.	■ Lightens or even removes fine lines and smoothes out the skin. If a strong enough acid is used, it can lighten or remove liver spots and freckles, too.
Laser resurfacing	■ A beam of light vaporizes a few layers of skin (more when the laser passes over several times) to remove discolorations, wrinkles, and surface irregularities. Laser resurfacing also may stimulate collagen growth so wrinkles and depressions fill in naturally, leading to smoother skin.	■ You get results with a speedy, in-office procedure.
Line fillers	■ Collagen extracted from cow tissue or grown from your own tissue in a lab is injected into facial lines, smile creases, and acne scars to make skin appear smoother. The same material can also be used to plump lips.	■ Injections in the doctor's office are quick and require only a topical anesthetic. Results last up to a year.

of all are chemical peels and Botox injections. In 1999, nearly half a million people underwent Botox treatment—about 11 percent of them male.

What's the best procedure for you? Here are five of the top options. Your choice depends on the depth of your wrinkles—and your pockets, since cosmetic surgery is rarely covered by insurance. Make sure you discuss all the pros and cons of any procedure with your dermatologist before moving ahead.

CONS	COST	BOTTOM LINE
It's disconcerting, to say the least, to think that you're being injected with a deadly toxin which, in much larger doses, can paralyze you from head to toe. Poor placement can lead to droopy brows or lids, though this occurs in only 2 percent of cases and can be corrected.	Typical treatment is about $500.	Injections last three to four months and then must be repeated, so over time you may spend more than you would on a face-lift.
Can cause some redness, lasting only about 10 minutes. Don't even think of combining this with an acid peel on the same day.	$125 to $250	Makeup goes on smoother, surface lines disappear, and any discoloration is evened out.
Recovery can take a while for deeper peels. Skin may remain crusty for two weeks and then red and unnaturally shiny for several months. Pain, infection, and scarring are possible side effects. Not everyone's skin is tough enough to handle the assault. (People with sensitive skin should consider a gentler, less expensive option, the glycolic peel, at $50 to $170.)	$200 to $300 for acid peel	This procedure may be for you only if you can afford to go into hiding for at least two weeks while your skin recovers.
Overaggressive blasting can burn and scar. It does not correct sagging, and redness can last for up to three months, no matter how skilled the expert treating you.	$800 (upper lip) to $4,000 (full face)	This procedure is now considered safer and more effective than dermabrasion, but it's more expensive. And you'll still want to make sure you choose a highly qualified doctor to perform it.
Allergic reactions are possible unless your own tissue is used. If you go too far in the quest for youth, you may remind yourself of an aging starlet.	$350 to $600, (consultation, allergy test if bovine collagen is being used, and treatment). Higher cost if your own tissue is used.	The results depend on the doctor's skill, so to avoid lumps and bumps, seek out an expert.

Perfecting Your Smile

Are you sure you don't have gum disease? Now that it's considered a risk factor for heart attacks, it's high time to find out.

It's easy to skip brushing and flossing your teeth. After all, it's not like those 5 to 10 minutes a day can save your life, right? Wrong. What you can't see can hurt you—and maybe already has.

The Heart of the Matter

According to the Canadian Dental Association, 9 out of 10 Canadians will develop gum disease at some point in their life. Early gum disease, or gingivitis, starts as plaque, a colorless film made of bacteria, mucus, and food particles that forms around the gums and on teeth. Plaque can irritate the gums, causing swelling and infection. Once the gums swell, a pocket forms between the gum and the tooth that becomes a trap for

more plaque. If left untreated, gingivitis may extend below the gums and eat away at the bone that surrounds your teeth. This advanced stage is called periodontitis.

Periodontitis may result in lost teeth—and that's not the biggest health threat it poses. Gum disease is also linked to our three principal killers: heart disease, diabetes, and lung disease. In fact, it doubles your risk for heart attack, making it the second leading risk factor behind smoking, as reported in *The New England Journal of Medicine*.

How can periodontitis affect your heart? The bacteria that attack your teeth also enter the bloodstream, possibly leading to infection of the heart. As part of the body's attempt to destroy the bacteria, it forms

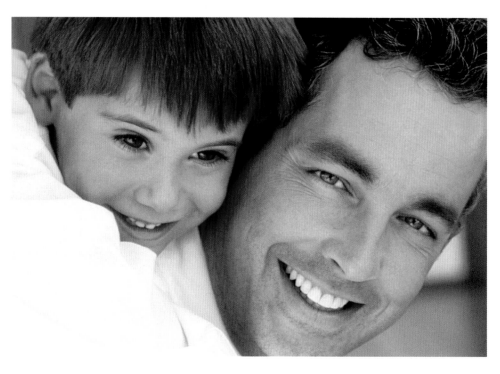

Want a winning smile? Ask your dentist about prescription-strength fluoride rinses and treatments. Studies show they are just as effective in adults as in children and adolescents at keeping teeth and gums healthy.

blood clots, which can block arteries and cause a heart attack or stroke.

Advanced gum disease can also exacerbate type 2 diabetes by impairing insulin processing, making blood-sugar levels more difficult to control. (Diabetes also increases the risk for gum disease.) Periodontitis has also been associated with a sevenfold rise in osteoporosis and a twofold hike in bronchitis.

Could you have gum disease and not know it? Check out the symptoms and risk factors on page 348.

Polish Your Technique

To save your teeth (and maybe your heart), you don't have to go far—just to your bathroom cabinet. Brushing and flossing prevent tooth loss and, if done well, can keep gum disease at bay. For best results, follow these tips:

● Get a dental checkup and a professional cleaning to remove hardened plaque every six months (or more often if your dentist recommends it for you).

● Hold your toothbrush at a 45-degree angle to your teeth and gums and use gentle back-and-forth strokes. Hold it vertically to clean the inside surfaces of your front teeth. Don't forget to brush your tongue to remove odor-causing bacteria.

● Use a tartar-control toothpaste that contains fluoride and triclosan (an antibacterial ingredient) if your dentist advises. Pastes with chlorine dioxide or tea tree oil also have germicidal properties.

● Use floss and rubber tips to remove the plaque that builds up around gums. To get the most out of flossing, curve the floss in a C shape against your tooth when

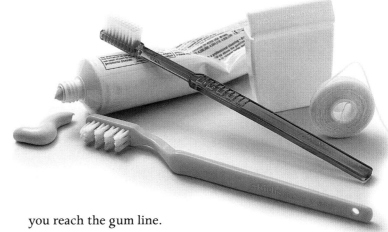

you reach the gum line. Gently slide the thread into the space between tooth and gum, holding the floss snugly against the tooth and moving it up and down. Remember to floss the backside of your back teeth.

Repairing the Damage

If you already suffer from advanced gum disease, your dentist or periodontist may give you oral or local antibiotics. He may also perform scaling and root planing, a technique in which the gum is moved back so that hardened plaque can be removed from roots and inflamed gums. These procedures can reduce the need to extract teeth from diseased jaws by 88 percent.

There's also a new technique that allows dentists to remove diseased gum without losing as much healthy tissue as in the past. Called laser excisional new attachment procedure, or LENAP, it costs up to $2,000 for each arch, or set, of upper and lower teeth.

If you've already lost some teeth, dental implants can bridge the gaps, provided you have enough bone left to support them. Comfortable and natural looking, these metal (usually titanium) implants are anchored permanently into the jaw by your

Brush thoroughly for two to three minutes using a soft-bristled brush with a small head that reaches easily into the corners of your mouth. Replace your toothbrush when the bristles begin to fray or after you've had a cold.

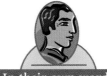

In their own words

"Some day not too far from now, the American Heart Association will add gum disease to the list of risk factors for heart disease. It is up there with smoking."
—Fredric Pashkow, M.D., Professor of Medicine, University of Hawaii

WARNING

According to the Canadian Dental Association, bleaching kits sold OTC in stores stay on your teeth longer than whitening toothpaste. However, these kits do not come with the added safety of having a dentist monitor any side effects. And the one-size-fits-all mouth trays can allow the chemical to seep into gums and cause irritation.

natural bone and are taking the place of traditional bridges and dentures for people who can afford them. A bonus: They prevent the bone loss and visible aging associated with dentures.

A Whiter Smile

It isn't just the pages of a book that yellow with time. Teeth can turn an unattractive shade that can make you look older. How does it happen? The tooth's protective colorless enamel thins with each passing year, allowing the yellow dentin underneath to show through. Eating sugary foods speeds the process by turning your saliva more acidic, which makes the enamel more porous. This permits residue from berries, colas, coffee, tea, and red wine to seep through and stain the teeth. Tartar deposits can also cause discoloration, as can smoking.

If you are dreaming of a whiter smile, you're not alone. The American Academy of Cosmetic Dentistry reported the number of patients requesting whitening procedures has tripled over the last five years. To brighten your pearly whites, you have several options. Note that these cosmetic procedures are not usually covered by insurance.

● **Power bleaching,** also called "chairside bleaching," is the most popular whitening procedure. Your dentist shields the inside of your mouth and gums with a protective barrier, applies a whitening gel (containing 20 to 35 percent hydrogen peroxide) to the teeth, and may use a powerful light source to activate the bleaching agent. (Lasers are also approved for in-office whitening, but many dentists are waiting for long-term safety and effectiveness data before using them.) Brown and yellowish stains respond best; gray tetracycline stains respond poorly. People with hypersensitive teeth and mouth tissue are probably not good candidates. The total cost is $600 to $1,500, and results last one to three years.

● **Home bleaching,** or "nightguard bleaching," can be done at home with your dentist's help. He'll take impressions of your upper and lower teeth and fashion molds or trays that resemble an athletic mouthguard. You'll receive a supply of whitening solution to apply to the trays. It's a less concentrated form of the in-office bleaching solution, usually 10 percent carbamide peroxide, which becomes 3 percent hydrogen peroxide in the mouth. You wear the trays for an hour or two a day, or overnight, depending on your sensitivity to the procedure. The treatment takes about two weeks (longer for tobacco

Preview the New You

You don't have to guess how you'd look after braces or bleaching or caps. Hundreds of cosmetic dentists and orthodontists now offer high-tech computer imaging that gives you a preview of your new look, usually at no fee. You can also mail in photos showing your smile in front and side views to the American Association of Orthodontists (AAO), and they'll send you back an altered view. To learn more, contact the AAO at 800STRAIGHT or find them online at www.braces.org.

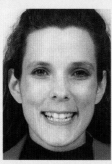
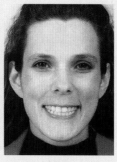

Before   **After**

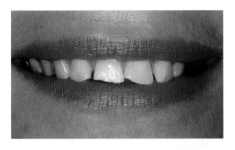

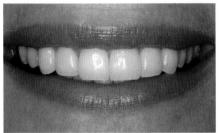

Amazing transformation: Say goodbye to chipped or uneven teeth with the help of caps, also called laminates or veneers.

stains). The price tag: $300 to $800. Results are about as long-lasting as with power bleaching, but you can reuse the molds later for at-home touch-ups.

● **Whitening toothpastes** contain chemical or polishing agents to remove surface stains from the teeth. The Canadian Dental Association gives its seal to a number of these products on the basis that they will help with caries control, and prevention and reduction of gingivitis.

Cap It Off

Ever wonder how celebrities achieve their million-dollar smiles? Many are fitted with porcelain veneers, also called laminates or "caps." Like fake nails for the teeth, these thin, custom-made shells of tooth-colored material are bonded permanently to your true ivories. Teeth must be filed and prepared to accommodate these shells, an irreversible process. Veneers

last about 15 years and are a dramatic solution for gaps, crooked teeth, and discolored teeth. They can even correct sunken cheeks or make lips appear fuller. Call it plastic surgery without a knife. It's about as expensive: about $800 to $2,000 per tooth.

A Bonding Experience

Another way to fix gaps is with bonding. In this procedure, a cosmetic dentist trims or builds up your teeth with composite resin that looks like natural tooth enamel. Bonding can be used to close gaps, even tooth length, and repair chipped teeth. It's a more conservative procedure than veneers and costs less, about $300 to $700 per tooth. It can last five years or more before needing repair. One negative: You can't whiten bonded teeth, which are susceptible to staining. If you choose bonding, have your teeth cleaned more frequently.

Brace Yourself

If you think braces are just for kids, think again. Today, about a third of people who opt for orthodontics are adults. One reason is that braces aren't nearly as noticeable as they used to be. Clear plastic wiring and tooth-colored ceramic brackets are now available to correct a bad bite and straighten crooked teeth. These braces cost about $300 more than traditional metal ones.

If you choose metal, new wiring made of nickel and titanium can cut straightening time by a third, to as little as six months, at no additional cost. Heat from the mouth strengthens the wire that is strung across all the teeth, making teeth move faster and more comfortably.

Fast Fact

Cosmetic dentists now are using lasers to even out, raise, and lighten gums. The transformation can take as little as 30 seconds and costs about $100 per tooth.

SimpleSolution

To avoid staining your teeth, use a straw to drink beverages such as iced coffee, iced tea, colas, and grape juice. Brush your teeth or rinse with water afterward. Using a straw also helps protect exposed tooth surfaces from decay caused by acidic and sugary beverages.

Great Hair Hints

If you prefer your silver in a jewelry chest, there's no reason to go gray. If you're happy with your steely shag, learn how to make it shine.

Most likely, you've noticed a gray hair or two—or 200. If you love your gray, great. After all, a silvery mane can be a stunning asset, a mark of distinction. But if you prefer your former color, you're not alone. According to some estimates, 64 percent of North American women between ages 35 and 49 color their hair specifically to cover gray. For women ages 50 to 69, the figure is 74 percent. And men represent the fastest-growing segment of the hair-care industry.

Color Me Younger

If you're ready for a change of hue and you're only partially gray, consider highlighting (which bleaches the gray and adds new color to it) or lowlighting (applying color to the gray). For best results, see a colorist. (For extra shine and conditioning, ask your hairdresser to add a light-reflecting cellophane gloss.) If you want to do it yourself, there are several brands of no-mess, mistake-proof coloring products that can also be used on beards and mustaches. Do an allergy patch test 48 hours prior to coloring and a strand test to determine timing and to judge the color against your complexion.

Best-Tressed Coloring Tips
Follow these pointers to ensure flattering, long-lasting hair color:
- Before coloring, wash your hair with a clarifying shampoo that removes mineral deposits, toxins, and styling-product residue and promotes better color absorption.
- If you want to cover your gray, choose a color a shade or two lighter than your natural color. (Skin tends to wash out with age and dark hair makes it look paler.)
- If you're left with a pinkish cast, the dye didn't fully penetrate the hair shaft. Don't panic. Just reapply, leaving the color on an extra 10 to 40 minutes. Also, choose a slightly darker and more ashen shade, rather than a copper, auburn, or golden hue.
- Use a color-extending shampoo and shield your hair from the sun, salt water, and chlorinated water.

If gray hair makes you feel old, get rid of it. Otherwise, show it off with a great haircut, and wear colors that flatter it.

Polish That Silver

To keep your gray from yellowing, avoid curling irons and hot rollers. To make your gray brighter and shinier, consider using a "gray-enhancing" shampoo. Look for one that contains essential oils of sweet violet, clover, or citric acid, all of which bring out the best in gray and neutralize any yellow.

Putting Moisture Back In

Like skin, hair loses moisture with age, and with it, luster and bounce. Here's how to counter these effects:

- **Use a mild shampoo** that contains fatty acids, balsams, moisturizers, or protein. Although these protein-rich products can't actually feed the dead keratin cells that make up your hair, they can "glue down" and protect the outer layer and help hair look shinier.
- **Switch shampoo brands** every six to eight months to avoid stripping away the same type of oil.
- **Don't shampoo twice**—this advice is geared only toward selling more product. You may even want to dilute the shampoo by half for gentler cleaning, and shampoo less often. Rinse well to avoid residue that can make hair limp.
- **Apply conditioner** only from the ears down, not on the scalp, where it can clog pores and overcondition hair, making it dull. Your scalp secretes enough oil to condition the first three inches of hair.
- **Seal hair cuticles** by rinsing with cold water.
- **Play it cool** by minimizing use of blow-dryers and curling irons to avoid drying out the hair and causing split ends. Hold your dryer 6 to 12 inches from your hair.

Dyeing to Try It?

Coloring your hair for the first time? You might start with temporary color before committing to a permanent change.

TYPE OF COLOR	FACTS AND TIPS
Temporary	■ Coats the surface of the hair with water-soluble pigment for a subtle change. ■ Won't cover gray. ■ Lasts for up to 3 washings.
Semipermanent	■ Contains no ammonia and no peroxide, so it's suitable for permed or chemically treated hair. ■ Boosts natural color, adds shine, and covers up to 50 percent of the gray. ■ To minimize the appearance of roots, choose a color within two shades of your own. Lasts 6 to 12 washings.
Demi-permanent	■ Contains a small amount of peroxide and no ammonia; it doesn't affect the condition of your hair. ■ Offers a greater selection of shades that will blend with and cover gray. ■ Goes deeper into the hair shaft than semipermanent color. May lighten hair. ■ Lasts about 24 washings.
Permanent	■ Contains peroxide and ammonia. ■ Changes or lightens color up to three shades. Hides even a full head of gray. ■ Adheres best to coarser hair. The ammonia softens the hair cuticle, helping wiry gray hairs blend in. ■ Grows out instead of washing out.

- **Avoid products that contain alcohol,** which parches the hair.
- **Limit use of shine products** that contain silicone, which over time creates a buildup that can leave hair dull and limp.
- **Trim hair** every four to six weeks to get rid of split ends.
- **Eat a diet** rich in zinc, magnesium, potassium, iron, and lean protein, all of which support healthy hair.

Battling Baldness

If your hairline seems to be retreating as fast as Napoleon's armies, don't give up— reinforcements are on the way.

Hair doesn't usually disappear overnight, though it may seem that way. Your hair growth actually starts to slow in your mid-twenties, whether you're a man or woman. About half of the men who eventually go bald experience serious hair loss before age 30, while only about 30 percent of women who lose some hair notice major thinning before age 50. For women, the positive difference is estrogen, which helps maintain hair growth.

Rogaine and Beyond

While they may not make the desert bloom, there are two medications currently available that seem to slow hair loss for about half their users. Minoxidil (Rogaine) is available over the counter for use by men with hair loss. It has not been approved in Canada for use by women. It can irritate the scalp, though, and if you stop treatments, the benefits will be lost.

For best results, start applying Rogaine before major hair loss has occurred. Note that it works best on balding spots. Consequently, it may

not do much to improve a receding hairline. In studies performed by the company that makes Rogaine, a quarter of men age 18 to 49 showed significant regrowth of hair on the crown of the head after four months.

Finasteride (Propecia) is a pill available by prescription only—and only for men. Like Rogaine, it must be continued indefinitely for lasting results. It may also lower libido.

Several new drugs are under development. Tricomin reportedly stimulates hair follicle growth and keeps existing follicles active. Another drug, diazoxide, dilates blood vessels on the scalp, much like Rogaine. In the pipeline are even newer products that are designed to stimulate a hair-boosting enzyme called aromatase.

WARNING

If you suffer sudden and severe baldness, consult a dermatologist, who may determine that illness, stress, hormonal changes—even antibiotics, anemia, or psoriasis—are behind it. Other possible causes are an excess of vitamin A in the diet or alopecia areata, a rare disorder that results in small bald patches.

Rogaine, applied twice a day, works best if you use it when you first begin losing your hair. It may not make all your hair grow back, but it may stop more hair from falling out.

A Permanent Fix

If serums and pills don't quite do the trick, you might consider surgical hair replacement. Each of these procedures uses your own hair and requires that you have healthy growth at the sides and back of your head. These treatments are sometimes used in combination, and while they won't restore a full head of hair, they will help fill in thinning patches.

With a hair transplant, hair is harvested from "donor" areas of the scalp and moved to the bald spots. Today's transplants look far better than those of a decade ago, when the first wave of "transplant fever" struck. That's because microsurgery techniques have improved, allowing a trained dermatologist or plastic surgeon to use more hairs on each skin graft so the grafts look more natural and less like "plugs." The main drawback? Price. One session lasting two to three hours, in which 300 to 500 grafts are removed and transplanted, costs $2,500 to $3,000, and your transplant may require several of these sessions.

In flap surgery, the surgeon first cuts away part of the bald section, then transplants to the area a flap of scalp on which hair is still growing. In tissue expansion surgery, a tiny balloonlike device is inserted under a bald patch of scalp near an area of good hair growth. As the balloon is gradually filled with salt water over a number of weeks, the skin bulges upward. Eventually, hair grows over the new skin, which is then used to repair the adjacent bald spot. In yet another surgical option, scalp reduction, the surgeon trims away bald patches of scalp and closes up the gaps between hair-growing areas.

Hair Loss Myths & Facts

MYTH	FACT
Hair loss is genetically determined, inherited from your father.	You can inherit thinning hair from either your mother's or father's side of the family. The more relatives you have who have experienced noticeable hair loss, the more likely you will, too.
Losing 50 to 100 strands of hair a day is cause for alarm.	Such hair loss is the norm. The average hair strand grows about a half-inch per month for about two years, then goes into a period of stasis and eventually falls out.
Hair thins all over your body as you age.	Hormonal changes in both men and women slow hair growth on the scalp, armpits, and pubis. However, these same hormonal changes can produce some unwelcome hair "growth spurts." Women may see some facial hair as they age, and men often experience hair growth on the eyebrows, in the ears and nostrils, and on the shoulders and back.
Hair loss is mostly a male problem.	By age 50, half of men will experience some hair loss, either at the top of the head or the temples. But one woman out of four will notice some all-over thinning due to the decline in estrogen that accompanies menopause.
Brushing the hair 100 strokes each night stimulates hair growth and the production of oil from the sebaceous glands.	This much brushing actually encourages hair loss.

Prior to any of these procedures, you will receive a local anesthetic to numb the scalp and a sedative to calm you. Of course, any type of surgery carries risks, such as scarring or infection. Be sure to discuss all of your options carefully with your doctor before you proceed.

PART 2

AILMENTS
A–Z

Allergies

SYMPTOMS

- ◀ Allergic rhinitis: itchy or watering eyes, stuffy or runny nose, sneezing, sore throat, plugged ears, and postnasal drip

- ◀ Allergic asthma: wheezing, coughing, chest tightness, or shortness of breath linked to certain times of year or environments

- ◀ Allergic contact dermatitis: red, dry, itchy skin patches and blisters

- ◀ Food allergies: swelling and tingling of the lips; itching, rash, or hives on any part of the body; abdominal cramps, gas, bloating, nausea, vomiting, or diarrhea. Severe cases can cause a rare but life-threatening reaction.

What is it?

Between 4.5 and 6 million Canadians—about one in five—are allergic to one or more things. Allergies occur when your immune system mistakes a usually harmless substance (allergen) for an intruder, then produces antibodies to defend the body against it. At the same time, cells in the affected areas produce histamine and other chemicals that rapidly cause sneezing, itching, hives, and other allergic reactions. These reactions almost always appear in or on the part of the body that had contact with the allergen—for example, breathing airborne pollen causes sneezing, and touching poison ivy causes a skin rash. Adults rarely outgrow allergies entirely, but symptoms occasionally become less severe with time. On the other hand, some people develop allergies in midlife.

TYPES OF ALLERGIC CONDITIONS

- **Allergic rhinitis** affects about one in seven Canadians. It can be seasonal (hay fever) or perennial—that is, year-round. Both have the same symptoms, but hay fever is caused by airborne pollen from trees, grasses, and ragweed, while perennial allergies are usually caused by such indoor allergens as dust mites, mold spores, feathers, and pet dander (dead skin scales).

- **Allergic asthma** is a potentially deadly disease that causes breathing problems on exposure to an allergen. Common triggers are pollen, mold spores, dust mites, pet dander, feathers, and cockroaches—especially their droppings. Five to 10 percent of Canadians have asthma, and 80 percent of asthmatics also have some type of allergy.

SELF TEST

What Is Your Risk for Allergies?

Heredity and your environment affect your chances of having allergies. Answer these questions to assess your risk:
◀ Did one of your parents have allergies? If yes, you have a 30 to 50 percent chance of having them, too.
◀ Did both your parents have allergies? If so, your risk increases to 60 to 80 percent—but you won't necessarily be allergic to the same things.

◀ Do you live in a house with high levels of cigarette smoke, mold, or other allergens? Or in a geographical area with high levels of pollen or air pollution (for example: road dust; diesel exhaust; or coal, gas, or wood smoke)? If so, your risk of developing an allergy to one of these substances is high—especially if you were exposed repeatedly in childhood.

- **Allergic contact dermatitis** is caused by skin contact with specific allergens like poison ivy, certain cosmetic ingredients, nickel (found in jewelry), or pet saliva.
- **Food allergies** kill approximately 100 North Americans each year. Fortunately, a true food allergy—the kind that can be life-threatening—occurs in only 1 to 2 percent of adults. In 90 percent of cases, the cause is one of the following foods: fish, shellfish, wheat, soy, milk, eggs, peanuts, or tree nuts, such as walnuts, cashews, and almonds. Peanuts and tree nuts are the number one cause of food allergy deaths—in the U.S. alone, for example, some 3 million people are allergic to them.
- **Drug allergies,** particularly to medications such as penicillin and similar antibiotics, are the most frequent triggers of reactions. They affect approximately 10 percent of the population and cause 2 to 3 percent of all hospital admissions.
- **Insect stings** provoke allergic reactions in about 15 percent of North Americans. Both drug and insect allergies can lead to life-threatening reactions (anaphylaxis); insect sting allergies account for at least 40 deaths a year in North America.

How is it treated?

The best treatment is to avoid the allergen. If that's not possible, the following treatments can help:

FOR ALLERGIC RHINITIS

- **Antihistamines** prevent allergy symptoms by blocking histamine release. Over-the-counter (OTC) brands such as diphenhydramine (Benadryl) and chlorpheniramine (Chlor-Tripolon) may cause drowsiness, but the newer antihistamines fexofenadine (Allegra), loratadine (Claritin), and cetirizine (Reactine) are less likely to. Antihistamines may make some elderly people feel excited, nervous, and irritable rather than sleepy.
- **Decongestants** reduce swelling in nasal passages after an allergy attack. Common OTC brands include oral pseudoephedrine (Sudafed) and xylometazoline (Otrivin). They can keep you awake, so take them only during the day. Don't use nasal sprays or drops for more than three or four days, because stopping them after prolonged use causes inflammation and congestion to return with a vengeance, a condition called rebound rhinitis.
- **Antihistamine/decongestant** formulations containing fexofenadine and pseudoephedrine (Allegra-D), pseudoephedrine and triprolidine (Actifed) and pseudoephedrine and loratidine (Claritin Extra).
- **Anti-inflammatory sprays** reduce swelling in nasal membranes. They include Cromolyn Nasal Solution and corticosteroid sprays like fluticasone (Flonase). They have few side effects but take several days to start working.

FOR ALLERGIC ASTHMA

- **Bronchodilators** like salbutamol (Ventolin) widen airways and stop sudden attacks. Corticosteroids like prednisone desensitize airways and prevent attacks. Antileukotrienes like montelukast (Singulair) and zafirlukast (Accolate) prevent inflammation and attacks. Anti-inflammatory sprays (see page 293) and oral prednisone decrease swelling.

FOR ALLERGIC CONTACT DERMATITIS

- **Corticosteroid** creams like 0.5 percent hydrocortisone (Cortate) are used for mild cases of allergic contact dermatitis. Severe cases may be treated with oral corticosteroids like prednisone. To prevent infection, keep the affected skin clean, cover it with dry bandages, and don't break any blisters. Besides reducing inflammation, corticosteroids relieve itching.

FOR FOOD, DRUG, AND INSECT STING ALLERGIES

- **Antihistamines** are used for mild reactions. Skin rashes may be treated with corticosteroid creams. Injectable epinephrine (EpiPen) is given for life-threatening reactions.
- **Allergy shots**—injections of minuscule, diluted doses of allergen—are used if drugs don't work or you can't avoid your allergen. This approach, sometimes called desensitization or immunotherapy, can decrease your reaction to dust mites, pet dander, pollen, and insect venom, but it's not used for food or drug allergies. Also, to be truly effective, allergy shots have to be given according to a strict schedule over at least a two-year period.

Your Prevention Plan

Diet ■ **Shun offending foods.** If you have a food allergy, scrutinize food labels and learn the scientific names for foods to which you react—for example, wheat may be called gluten, and egg white, albumin. Ask about food ingredients when you eat out.

■ **Eat high-C foods.** Vitamin C is said to be a natural antihistamine and some studies link low levels of C with allergies. Good sources are citrus fruits, tomatoes, green peppers, potatoes, and cabbage.

■ **Ask for yogurt.** A University of California study showed that 6 ounces of live-culture yogurt a day reduces the severity of hay-fever attacks.

Exercise ■ **Work out indoors.** If you have hay fever, exercise inside on windy days and during allergy seasons, especially in the early morning when pollen counts are highest.

■ **Plan ahead.** Exercising, especially in cold, dry air, can induce asthma. Inhale your medication 15 minutes before working out to help prevent symptoms.

■ **Do stay active.** Notwithstanding the precautions you might have to take, regular exercise clearly improves lung function in people with asthma. If you have severe, unpredictable attacks, ask your doctor if there are additional preventive measures that would let you be active safely.

Medical Options ■ **Be prepared.** Allergic to insect stings? Carry epinephrine at all times. Hay fever getting you down? Start taking antihistamines two weeks before allergy season and 30 minutes before going outdoors.

■ **Get tested.** If you aren't sure what's causing your allergy, an allergist can find out. Skin tests involve injecting tiny amounts of diluted allergens under your skin. If an injected area becomes red and swollen in 15 to 20 minutes, you're allergic to that allergen. Blood tests can be done while you're having symptoms. If white blood cells increase, your immune system is mounting an allergic response. A radioallergosorbent (RAST) blood test pinpoints the allergen by measuring levels of antibodies against it.

Supplements ■ **Take a multi.** Some experts recommend a multivitamin with 1,000 mg of vitamin C, 10,000 IU of beta-carotene, and 400 IU of vitamin E to ease allergy and asthma symptoms.

Natural Health ■ **Relax.** In one study, asthmatic adults who did yoga had less severe symptoms, fewer attacks, and better lung function than similar people who didn't practice the discipline. Any stress buster—like meditating, listening to music, or walking—can help control asthma symptoms.

■ **Consider acupuncture.** Studies show that it sparks production of endorphins, brain chemicals that help alleviate pain and stress. In one study, asthma patients reported that acupuncture improved their quality of life, even though their lung function stayed the same.

Lifestyle ■ **Allergy-proof your home.** If you're allergic to airborne particles, take these steps: Close your windows to keep out pollen. Because dust mites thrive in a warm, moist environment, an air conditioner can keep them at bay. So can washing bedding in hot water once a week and covering mattresses, box springs, and pillows with plastic coverings. Keep pets outside or at least out of your bedroom. Get rid of mold and mildew by airing out and cleaning kitchens, bathrooms, and basements regularly. Don't smoke or expose yourself to secondhand smoke, don't burn wood or use a kerosene heater, and, if possible, use electricity instead of natural gas for cooking and heating. Avoid aerosol sprays, perfumes, talcum powder, room deodorizers, and fresh paint.

■ **Look, but don't touch!** Learn what poison ivy, oak, and sumac look like. If you touch a plant, wash your skin with soap within 5 to 10 minutes to help prevent a reaction.

■ **Advertise your allergy.** Wear a medical alert necklace or bracelet if you've ever had a severe allergic reaction in the past.

WARNING

Anaphylactic shock is a deadly allergic reaction. It can occur within seconds of contact with any allergen, but foods, drugs, and insect stings are the usual culprits. Symptoms are mouth tingling, flushing, rash, breathlessness, vomiting, diarrhea, sudden drop in blood pressure, unconsciousness, and shock. Epinephrine must be given immediately to stop the reaction. If you're highly allergic to something, ask your doctor to prescribe a single-dose kit of injectable epinephrine—and always keep it with you. After self-injecting, go to the emergency room right away.

Alzheimer's Disease

◀ Early symptoms are memory loss, confusion and disorientation, difficulty completing simple or routine tasks, mood changes, social withdrawal, diminished judgment, and difficulty making decisions.

◀ Later symptoms include anxiety or anger in response to change or stress, difficulty with daily activities like dressing or eating, repetitive conversation, inability to find the right word, problems with reading and writing, trouble recognizing family and friends, sleep disturbances, wandering, and delusions.

◀ The severe stage produces weight loss, incontinence, and complete dependence on a caregiver.

What is it?

Alzheimer's is a brain disease that affects memory, thought, language, and reasoning. As brain cells are progressively destroyed, the disease becomes more and more disabling—eventually robbing you of the ability to think or speak coherently. Abnormal plaques and tangles form in the brain. Plaques are clumps of a sticky protein called beta amyloid, which builds up on neurons (nerve cells). Scientists believe that beta amyloid releases free radicals, which attack the neurons. Tangles occur when protein threads that normally support the neurons become twisted, damaging the neurons.

Alzheimer's disease can't be cured, and its symptoms can't be reversed. In 2001, an estimated 238,000 Canadians over the age of 65 suffer from it. Some experts say that the total number of Alzheimer's cases may triple in the next thirty years.

Age and heredity are the only known risk factors. You're at higher risk if you're over age 65, and your risk rises for each successive decade of life. Your risk is also higher if you have a close relative with Alzheimer's. More women than men are affected, but this may simply be because women live longer. A recent study showed that people who come from large families (five or more siblings) are at increased risk. Serious head injury, resulting in loss of consciousness, may also put you at risk.

Alzheimer's is difficult to diagnose because many of its symptoms can be associated with other disorders. Your doctor should ask about your medical history, perform a physical exam, and test your memory, attention, and problem-solving ability. Blood and urine tests and a brain scan may be

SELF TEST

Is It Alzheimer's?

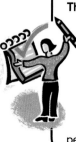

The Alzheimer's Association recommends that you consult a doctor if you or someone in your family has three or more of the following symptoms. Be alert for changes in the way the person usually acts.

Here's what to look for:

◀ memory loss that affects job skills

◀ difficulty performing familiar tasks

◀ problems with language, such as not remembering the right words

◀ disorientation about time and place

◀ poor judgment

◀ problems with abstract thinking

◀ tendency to misplace things

◀ changes in mood, behavior, or personality

◀ loss of initiative

What Causes Alzheimer's?

Research is ongoing into the factors that determine why some people develop Alzheimer's and others are spared. There are currently three principal avenues of investigation:

- **Is it hereditary?** As many as 15 percent of Alzheimer's cases have a genetic link. If one parent is affected, you have three times the risk of developing the disease. If both are, you have five times the risk. Alzheimer's is associated with the presence of the gene known as ApoE4. People with this gene have greater deposits of the protein beta amyloid—and almost twice the lifetime risk of developing the disease. But ApoE4 isn't a foolproof marker. Most people who have it don't develop Alzheimer's, and many who have the disease don't carry the gene. Most researchers believe that although genes have some role in Alzheimer's, your medical profile (for example, high blood pressure or past head trauma) is also a factor.

- **Is it environmental?** Some scientists had thought that exposure to aluminum, a mineral found in food additives, antiperspirants, some antacids, and household products such as cookware and aluminum foil, might lead to Alzheimer's. But recent research has yielded no proof of a link. The same applies to the mineral zinc. Some scientists believe that too much zinc may cause plaques to form, but that theory has not been confirmed.

- **Is it viral?** Some brain disorders are caused by a virus, and researchers have investigated whether this is true for Alzheimer's. The theory is that an infectious virus may incubate in the body for several decades before symptoms appear. But as yet there is no hard evidence to support this idea.

used to rule out conditions such as a vitamin deficiency, stroke, thyroid problems, or a brain tumor. While clinical diagnosis is 90 percent accurate, the disease can be confirmed only after an autopsy. Researchers are working to develop better diagnostic tools, including more sophisticated brain imaging techniques and a test that measures spinal fluid levels of proteins associated with Alzheimer's.

How is it treated?

Several new drugs are being tested, but only two are currently available. Rivastigmine (Exelon) and donepezil (Aricept) slow the breakdown of acetylcholine, a brain chemical that helps transmit nerve signals. They can slightly improve memory and language skills for people with mild or moderate Alzheimer's. But they don't work for everyone. Common side effects of these drugs include nausea, vomiting, diarrhea, loss of appetite, and fatigue.

Other treatments are aimed at helping some of the behavioral symptoms of Alzheimer's. Here are some common prescription drug treatments:

Fast Fact

Unless a cure is found, the number of people with Alzheimer's is expected to surge. Because of the rapidly increasing population of seniors, the number might reach 600,000 by 2030.

Fast Fact

Although identical twins carry the same genes, in half of the cases in which one twin developed Alzheimer's, the other didn't.

- Anxiety and agitation may be eased with the anti-anxiety agents clonazepam (Rivotril), diazepam (Valium), lorazepam (Ativan), or oxazepam (Serax), or with sedatives such as chloral hydrate.
- Depression is typically managed with selective serotonin reuptake inhibitors (SSRIs), including fluoxetine (Prozac), fluvoxamine (Luvox), paroxetine (Paxil), and sertraline (Zoloft).
- Sleep problems are sometimes treated with the hormone melatonin.

Nondrug treatments include massage, aromatherapy (the use of essential oils to affect mood), music therapy, and pet therapy.

If You're Caring for a Person with Alzheimer's

Since Alzheimer's impairments can progress slowly, most people with the disorder continue to function at home with help from family. Experienced caregivers offer these tips:

- **Accept the person's own reality.** A person with Alzheimer's feels anxious and demoralized and is more likely to withdraw from social contact when you continually correct her memory lapses or challenge her factual errors. Enhance her self-esteem by tapping into her subjective world and supporting her version of reality. Simple behaviors, such as cuddling a doll or playing children's games, may give pleasure to a person with Alzheimer's. By recognizing that her personality changes aren't willful but the result of damage to the brain, you can better accept these behaviors as a creative way of coping with the disease.
- **Walk with her.** Wandering, a common symptom of Alzheimer's, may be random behavior or may signify an attempt to escape what seems like an unfamiliar environment. Many nursing homes now provide enclosed circular walkways for Alzheimer's patients. If someone with Alzheimer's is living with you, provide opportunities for exercise and accompany her on walks around the neighborhood.

- **Provide calming influences.** Music therapy, aromatherapy, and massage may improve behavior and induce more restful sleep in a person with Alzheimer's.
- **Reminisce.** While a person's short-term memory may fail, long-term memory remains intact for a longer period and can be a source of consolation. Spend time going through photo albums, family movies or videos, and memento-filled scrapbooks and memory boxes. Or help the person compile a photographic collage picturing people and events in her life. These activities reduce anxiety and frustration by validating her life and achievements and reminding her of who she is.
- **Listen.** Someone with Alzheimer's typically has trouble making herself understood. Maintain eye contact and show that you're listening. Don't rush the conversation or interrupt or criticize. Speak gently, slowly, and clearly.

DRUG CAPSULE

Recent research with animals holds promise for a human vaccine against Alzheimer's. Scientists genetically engineered mice to produce too much beta amyloid, the protein that forms plaques in the brain. They then injected the mice with an experimental vaccine. Not only did the vaccine stop plaques from developing in young mice, but it also reduced plaques in older mice that already had some.

Your Prevention Plan

Diet
Favor nutrient-rich foods.
Pack your diet with foods rich in antioxidant vitamins C, E, and A, and the mineral selenium to help fight free radicals. Top food choices include prunes, raisins, blueberries, blackberries, strawberries, raspberries, kale, spinach, and Brussels sprouts.

Forgo the fat. Cut back on your consumption of animal fat and you may reduce your chance of developing Alzheimer's. Around the world, the disorder is less prevalent in countries where fat intake is low.

Feed on fish. Increase the amount of cold-water, deep-sea fish in your diet, and you'll be getting the protective benefits of omega-3 fatty acids. Their anti-inflammatory properties may help prevent the formation of plaques and tangles in the brain. Aim for three to six ounces of tuna, halibut, sardines, or mackerel per week.

Exercise
Keep moving. A 1998 study showed that regular exercise can reduce your risk for developing Alzheimer's. Researchers analyzed the long-term exercise habits of 373 people, 126 of whom had Alzheimer's. The rest were healthy. The study showed that those who had maintained consistently higher levels of physical activity earlier in their lives were less likely to have the disease.

Medical Options
Protect with non-steroidal anti-inflammatory drugs.
Research suggests that a therapeutic dose of a nonsteroidal anti-inflammatory drug (NSAID) like ibuprofen (Motrin IB, Advil) may help slow the progression of Alzheimer's disease. In one study, people who took a 400 mg dose three times a day for at least two years were 30 to 60 percent less likely to develop the disease. Severe arthritis sufferers who took NSAIDs regularly also had a lower risk. Other NSAIDs include aspirin, naproxen (Naprosyn), and indomethacin (Indocid). Acetaminophen (Tylenol) had no effect on the disease. Be aware, however, that long-term NSAID use can cause gastrointestinal bleeding and kidney problems, so check with your doctor before taking any of these drugs.

Supplements
Try vitamin E.
A study in *The New England Journal of Medicine* reported that large doses of vitamin E, an antioxidant that neutralizes free-radical damage, slowed the progression of Alzheimer's in people with the disease by about seven months. Ask your doctor about the dosage that's appropriate for you.

Natural Health
Go with ginkgo.
European studies have shown that ginkgo can help prevent memory loss in the elderly. A 1996 German study of 154 people with Alzheimer's or another form of dementia showed significant gains in mental function after 24 weeks of herbal therapy. In one study, a dose of 120 mg daily for a year yielded improvements. Talk to your doctor before taking ginkgo because it can interact with other medications.

Keep your eye on other herbs. Chinese club moss contains huperzine, a substance that slows the breakdown of acetylcholine, the brain chemical vital for maintaining memory. It can be found in health stores, sometimes in combination with ginkgo and vitamin E. Rosemary also contains compounds that may prevent acetylcholine breakdown. (It's available in teas, too.)

Lifestyle
Use it or lose it. Keeping your mind sharp may help save it from Alzheimer's. Several studies reveal that the intellectual activity of education may help reduce the risk of mental impairment later in life. Formal education or even the mental calisthenics of traveling, reading books, learning new skills, working out puzzles, taking adult education classes, pursuing hobbies, and even performing familiar activities in novel ways can increase the number of neural pathways in the brain.

Arthritis

◀ OA may be so mild that it never causes noticeable symptoms. Or symptoms may range from mild aching and stiffness, especially in the morning, to severe pain, deformity, and disability.

◀ OA mostly afflicts weight-bearing joints (hips, knees, and spine), although it may affect other joints, especially in women's hands.

◀ RA tends to affect more joints than OA and is symmetrical: If your left wrist hurts, the right one will, too.

◀ RA may also cause fever and fatigue.

What is it?

Arthritis literally means inflammation of a joint. The term comprises more than 100 different rheumatic diseases that cause pain, swelling, inflammation, and impaired movement in joints and connective tissue throughout the body. Most are chronic—once you develop arthritis, you have it for life—and your genes may add to your risk. But aggressive treatment can help you manage your arthritis and prevent pain, disability, and deformity. That's why the sooner the condition is diagnosed, the better. If you experience any joint or muscle pain, stiffness, or swelling that lasts more than a few weeks, see your doctor.

The most common type of arthritis is osteoarthritis (OA), which afflicts about 1 in 10, or 3,000,000 Canadians. OA, a degenerative joint disease, is most common in people over age 45. The condition develops as protective cartilage—the rubbery cushioning material that covers the ends of bones at the joint—gradually wears away. The joint's inner bone surfaces eventually are exposed and rub together, causing pain and damage to the joint.

Rheumatoid arthritis (RA) is a more serious disorder and can strike people of any age. It is an autoimmune disease in which the immune system runs amok, attacking joints and connective tissue as if they were foreign invaders. It can cause inflammation throughout the body.

How is it treated?

Cutting-edge treatment involves a combination of therapies. You may need several drugs plus special exercises, rest, use of heat and cold, dietary changes, and/or nutritional supplements. Surgery is an option of last resort, to repair or replace damaged joints.

DRUGS

For OA, Synvisc (hylan G-F 20) is a new drug derived from hyaluronic acid, a component of joint fluid. Injected directly into the knee once a week for several weeks, Synvisc can banish pain for up to 26 weeks more. Originally developed for the treatment of knees, Synvisc is now being tested in people with arthritic hips.

For some people with OA, simple painkillers such as acetaminophen (Tylenol, Tempra) may be enough. More severe pain and inflammation calls for nonsteroidal anti-inflammatory drugs (NSAIDs) such as ibuprofen (Advil, Motrin, and others) or aspirin.

Use NSAIDs with caution because they pose a risk of ulcers and internal bleeding. Risk is highest in older adults. One solution: Use new versions called COX-2 inhibitors, such as celecoxib (Celebrex) and rofecoxib (Vioxx). They are about as potent as ibuprofen but are gentler on the stomach. Another way to make NSAIDs safer is to apply them topically. Under clinical investigation is a gel containing diclofenac (Pennsaid) that significantly relieves the pain and stiffness of knee OA. It causes only minor local irritation and no stomach problems.

For RA, beyond NSAIDs there are disease-modifying antirheumatic drugs (DMARDs) that help slow joint damage. The immune suppressant methotrexate (Rheumatrex) is the current leader, but older drugs, some with fewer risks, help many people. They include hydroxychloroquine (Plaquenil), sulfasalazine (Salazopyrin), azathioprine (Imuran), auranofin (Ridaura), and corticosteroids such as prednisone. Any of these may soon be supplanted by more potent drugs with fewer side effects, such as leflunomide (Arava) or injected medications.

Most exciting are shots that target only certain inflammation-promoting chemicals rather than damping down the whole immune system. You can self-inject etanercept (Enbrel) twice a week. Or receive infliximab (Remicade) as an intravenous infusion (a two-hour outpatient procedure) every four to eight weeks. Be patient, though. These newest drugs may take weeks or months to help you feel better. But they deliver more than pain relief—they can slow or halt joint damage. And they last: Improvement may continue for months after a course of shots, or you may need the drug only once every few months.

BLOOD FILTERING

A procedure involving a device called the Prosorba Column may help the 5 to 10 percent of RA sufferers who don't respond to drugs. It's a form of blood cleansing, similar to kidney dialysis, that filters out antibodies that aggravate RA symptoms. After 12 weekly three- to four-hour treatments, about half of patients typically experience a substantial (at least a 20 percent) improvement in symptoms. Benefits usually last about nine months, but sometimes can last as long as a year and a half.

AUTOLOGOUS CHONDROCYTE IMPLANTATION

This procedure, known as ACI and already used for small injuries, may soon be used to repair larger OA-damaged areas. Doctors withdraw healthy cartilage cells from your knee, speed up their growth in the laboratory to produce millions of cells, then insert them a few weeks later into the damaged area of the joint.

SURGERY

When is it time for joint surgery? Consider it if your pain has become so severe that it wakes you at night or makes you unable to perform normal daily activities comfortably. Surgical options include joint repair and replacement.

See *Your Prevention Plan* (pages 302-303) for practical ways to manage the symptoms of arthritis and slow down its development.

Your Prevention Plan

Diet

■ **Lean toward vegetarian.** Since animal fats may exacerbate inflammation, a largely vegetarian diet can reduce joint pain and swelling, often enabling people with RA to cut back on their arthritis medications.

■ **Get extra vitamin C.** In a 10-year study, participants with knee OA who consumed the most vitamin C (between 150 and 450 mg daily) were three times less likely to have the condition worsen than those who consumed the least. Adding even just 100 mg of vitamin C, or one or two oranges, to your daily diet can make a difference.

■ **Bag the extra baggage.** Losing as little as 10 pounds of excess weight may help prevent OA or slow its progression. While weight loss can reduce joint stress and ease pain in all types of arthritis, it seems to be especially important for preventing and relieving OA.

Exercise

■ **Get moving.** People with all types of arthritis who exercise regularly experience less pain, joint deformity, and disability than people who don't. Start your exercise program slowly, with frequent 10-minute walks or swimming in a heated pool. Increase gradually to 30 to 60 minutes of daily activity. Ask your doctor to refer you to a physical therapist who can plan a safe regimen for you.

■ **Make a muscle.** Work with light weights (one to five pounds) to build your strength, since strong muscles support—and reduce stress on—joints. People with knee OA are more apt to have weak quadriceps and hamstring muscles in their thighs. Strengthening these muscles may reduce your risk of developing OA or reduce the stress on affected joints if you already have it.

Medical Options

■ **Zap your pain.** Bionicare 1000, a portable battery-operated device, sends pulsed electrical stimulation into your joints while you sleep. FDA-approved in the U.S. for OA, it can reduce pain, swelling, and stiffness and increase joint function within a month of nightly use. One study showed that using the device for six months to a year eliminated the need for joint replacement surgery in 75 percent of users.

Supplements

■ **Take your vitamins.** Studies have shown that people with some types of arthritis have underlying vitamin and/or mineral deficiencies, so taking a multivitamin with minerals can help.

■ **Bone up on calcium.** Long-term use of corticosteroid drugs increases your risk of osteoporosis, so if you take them, bone-building supplements are essential. Aim for 1,500 mg of calcium and 800 IU of vitamin D daily.

■ **E is for easing pain.** People with the highest blood levels of vitamin E are at lower risk of OA. What's more, a German study showed that taking 1,500 IU of E daily decreases pain and morning stiffness and improves grip strength in people with RA as well as the drug diclofenac does—without the stomach upset. Shopping tip: Choose vitamin E supplements containing pure alpha tocopherols instead of gamma tocopherols, which may increase your risk of knee OA. Also avoid the gamma tocopherols found in palm, soybean, corn, and cottonseed oils.

■ **Give glucosamine a try.** Many European studies have shown that people with OA who took glucosamine and chondroitin sulfates—the building blocks of cartilage—showed improvement. Recent research offers X-ray evidence that the supplements seem to halt joint damage. To see results, you need to take 1,500 mg of glucosamine and/or 1,200 mg of chondroitin daily. Benefits usually kick in after four to eight weeks.

■ **Add fatty acids.** Because some people with RA have low fatty-acid levels, supplements of omega-6 polyunsaturated fatty acids, such as those found in evening primrose and borage oils, may help. Check the label for gamma linolenic acid (GLA), which helps quiet inflammation. Improvement won't start until you've been taking high doses (1,000 to 2,000 mg of GLA daily) for at least four to eight weeks. Eicosapentaeonic acid (EPA) and docosa-hexaenoic acid (DHA)—omega-3 fatty acids found in fish oil—also can help reduce RA symptoms. Take 3,000 mg daily, or eat more oily fish, such as salmon, sardines, or tuna.

■ **Curtail with copper.** Copper supplements may help quell inflammation. In one study, adults with knee OA took 0.3 mg of copper—about the same amount in most multivitamins—three times a day. Within a month, although improvements were modest, people taking copper had less pain than those in the placebo group.

■ **Consider SAMe.** Research has shown that some OA pain is managed nearly as well with supplements of SAMe (S-adenosylmethionine, a natural substance found in the body that has anti-inflammatory effects and may be important in cartilage repair) as with NSAIDs (drugs such as aspirin), without the risk of upset stomach, ulcers, and other drug-related side effects.

■ **Try type II collagen.** Some studies show that oral doses (about 500 mcg) may relieve RA symptoms. Discuss this supplement with your doctor, and ask about possible interactions with other drugs that you're taking.

Natural Health ■ **Therapy with a point.** Studies have shown that a month of twice-weekly acupuncture treatments relieves pain and aids movement in OA. Benefits may last for weeks or months after a course of therapy.

■ **Look to India.** In one study, people with RA showed decreases in pain, stiffness, joint tenderness and swelling, and inflammation, and improvement in grip strength after four months on an Ayurvedic combination of four plant extracts: boswellin, ginger, curcumin (the active component in turmeric), and withania somnifera (also known as ashwagandha).

■ **Go green.** Green tea contains compounds called polyphenols, which may help relieve RA inflammation. In one study, green tea extract was found to cut the rate of arthritis in animals taking it. Green tea is available in capsules, or drink it the old-fashioned way. Skip the milk, though—it may block the effects of polyphenols.

Lifestyle ■ **Just relax.** Learn a relaxation technique, such as meditation, deep breathing, or progressive muscle relaxation, and practice it every day for at least 30 minutes.

■ **Picture yourself well.** Psychological factors can play a significant role in RA flare-ups. During your daily relaxation, imagine yourself completely well again—doing the things you love to do. Believe that you can get there again.

Back Pain

◀ Pain or stiffness in your lower back

◀ Reduced flexibility in your spine

◀ Pain may radiate from your back down through your buttock to your lower leg. If numbness, tingling, or muscle weakness in one or both legs occurs, call your doctor.

◀ See your doctor immediately if the pain is accompanied by a loss of bladder or bowel control.

What is it?

After the common cold, back pain is the second leading reason Canadians visit their doctors. And it's no wonder, given the spine's complex structure of vertebrae, disks, nerves, and numerous muscles and ligaments. Pain can occur at any point on the spine. The most common site is the lower back because it bears most of your weight. Back pain can be caused by:

● Stress or injury from weak, tight, or tense back muscles, ligaments, and tendons. Back muscles may even throb from the strain of supporting a sagging belly.

● Damage to one or more of the small, cushiony disks that act as shock absorbers between the spinal vertebrae. When a disk herniates, its soft rubbery center squeezes through a weak point in the hard outer layer, creating a bulge that presses against nearby nerves and causes severe pain. Bony outgrowths (spurs) may develop on aging vertebral joints, adding to the pain.

● Normal aging, which can cause fluids in the spinal disks to dry out so that they shrink and weaken.

● Arthritis, osteoporosis, or other conditions that affect the spinal nerves or the vertebrae.

Sciatica—severe pain along the sciatic nerve that extends down each leg from your hip to your heel—affects about 10 percent of people with back pain. It may produce tingling, numbness, or muscle weakness in the affected leg. Coughing, sneezing, or other activities that exert pressure on the spine can make it worse.

Your doctor will ask if your pain began all at once or slowly, whether it occurs when you do certain activities, what makes it feel better or worse, and how long you've been suffering. She'll also ask about other symptoms, such as numbness or tingling, leg irritation, fever, fatigue, or bladder or bowel incontinence. She'll examine your back muscles and spine and test your muscle strength and arm and leg reflexes.

Diagnostic tests are generally overprescribed, often ordered by doctors eager to show patients that they are doing *something*. Acute back pain generally results from a strain, or minor tear, of the muscles and ligaments that support the lower back. Such strains never show up in X rays and rarely are detected by magnetic resonance imaging (MRI). These imaging tests can add significantly to the cost of care, and it's never a good idea to expose yourself to unnecessary X rays.

However, one or more tests may be in order when back pain is the result of an accident or is accompanied by fever, sudden weight loss, or severe or progressive leg weakness—and doesn't improve with rest, pain-

Fast Fact

Eighty percent of us will suffer back pain at some time in our lives.

killers, and follow-up back-strengthening exercises prescribed by your doctor. An X ray is often used to rule out a fracture, bone tumor, infection, and arthritis. A computerized tomographic (CT) scan, which renders a detailed computerized X-ray image of your spine, can indicate spinal arthritis and spinal stenosis (bony overgrowths that press on the spinal canal). An MRI uses sound waves to produce a similar image and is most useful in viewing disks and nerves. Electromyography measures the electrical activity in your muscles, helpful in checking neuromuscular function. If a disk problem is suspected, your doctor may order a blood test to detect the presence of the chemical phospholipase A, which spills into the bloodstream when a disk is crushed.

How is it treated?

Usually the pain from strains, sciatica, and minor disk injuries resolves on its own in about a week, with a combination of painkillers, icing and heat, and gentle exercise. Proper rest is the best prescription—but not too much of it. Doctors now know that more than two days of bed rest can cause muscles to weaken and exacerbate the problem. If you have a herniated disk, you may feel better after several days of sleeping on your back (place a pillow under your knees) on the floor or on an extra-firm bed (put a board under the mattress).

Depending on your pain, muscle relaxants, anti-inflammatory drugs, or painkillers such as aspirin (with or without codeine) are used. PENS, or percutaneous electrical nerve stimulation, delivers short-term pain relief. It involves inserting electric needle probes into the soft tissue of the lower back. Another procedure called TENS (transcutaneous electrical nerve stimulation) involves attaching electrodes to the skin and and sending mild electric impulses to the nerves. Steroids injected into the space near a herniated disk can control pain and inflammation. Surgery is rarely necessary and is viewed as a last resort.

For easy at-home care, apply a cold pack often in the first day or two to relieve pain and reduce swelling. Follow up with the application of gentle heat (use a moist hot pack, a whirlpool, or a heating pad on low) to increase blood flow to the injured area. Salt baths can be helpful, and some people get limited relief with OTC deep-heat creams, but do not use these creams simultaneously with heating pad treatment.

Although rigorous scientific studies are limited, many back pain sufferers report good results from a variety of hands-on treatments including osteopathic or chiropractic manipulation and deep-tissue massage by a skilled massage therapist. *The New England Journal of Medicine* reported one 12-week study in which 155 chronic back pain sufferers who received manual therapy by an osteopath needed fewer pain-relieving drugs and required less physical therapy than those treated with conventional means.

As your pain subsides, your doctor may suggest a program of physical therapy and exercises to stretch and strengthen your lower back muscles to help prevent future problems.

WARNING

You could worsen your back problem—or cause permanent damage—by returning to your previous activity level too soon. You're not fully healed until you can do all of your rehabilitation exercises without pain. You should have full range of motion in your back and no shooting pain in your legs or arms. You should also be able to run, jump, and twist without discomfort.

Your Prevention Plan

Diet ■ **Lighten up.** Excess weight, especially when carried around the middle, taxes the back muscles and disks, causing tension, spinal misalignment, and pain. (See Chapter 2, *Watching Your Weight*, for helpful weight-loss tips.)

■ **Produce power.** Studies have shown that cultures in which people consume the highest amounts of vegetables have the lowest rates of back problems. Why? Vegetables contain vitamins (including C, E, and B complex), minerals (such as calcium and magnesium), fiber, water, carbohydrates, and protein—all of which are essential for maintaining healthy muscles and strong bones.

Exercise ■ **Get with a program.** A study in the *British Medical Journal* indicated that people age 18 to 60 who had suffered lower back pain for periods ranging from four weeks to six months, and who attended exercise classes led by a physiotherapist for six months, experienced significantly less back pain than those who didn't attend the classes.

■ **Stomach this.** Strong stomach muscles can stabilize your spine and help protect it from injury. Maintain strong stomach muscles by using an abdominal roller or performing other stomach-strengthening exercises, like crunches. (See the best way to do crunches in Chapter 4, page 133.)

■ **Stretch your limits.** Gain more flexibility in your spine with stretching exercises, such as the cat stretch, described on page 137.

■ **Go the distance.** Walking and swimming can help strengthen and protect your spine without placing undue stress on the vertebrae.

Medical Options ■ **Consider a physiotherapist.** Physiotherapists take an active approach and teach their patients how to manage their pain with exercise, manipulation, passive traction, and education. Most episodes of back pain respond well to an active approach, so short-term physiotherapy is a wise investment in good back health.

■ **See an osteopath.** Osteopaths manipulate the soft tissue around the spine to help improve blood circulation and maintain or restore health. According to a study in *The New England Journal of Medicine*, individuals who suffered from low back pain and received osteopathic manipulation improved as much as those who received standard treatment.

■ **Consider a chiropractor.** A chiropractor applies gentle force to the spine with the hands to adjust and align the vertebrae. According to the U.S. Agency for Health Care Policy and Research (AHCPR), spinal manipulation is most likely to help people with short-term low back pain and no complicating factors. People with sciatica or herniated disks may benefit from spinal manipulation, but AHCPR advises caution because further neurological damage may occur.

Natural Health

■ **Massage yourself.** Be your own masseuse. Extend your arms behind you, and press the fingers of both hands firmly against your lower back muscles about an inch away from your spine. Work out the kinks by making small, deep circles, moving your fingers up slowly as far as you can reach.

■ **Rub it in.** Pain balms can soothe tired muscles by creating a sensation of heat, which dilates blood vessels and improves blood flow where applied. Look for brands that contain capsicum (the substance that makes hot peppers hot) and menthol.

■ **Try acupuncture.** In 1998 the National Institutes of Health (NIH) in the U.S. agreed that evidence shows acupuncture helps relieve the chronic pain of low back disorders. Note that if you don't see an improvement after six to eight sessions, this type of therapy probably won't help.

■ **Look into natural supplements.** Bromelain, an enzyme found in pineapples, is now used in some hospitals to reduce inflammation and treat pain from trauma, sports injuries, and arthritis. Arnica ointment can be applied topically to reduce inflammation and back pain while stimulating healing.

Lifestyle

■ **Stand up straight.** Keep your shoulders back and your abdomen pulled in. When standing for long periods of time, move around frequently and shift your weight from one foot to the other. If you're standing a lot in one spot—say, doing the dishes—place one foot on the rung of a stool or a small step to take the pressure off your lower back.

■ **Sit pretty.** Choose a chair with good back support and a firm seat. Armrests help, too. Insert a pillow in the small of your back, or use a lumbar roll or rolled-up towel. Whenever sitting for a long time, get up every 20 minutes or so to stretch.

■ **Lift like the pros.** When lifting objects, don't bend over from the waist. Instead, kneel or squat beside the object, then use your thigh muscles to do the lifting while keeping your stomach muscles tight. Once you've lifted the object, don't twist your back to put it where you want it. Instead, turn your whole body.

■ **Sleep right.** Sleep on a firm mattress or one with a bed board under it. Lie on your side—never on your stomach—with your legs bent and a small pillow between your knees. Or lie on your back with a large pillow under your knees.

■ **Chill out.** Severe emotional stress can exact a physical toll, even throwing your back muscles into spasm. Make stress-reduction techniques (such as yoga, deep-breathing exercises, and meditation) part of your personal health maintenance plan.

Fast Fact

A study in the medical journal Spine reminds us that at least one physical activity can cause lower back pain: lifting a cigarette. Smoking impairs blood circulation, even in the lower spine. Reduced circulation increases your risk for back pain and slows healing.

Breast Cancer

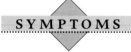

SYMPTOMS

◄ A lump or thickening in your breast or armpit

◄ A retracted or inverted nipple

◄ Clear or bloody discharge from your nipple

◄ A change in your breast size, contour, or color

◄ Pitting or dimpling of your breast skin, resembling the skin of an orange

What is it?

Breast cancer is a malignancy that begins as a single abnormal cell, which multiplies uncontrollably. It usually forms in the ducts that carry milk to the nipple or in the small sacs that produce milk. Breast cancer can grow slowly or spread aggressively to nearby lymph nodes or more distant areas. It's second to lung cancer as the leading cause of cancer death among Canadian women. It can occur in men, but this is rare.

How is it treated?

More than 95 percent of early-stage breast cancers are curable. Treatment depends on the cancer type and stage of development, the characteristics of the cancer cells, and the involvement of the other breast. Your age, weight, general health, and menopausal status also affect treatment choices. Typically treatment involves a combination of surgery—lumpectomy (removal of only the lump), mastectomy (removal of the entire breast), and/or lymph node removal; radiation therapy; chemotherapy; and hormone therapy with the drug tamoxifen, which may prevent recurrence.

SELF TEST
What Is Your Risk for Breast Cancer?

Here are the factors that put you at greater risk. If you have several factors in the first group, be diligent about self-examination and mammography, and ask your doctor about preventive medication. You can take specific action to eliminate the risks in the second group.

What you can't control:

◄ **Advancing age.** Probability of developing breast cancer: age 30: 0.4%, age 40: 1.3%, age 50: 2.3%, age 60: 2.9%, age 70: 3.2%.

◄ **Family history.** The more family members who've developed breast (or ovarian) cancer, the greater your risk.

◄ **Age of menstruation or menopause.** You're at higher risk if you began menstruating before age 12, or if you reached menopause after age 51.

◄ **Reproductive history.** Your risk climbs if you gave birth to your first child after age 30, or if you have few or no children.

What you can control:

◄ **Hormone replacement therapy (HRT).** HRT may raise your risk slightly, but it returns to the previous level when you stop.

◄ **Your weight.** Risk increases if you're overweight, especially after menopause.

◄ **Alcohol consumption.** Having three or more alcoholic drinks a day doubles your risk.

Fast Fact

Up to 20 percent of women have a family history of breast cancer. But only 5 percent of women have a history that suggests they have inherited a gene defect that puts them at greatly increased risk of breast cancer.

Your Prevention Plan

Follow the recommendations in *Cancer*, pages 310-311, plus these suggestions:

Diet ■ Be choosy about fats.

Certain types of fats seem to increase estrogen levels, which in turn raise breast cancer risk. A recent Swedish study has suggested that monounsaturated fats may help reduce risk and polyunsaturated fats may increase it. Lean toward monounsaturated oils like olive and canola, and omega-3 fatty acids, found in salmon, sardines, and herring. Steer clear of trans fats, found in stick margarine, packaged baked goods, and snack foods (check for *partially hydrogenated* on the label), and the polyunsaturated fats abundant in corn, sunflower, and safflower oils.

■ **Bring on the fiber.** Fiber binds up excess estrogen and carries it away through your intestinal tract. Good sources include beans, brown rice, whole-grain breads and cereals, and many fruits and vegetables.

■ **Eat your fruits and veggies.** In particular, get enough cruciferous vegetables—such as broccoli, cabbage, and cauliflower—all of which can boost cancer-fighting enzymes.

■ **Savor soy.** Isoflavones in soy foods are weak estrogen-like compounds that block the action of estrogen, which may contribute to breast cancer. Use soy flour in recipes, add tofu to soups or main dishes, eat green soybeans, or drink soy milk.

■ **Avoid additives.** When possible, buy hormone-free organic meats, poultry, and dairy foods. Be sure to wash fresh produce and, when feasible, remove peels to get rid of pesticide residue.

Exercise ■ Get active. Studies

show that women who exercise at least four hours a week reduce their breast cancer risk by 37 percent as compared with less active women. Exercise may cut estrogen production by burning calories and reducing fat.

Medical Options ■ Keep on top

of it. Mammograms can detect breast cancer two to five years before you can feel a lump. If you're age 50 to 69, have a mammogram—and a clinical breast exam—at your doctor's office every two years. (high-risk women may need more frequent mammograms.) Also, if you're still menstruating, be sure to do a monthly breast self-exam 7 to 10 days after the beginning of your period. If you're postmenopausal, do your self-exam on the same day each month. It is estimated that if every woman examined her breasts monthly and had mammograms at the recommended times, it would save more than 15,000 lives in North America each year.

■ **Consider a SERM.** Tamoxifen—a common breast cancer treatment—may also help prevent the disease. But many doctors believe its side effects (increased risk of endometrial cancer and blood clots) outweigh its benefits. It should be considered only for high-risk women. Researchers are now studying a newer selective estrogen receptor modulator, Evista, which may have similar benefits but fewer side effects.

Supplements ■ Try vitamin E.

In a small study at SUNY at Buffalo, participants with a family history of breast cancer had an 80 percent lower risk for developing breast cancer if their diets contained 10 or more IU per day of vitamin E. Ask your doctor or nutrition counselor about the dosage that's safe for you. (See supplement guidelines in *Cancer*, page 311.)

Lifestyle ■ Go slow on alcohol.

Too much alcohol is linked with increased risk. Limit yourself to no more than two or three drinks a week.

Cancer

SYMPTOMS

The watchword is CAUTION. Call your doctor right away if you notice any of these general signs of cancer:

◀ **C**hange in bowel or bladder habits

◀ **A** sore throat that doesn't heal

◀ **U**nusual bleeding or discharge

◀ **T**hickening or lump in the breast or elsewhere

◀ **I**ndigestion or trouble swallowing

◀ **O**bvious change in a wart or mole

◀ **N**agging cough or hoarseness

While some of these symtoms signal cancer, they are also associated with other diseases. See *Breast Cancer, Colorectal Cancer, Lung Cancer, Ovarian Cancer, Prostate Cancer,* and *Skin Cancer* for information about specific symptoms.

What is it?

Cancer is the uncontrolled multiplication of a single abnormal cell. As disease cells relentlessly copy themselves, they form tumors that compress, invade, or destroy normal tissue. If tumor cells break away, they can travel through the bloodstream or the lymph system to other areas of the body. At these new sites they may form "colony" tumors and continue to grow in a process known as metastasis. If the spread isn't controlled, it will eventually cause death.

Cancer can result from genetic, lifestyle, and environmental factors. About 70 percent of new cases are diagnosed in people who are at least 60 years old. If your family has a history of cancer, a faulty gene passed from generation to generation may increase your chances of developing a particular cancer. Heredity, however, is the central cause of only about 5 to 10 percent of cancers. The vast majority of cases—about 75 percent—are caused by things that you can control, such as smoking, a poor diet, significant overweight, alcohol abuse, and exposure to various cancer-causing substances, also called carcinogens, such as pesticides, asbestos, and radon. Some experts contend that bad eating habits are responsible for approximately one-third of cancer deaths in North America.

How is it treated?

Treatment depends on the type of cancer, how far it has spread, and how fast it's growing. Medical and pharmaceutical research and technology have advanced so far so fast that more and more people are surviving cancer, thanks to carefully targeted interventions. It's always wise to get a second opinion before starting any anticancer therapy, but do not delay treatment. Your treatment options include:

● **Surgery,** which about 60 percent of people with cancer will undergo, often in combination with other treatments.
● **Radiation therapy,** which kills or damages cancer cells by exposing them to X rays or gamma rays.
● **Chemotherapy,** which uses drugs to poison cancer cells and block their reproduction.
● **Hormone therapy,** which works by disrupting the production or action of hormones, chemical messengers that perpetuate the reproduction of some types of cancer cells. Sometimes hormone therapy involves surgical removal of hormone-producing glands to kill cancer cells or slow their growth.
● **Immunotherapy,** which supports the body's immune-system defense against cancer.

Fast Fact

Cancer is the second leading cause of death in Canada, claiming the lives of 65,000 Canadians.

Your Prevention Plan

Diet
■ **Limit fat.** Keep your fat intake to 20 percent of your diet. Avoid saturated fats (those that are solid at room temperature) and trans fats (found in margarine and many processed foods, especially snack foods and baked goods and anything with the words *partially hydrogenated* on the label). Use monounsaturated oils like olive oil or canola oil (organic canola oil is ideal) instead of vegetable oils that contain polyunsaturated fats.

■ **Favor fish.** Replace red meat with white meat or fish, especially fish rich in omega-3 fatty acids—salmon, sardines, herring, and anchovies. Just one serving a week can lower your risk of colorectal, esophageal, and stomach cancers.

■ **Go for five.** Eat at least 5 servings a day of fruits and vegetables, which are packed with cancer-preventing substances. The cruciferous vegetables (including broccoli, kale, Brussels sprouts, and cauliflower) are particularly rich in these compounds. Tomatoes also have anticancer properties; to reap the greatest benefit, eat them cooked, in sauces, soups, and even catsup. Garlic and onions have cancer-fighting properties, too.

■ **Increase fiber.** Eating plenty of fiber replaces excess fat in your diet and may help prevent certain cancers. Whole-grain cereals, beans, and other legumes are great fiber sources.

■ **Eat soy.** Soy contains substances that are thought to cut cancer risk. Have some soy milk, miso, or green soybeans (available frozen). Try soy flour in your pancake recipes, or add tofu chunks to your stir fry or soup.

■ **Ban barbecue.** Charcoal-grilled foods may be carcinogenic, so choose another cooking method whenever you can. Marinating meat before putting it on the grill may cut down on carcinogens. Or cook it partially in the microwave first so it spends less time on the grill.

■ **Nix nitrites.** These food additives, which have an extensively documented link to cancer, are found in smoked meats and fish, bacon, ham, hot dogs, sausages, and luncheon meats.

Exercise
■ **Get in shape.** Even moderate physical activity can help protect against colorectal cancer and cancers of the lung, breast, prostate, and uterus. Another advantage: Exercise helps you keep off extra weight, which increases your risk.

Medical Options
■ **Catch it early.** Learn more about the symptoms of various cancers and discuss your risk factors with your doctor. Then schedule appropriate screening tests such as mammography (to detect breast cancer) and colonoscopy (to detect colorectal cancer). Ask your family doctor or dermatologist to check your skin annually for suspicious growths.

Supplements
■ **Arm yourself with antioxidants.** Andrew Weil, M.D., head of the complementary medicine program at the University of Arizona, Tucson, recommends a daily regimen of 250 mg of vitamin C and 25,000 IU of mixed carotenes (beta-carotenes and other nutrients in the carotene family) at breakfast; 400 to 800 IU of natural vitamin E and 200 mcg of selenium at lunch; and 250 mg of vitamin C at dinner. However, no clinical trial data support these dosage recommendations.

Natural Health
■ **See green.** Green tea contains a powerful antioxidant called EGCG, which scientists believe may help fight cancer. Studies suggest that drinking green tea may lower the risk for colorectal, breast, stomach, and skin cancers.

Lifestyle
■ **Limit alcohol.** Excessive alcohol consumption increases your risk of certain cancers. Have no more than one drink a day for women or two drinks a day for men.

■ **Stop smoking.** Countless studies have confirmed the harmful effects of tobacco products. They cause not only lung cancer, but also cancers of the mouth, throat, esophagus, bladder, and pancreas.

Cataracts

What is it?

A cataract impairs your vision by causing your eye's normally clear lens to grow murky or opaque. The lens directs light onto the retina, but if you have a cataract, the light is obstructed or distorted. About half of all people between ages 52 and 64 have cataracts, and almost everyone has them by age 75. Cataracts are painless and develop slowly, so you probably won't notice vision changes until you're in your sixties.

You are more likely to develop cataracts if you:
- have a family history of cataracts
- smoke
- have diabetes
- have injured your eye
- use corticosteroids
- have had long-term sunlight exposure
- drink alcohol to excess
- are a woman
- are of African descent.

How is it treated?

At first, all you may need to do is get stronger eyeglasses and brighter home lighting, wear sunglasses outside, and avoid night driving. But a cataract will eventually get worse, so you'll probably need to have it removed. The surgeon will make a small incision in your eye, remove the cloudy lens, then replace it with a permanent plastic or silicone implant. The procedure, which takes less than an hour, is done on an outpatient basis under local anesthesia. It's at least 90 percent effective in improving vision.

SYMPTOMS

◄ Reduced distance and night vision and double vision in the affected eye

◄ Sensitivity to light and glare, or seeing halos around lights

◄ Feeling of a "film" over your eye

◄ Frequent changes in your eyeglass prescription and the need for brighter light for close work

WARNING

If you've been on high-dose corticosteroids (10 to 15 mg/day) for one to two years, you're at high risk for cataracts. See your eye doctor every three to six months.

Cataract Q & A

Are lasers used to remove a cataract?
No. A cataract is removed through a surgical incision. But lasers are used weeks or even years after surgery to open the membrane behind the implanted lens if it, too, becomes cloudy.

Can the cataracts in both my eyes be removed at once?
No. Your eyes will be operated on separately, about six weeks apart. This way, if you have complications during or after surgery, your doctor can consider a different approach. It's also more practical because you'll need to wear an eye patch for 24 hours after surgery, and the vision in your affected eye will take time to improve.

Will my vision be 20/20?
Not necessarily, but it will be much better than it was before. To read or see well at a distance, most people must continue to wear glasses or contact lenses.

Your Prevention Plan

Diet ■ **Control the damage.** Research shows that antioxidants block free radicals (unstable oxygen molecules) from accumulating in the eye, where they can cause cataracts. Good food sources are citrus fruits, strawberries, purple grapes, blueberries, broccoli, tomatoes, cantaloupe, red and green peppers, corn, carrots, and dark-green leafy vegetables. Foods that contain selenium, iron, zinc, niacin, thiamine (vitamin B₁), and riboflavin (vitamin B₂) also guard against free-radical damage. Good food sources include meat, poultry, seafood, soybeans, fortified cereals, legumes, potatoes, eggs, milk, and cheese. Foods rich in vitamin A—which promotes normal vision—include beef liver, egg yolks, and yellow and dark-green leafy vegetables.

■ **Have a bowl.** Many of today's cereals are fortified with vitamins. Look for ones with close to the recommended daily allowance of nutrients you don't get enough of through diet.

Medical Options ■ **Get checked.** If you are between ages 40 and 59, have a complete eye exam every one to two years. People over age 60 should be checked annually.

Supplements ■ **Take a multivitamin.** It can't hurt, especially if you don't eat the recommended five servings of fruits and vegetables per day.

■ **Consider C.** Several studies suggest that taking vitamin C for at least 10 years can prevent cataracts. But dosage recommendations range from 250 to 1,250 mg a day. Ask your doctor for advice.

■ **Look to A and E.** Vitamin A can help support healthy vision. Vitamin E, like other antioxidants, may help prevent cataracts. In a four-year study, researchers found that vitamin E decreased the risk of developing a cataract by 50 percent. A safe dosage is 200 IU per day.

Lifestyle ■ **Protect your eyes.** Ultraviolet light causes free-radical formation. Wear sunglasses and a visor or wide-brimmed hat on sunny days. Shop for sunglasses that filter out at least 99 percent of the harmful UVA and UVB rays, a feature available in both high-priced and less expensive pairs. If you work on do-it-yourself projects or participate in sports that might cause an eye injury, be sure to wear safety glasses.

■ **Control diabetes.** Uncontrolled diabetes can lead to various eye diseases, including cataracts—and even blindness.

■ **Stop smoking.** Another reason to quit: People who smoke have a much higher incidence of cataracts and develop cataracts about 10 years earlier than nonsmokers.

■ **Steer clear of toxins.** Guard against exposing your eyes to toxic substances and radiation from X rays or infrared light. Both have been implicated in the formation of cataracts.

Nutrition Note

Two recent Harvard studies show that eating kale, broccoli, spinach, and other dark-colored greens may cut your risk of cataracts. Researchers tracked more than 77,000 women and 36,000 men for 8 to 12 years. Altogether, the group had 2,311 cataract surgeries. But women who ate spinach and other greens twice a week had 18 percent fewer cataracts than those who ate these foods less than once a month. Men who ate broccoli twice a week had 23 percent fewer cataracts than those who ate it less than once a month.

Colorectal Cancer

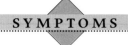

SYMPTOMS

◄ None in the early stages

◄ Persistent constipation or diarrhea

◄ Unusual abdominal cramping or gas

◄ Unexplained fatigue

◄ Loss of weight or appetite

◄ Bloody stools or rectal bleeding

◄ Narrow stools about the diameter of a pencil

◄ Pain and tenderness in the lower abdomen

◄ Any change in the color, diameter, or frequency of bowel movements that lasts more than two weeks

What is it?

Colorectal cancer is cancer of the colon and/or rectum, the two structures that make up the large intestine. It usually develops over many years, starting as a polyp (a small noncancerous growth) and gradually mutating, usually over the course of about 5 to 10 years, into a malignant tumor. About one-quarter of colon cancer patients—specifically, those who develop the disease in their thirties and forties—are genetically predisposed to the disease.

The cause of most cases is unknown, but a diet lower in fruits and vegetables and high in red meat seems to increase risk.

Colorectal cancer is the second leading cause of cancer-related deaths in Canada. But it needn't be. When polyps and early-stage cancers are found and removed before they've produced any symptoms, the cure rate approaches 100 percent. See *Your Prevention Plan* (opposite) for screening recommendations.

To diagnose colorectal cancer, your doctor should test your stools for hidden blood every year. She may also perform a sigmoidoscopy, in which a flexible, lighted tube with a camera on its tip is inserted into the lower third of your colon. Nearly half of all colon cancers are found in this area. To check for growths in the rest of the colon, colonoscopy is performed. It is the same as sigmoidoscopy except that the viewing instrument is advanced through the entire length of the large intestine. Alternatively, you can have an X-ray examination of the colon after you receive a barium enema, which fills the rectum and colon with an opaque liquid that is visible on X-ray film.

SELF TEST

What Is Your Risk for Colorectal Cancer?

You're at greater risk if you have one or more of these factors:

What you can't control:

◄ **Age.** Your risk increases significantly after 50.

◄ **Family history.** A history of colon cancer in your immediate family triples your risk. Your chances of developing the disease are also well above average if any second-degree relatives (aunts, uncles, cousins) have had it.

◄ **Predisposition.** You're at greater risk if you have (or have ever had) ulcerative colitis.

What you can control:

◄ **Diet.** Although the jury is still out on whether or not a low-fat, high-fiber diet helps prevent colon cancer, it provides so many other health benefits that most experts still highly recommend it.

◄ **Screening.** Doctors recommend colorectal cancer screening beginning at age 50 (earlier if you have a family history), including annual fecal occult blood testing and sigmoidoscopy or colonoscopy every three to five years.

◄ **Smoking.** Smoking raises your risk.

How is it treated?

DRUGS

Chemotherapy—anticancer drugs—may be recommended for people with advanced cancers.

SURGERY

The doctor removes any polyps during colonoscopy. If a tumor is found early, the section of colon containing it is surgically removed and the colon functions normally—a complete cure. But if the cancer has penetrated the colon wall and reached the lymph and blood vessels, chemotherapy is necessary. Removing a large tumor may also require a temporary or permanent colostomy, in which the colon is rerouted through an opening in the abdomen. Feces pass through the opening into a pouch outside the body. Thanks to improved surgical techniques, colostomies are needed in only 2 percent of cases compared with 20 percent two decades ago.

Your Prevention Plan

Follow the guidelines listed in *Cancer*, pages 310-311, in addition to the ones below.

Diet ■ **Fight free radicals.**
Studies show that consuming broccoli, spinach, carrots, and orange juice reduce your risk, perhaps because they all contain a compound that neutralizes cancer-causing free radicals. Research to date has shown no benefit in taking antioxidant supplements.

■ **Fill up on fiber.** Scientists have long thought that a high-fiber, low-fat diet reduces the risk of colorectal cancer by speeding waste—and cancer-causing toxins—through the colon. But studies by the National Cancer Institute and the University of Arizona cast doubt on that assumption. Although the studies showed that dietary changes did not lower risk in people who had already developed at least one polyp, scientists left open the possibility that fiber might still be protective before a polyp develops. A high-fiber, low-fat diet is good for you for so many other reasons that most experts still recommend it.

■ **Drink more water.** Water helps dilute cancer-causing toxins and speeds their excretion from the body. In one study, men who drank at least 32 ounces of water daily had a 92 percent lower risk than men who drank 10 ounces or less.

Medical Options ■ **Get checked.**
If someone in your family has had colorectal cancer or ulcerative colitis, ask your doctor about starting screening tests in your thirties or forties. Otherwise, beginning at age 50, discuss with your doctor how often you should have a test to detect hidden blood in the feces, a sigmoidoscopy or a colonoscopy.

■ **Look at estrogen.** Studies show that postmenopausal women on estrogen replacement therapy have a below-average risk of colorectal cancer.

■ **Ask about aspirin.** Studies have shown that long-term use of aspirin and other nonsteroidal anti-inflammatory drugs (NSAIDs), at doses used for arthritis pain, significantly lowers risk. There are possible side effects, so talk to your doctor first.

Supplements ■ **Value in vitamins.**
Consider taking 400 mcg of folic acid. In a study of 90,000 nurses, folic acid lowered risk 75 percent over 15 years.

■ **Try calcium.** Calcium helps reduce the formation of precancerous polyps according to researchers at Dartmouth Medical School. Get 1,000 mg of calcium daily through diet or supplements.

Congestive Heart Failure

◆ SYMPTOMS ◆

- ◀ Rapid weight gain
- ◀ Swelling in the feet, ankles, legs, or abdomen
- ◀ Fatigue
- ◀ Shortness of breath, especially when lying down or trying to sleep
- ◀ Clammy, pale skin that may turn blue
- ◀ Muscle loss
- ◀ Wheezing or a dry cough (which may produce a pinkish froth) that starts when you lie down but stops when you sit up

What is it?

Congestive heart failure (CHF) is a chronic condition in which the heart loses its ability to pump efficiently. It develops when disease weakens the heart muscle or when the valves that control blood flow out of the heart close improperly. Because each heartbeat now pumps out less blood, the oxygen-depleted blood returning to the heart from the rest of the body backs up, collecting in the lungs and leaking into tissues. Many symptoms of CHF result from this fluid buildup. The underlying cause, however, is usually heart disease, high blood pressure, diabetes, or an abnormal heart rhythm. Untreated CHF can cause body systems to shut down.

CHF is most common on the left side of the heart, which receives freshly oxygenated blood from the lungs and does most of the work to pump it out to your organs, but it can also occur on the right side, which receives oxygen-depleted blood and sends it to the lungs to be reoxygenated. Because the two sides are codependent, failure on one side usually leads to failure on the other.

About 5 million North Americans have CHF, and the number is growing because people are living longer and surviving conditions (such as heart attacks) that increase the risk for CHF. To diagnose CHF, your doctor may use lung X rays, echocardiography (heart ultrasound), and a physical exam.

How is it treated?

CHF can sometimes be corrected by treating the underlying disease that has damaged your heart. Drugs can slow the condition's progression.

DRUGS

Medications can help your heart pump more effectively and prevent further damage. Four types are used. *Vasodilators* widen your blood vessels,

SELF TEST

What Is Your Risk for Congestive Heart Failure?

You are at greater risk if you:

- ◀ are over age 70. People over age 70 have a 10 percent chance of experiencing heart failure.

- ◀ are of African descent. Your risk is 25 percent higher than that of Caucasians.
- ◀ have high blood pressure, which doubles your risk.

- ◀ have had a heart attack, which puts you at five times greater risk.
- ◀ have a family history of early heart failure

caused by diseases that damage the heart.
- ◀ smoke.
- ◀ are sedentary.
- ◀ drink too much alcohol.

allowing blood to flow more easily from your heart. The most common are angiotensin-converting enzyme (ACE) inhibitors, such as quinapril (Accupril), which in some people cause an irritating cough. ACE inhibitors were the first drugs proven to prolong life and reduce hospitalizations in people with CHF. *Diuretics*, such as furosemide (Lasix), make you urinate more, which helps prevent fluid from collecting in your lungs and allows you to breathe more easily. *Digoxin* (Lanoxin), a digitalis derivative, boosts the strength of heart contractions. *Beta-blockers*, such as propranolol (Inderal), improve blood flow and prevent some heart-rhythm problems. Adding a beta-blocker to an ACE inhibitor, a diuretic, and digoxin greatly improves survival rates and slows the progression of the disease.

WARNING

Studies show that doctors aren't prescribing ACE inhibitors as often as they should. Women and nonwhites are less likely to get them than white men. Ask your doctor if these drugs could help you.

SURGERY

If drug therapy doesn't help and you are under age 65, your doctor may suggest a heart transplant. Survival rates and quality of life after this operation are excellent, but there is a shortage of donors. A tiny mechanical pump once used to temporarily help people awaiting a transplant may actually help the heart regain strength. Called a left ventricular device, it is implanted in the chest to increase your heart's pumping action.

Your Prevention Plan

Whether you are at high risk for CHF or already have it, follow the recommendations in the *Prevention Plan* in *Heart Disease*, pages 362-363, regarding exercise, diet, weight control, blood pressure control, diabetes control, and smoking, as well as the ones below.

Diet ■ **Reduce salt.** It causes your body to retain fluids, so limit your intake to less than 4 to 6 grams a day.

■ **Limit alcohol.** Drink no more than one alcoholic beverage a day. Excessive alcohol consumption can reduce your heart's pumping ability.

Exercise ■ **Get going.** Exercise helps prevent CHF. And while it was once forbidden for those with CHF, studies show that moderate exercise strengthens your heart. Talk to your doctor before starting.

Natural Health ■ **De-stress.** Reducing stress may lower the levels of certain hormones in your body that can have a negative impact on your immune system and heart. Try yoga, tai chi, guided visualization, or meditation.

Lifestyle ■ **Step on the scale.** If you're already taking medication for CHF, weigh yourself daily before breakfast (after you've urinated). If you suddenly gain more than two pounds, you may be accumulating fluids. Call your doctor immediately.

■ **Ask for help.** If you live alone or lack support at home, you're at greater risk for readmission to the hospital or death from uncontrolled CHF. Many hospitals offer follow-up programs to help you make positive lifestyle changes and take your medications as directed.

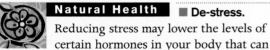

Constipation

SYMPTOMS

◀ Infrequent bowel movements and small, hard stool that is difficult to pass

◀ Abdominal fullness or bloating, gassiness, rectal discomfort, and incomplete elimination

◀ Weight loss, severe abdominal pain, or rectal bleeding may signal a more serious condition.

What is it?

Constipation is a condition in which you can't move your bowels on a regular schedule, resulting in dry, hard stool that is difficult to pass. Normal bowel habits differ among healthy people. Some people have one or more bowel movements daily, while others may have just two to three a week. You are said to be constipated when your normal pattern slows dramatically.

Any change from your regular diet may cause your stool to lose water and dry out as it moves through the large intestine (colon). Other constipation triggers include changes in exercise habits or lifestyle, a lack of dietary fiber, unrelieved stress, and delaying bowel movements for the sake of convenience.

If you don't eat normally for a few days, your digestive tract may take time to catch up when you're back on track, and you may not have a bowel movement right away. Don't worry. Once your system captures the nutrients it missed, it will pass the excess.

Certain medications, including iron supplements, calcium channel blockers, narcotic painkillers, antacids that contain aluminum, and blood pressure medication can produce constipation by sapping moisture from your colon. Endocrine disorders such as diabetes or thyroid disease may also affect bowel habits.

If you consult your doctor, he'll ask how long you've been constipated, when you last moved your bowels, what your stool consistency was, and whether you've passed blood.

How is it treated?

Because eating habits are often to blame for constipation, adding fiber to your diet is a good first step. The average North American eats only 10 to 20 grams of fiber a day. You should aim for 25 to 35 grams daily. And always try to get fiber from foods first. Bran is an excellent source. (See *Your Prevention Plan* at right for more good sources.) Adding mild natural laxatives to your diet may be all you need to correct the problem. Try prunes, sauerkraut, rhubarb, or green sprouts.

A suppository or gentle enema can offer immediate relief. If you're shopping for an over-the-counter laxative, first try the mildest product you can find—and don't make a habit of using it. (See Chapter 6, *Avoiding Common Health Traps*, for more details.)

Your doctor may prescribe a stool softener. If constipation is a side effect of a medication you're taking, he might suggest a change in dosage or an alternate drug.

SimpleSolution

When you have to go, then go. Ignoring this important message from your digestive tract may lead to hard stools— and may eventually make your bowel insensitive to the urge.

Your Prevention Plan

Diet ■ **Bulk up with fiber.** Fiber is the indigestible part of plant food. By helping the stool retain water, it adds bulk. This stimulates the natural contraction of the intestines and provokes a bowel movement. Insoluble fiber from whole grains can also accelerate the stool's passage through the colon. Fruits, vegetables, beans, and whole grains are excellent sources of fiber. So is bran. Switch to a bran cereal, or buy the unprocessed form (available in health food stores) and add a little to casseroles and baked goods. Also try substituting brown rice for white—it has three times the fiber. Boost your fiber intake gradually or you may experience gas, bloating, and abdominal pain.

■ **Founts of Fiber**

Food	Serving	Fiber in Grams
Raspberries	1 cup	6
Pear with skin	1 medium	4
Apple with peel	1 medium	3
Acorn squash	3/4 cup	4
Brussels sprouts	1/2 cup	3
Black-eyed peas	1/2 cup	4
Lima beans	1/2 cup	4
Lentils	1/2 cup	4
Brown rice	1 cup	3
Oatmeal	2/3 cup	3
Whole-wheat cereal	1 cup	3
100% bran cereal	1/3 cup	8
Baked potato with skin	1 medium	4

■ **Wash it down.** Drink plenty of fluids—at least eight 8-ounce glasses of water daily—to soften the stool. If you make the mistake of increasing your fiber intake without drinking enough, the extra bulk may slow or block bowel function.

Exercise ■ **Get a move on.** Regular exercise promotes proper bowel function. Studies have shown that exercise accelerates the stool's transit time through the large intestine. Faster transit time means less time for the stool to lose water, resulting in stools that are easier to pass.

Supplements ■ **Fortify yourself.** Until you change your eating habits to include more fiber, you might consider a fiber supplement, such as Metamucil. Take it with meals for best effect. These products can be helpful but, unlike the natural fiber you get from whole foods, they contain no nutrients.

Lifestyle ■ **Aim for consistency.** Try to maintain a regular routine as much as possible. A sudden change in activity level or eating habits, as might occur during an illness or on a relaxing vacation, can result in constipation.

WARNING
Never take a stimulant laxative (such as Correctol or Ex-Lax) for more than three consecutive days. Overuse can cause intestinal damage and "lazy bowel syndrome," in which the bowel can't function normally without a laxative.

Depression

SYMPTOMS

◄ Daily preoccupation with sad thoughts; frequent crying

◄ Loss of interest in pleasurable activities

◄ Loss of energy

◄ Guilt

◄ Insomnia or excessive sleepiness

◄ Slowed reactions

◄ Weight gain or loss (apart from dieting)

◄ Difficulty concentrating or making decisions

◄ Thoughts of suicide

What is it?

Depression is a disease of varying intensity. Bereavement, a normal reaction to loss or death, is sometimes a cause of depression and may be referred to as situational depression. But the symptoms of bereavement, which can be identical to those of depression, dissipate in a few weeks or within several months. Chronic low-level depression that doesn't prevent you from functioning but steals the joy from daily life is called dysthymia. Major or clinical depression is signaled by debilitating symptoms that interfere with normal activities. Suicidal feelings indicate serious depression.

Researchers believe that depression occurs when the mood-regulating brain chemicals (neurotransmitters) serotonin, dopamine, and norepinephrine swing out of balance. This can result from biological or environmental triggers. If you have a medical condition or painful illness, depression makes you feel worse. It can masquerade as migraine headache, overall body pain, or digestive problems. Or it can show up as a contributing factor in poorly understood conditions such as chronic fatigue, irritable bowel syndrome, or fibromyalgia.

How can you tell if you're depressed? The American Psychiatric Association says to watch for the signs and symptoms listed at left. If you have either of the first two, plus four others, on most days (for most of the day), for at least two weeks, you are probably suffering from major depression.

How is it treated?

Treatment depends on the factors that have made you depressed and on the severity of your symptoms. Before starting therapy, your doctor will determine if there is a physical cause for the depression. Ten to 15 percent of cases stem from an underlying medical condition, such as undetected

SELF TEST

What Is Your Risk for Depression?

About 11 million North Americans suffer from depression. You're at higher risk if you:
◄ are a woman
◄ have been depressed before
◄ lack an adequate

social support system
◄ have ongoing stresses in your life, such as illness in the family or financial burdens
◄ have an illness associated with depression, such as Alzheimer's

disease, arthritis, cancer, diabetes, heart disease, Parkinson's disease, stroke, or a thyroid disorder
◄ take medications that may cause depression—for

example, beta-blockers, sleep medications, narcotics, benzodiazepines, corticosteroids, sedating antihistamines, and tranquilizers.

hearing loss, diabetes, cancer, or underactive thyroid. Although treating the condition is essential, the "secondary" depression usually requires drug treatment. Your doctor will also review your medications to see if one of them is the culprit.

For sad feelings without diagnosed major depression, you may benefit from talk therapy or the herbal supplement St. John's wort. Exercise, acupuncture, and biofeedback are also sometimes effective. Maintaining strong family and social ties, worshipping, or exploring your spirituality can also help. If your depression coincides with a wintertime decrease in daylight (see *Shedding Some Light on SAD*, page 323), light therapy should brighten your mood.

When major depression occurs, your doctor should suggest one or more of the following:

- **Antidepressant drugs:** Most people take these drugs for about a year, but some people stay on them indefinitely. See *Choosing the Right Antidepressant*, below.
- **Talk therapy:** Talking about your problems, especially with a professional therapist, has helped millions of people overcome depression. Cognitive-behavioral therapy is particularly effective in treating depression. The goal is to help you identify and consciously change patterns of negative or counterproductive "self-talk" and replace them with positive thought patterns and behaviors. In older people, talk therapy alone—without also taking antidepressants—is not very effective.
- **Electroconvulsive therapy (ECT):** ECT can break through depression when other therapies fail. Formerly known as "shock treatment," ECT uses an electrical charge to produce a momentary intense discharge of neurotransmitters (brain chemicals) that results from alteration of the brain's electrical environment. The treatment has been refined greatly in the past 20 years. Today, for example, patients receive a pre-ECT muscle relaxant and sedative to eliminate muscle spasms, which otherwise would be induced by the charge. How ECT cures depression is poorly understood, but its effects are often immediate and dramatic.

CHOOSING THE RIGHT ANTIDEPRESSANT

More than 20 different drugs are currently available for treating depression. Although they fall into four general categories, each individual drug has a unique chemical structure, so there are subtle differences in effects and side effects. Some drugs, for example, tend to energize people whose depression makes them sluggish and sleepy, while others are good for quelling the anxiety and agitation that often accompany depression. Likewise, different people, because of their unique body chemistry, can have different responses to the same drug. This means you may have to work with your doctor to find the treatment that best addresses your symptoms.

Selective serotonin reuptake inhibitors (SSRIs) such as fluoxetine (Prozac), paroxetine (Paxil), and sertraline (Zoloft) usually take a few weeks to become effective and can cause dry mouth, constipation, dizziness, weight gain or loss, and sexual dysfunction. These drugs (especially

Fast Fact

Brown University researchers suggest that antidepressant drugs and psychotherapy relieve chronic depression more effectively in combination than either treatment does alone. In a recent study, combining structured psychotherapy with a typical antidepressant regimen increased depressed patients' response to treatment by 30 percent.

fluoxetine) can interfere with the liver's ability to metabolize other drugs, so it's important for your doctor to review a list of all medications you take.

Tricyclic antidepressants (TCAs), such as desipramine (Norpramin), doxepin (Sinequan), and protriptyline (Triptil), take several weeks to become effective. TCA side effects may include problems with urination, unexpected weight gain, heart-rhythm disturbances, and dizziness when you stand up quickly.

Monoamine oxidase inhibitors (MAOIs) carry the potential for serious side effects—including extremely high blood pressure—if you eat foods that contain tyramine (such as red wine or pickles). Newer versions of these drugs eliminate the potential for food interactions, but they can cause impotence and insomnia. Your doctor may recommend that you try an MAOI if you haven't had any luck with other antidepressants.

Newer antidepressants such as nefazodone (Serzone) and venlafaxine (Effexor), and investigational drugs such as mirtazapine and reboxetine may be as effective as SSRIs but produce a variety of different effects, allowing for more precise tailoring of therapy to symptoms.

HERBAL ALTERNATIVE

St. John's wort, an over-the-counter herbal supplement, is a natural mood lifter. It seems to work by slowing the rate at which brain cells absorb serotonin, leaving more of the mood-enhancing chemical in the synapses between the cells. This is similar to the action of SSRIs. You may need to take the herb for three to six weeks before it starts working. Purchase pills that have 0.3 percent hypericin (the active ingredient) and take 200 to 300 mg three times a day.

St. John's wort got a seal of approval from the medical establishment in mid-2000 when the American College of Physicians–American Society of Internal Medicine told doctors that it could be effective for people

Depression in the Elderly

Many people think that depression is a natural part of aging. Not so! Even though older people face many changes and losses, coping skills actually increase with age. Still, about 3 percent of elderly people suffer major depression, and another 15 percent have depressive symptoms that don't meet the criteria for major depression.

Yet many doctors have not been trained to look for depression in seniors, even though antidepressant medication can renew the pleasure in life. By some estimates, fewer than one out of every six depressed older patients gets appropriate treatment.

Depression can accompany many of the chronic medical conditions older people may suffer. Loss of independence due to disability or illness can also contribute to an elderly person's depression. Finally, loneliness and isolation are exacerbated as friends and loved ones move away or die.

Taking multiple medications (called polypharmacy), which is common among the elderly, is another contributing factor. Certain drugs in particular (see *What Is Your Risk for Depression?*, page 320) tend to cause or worsen depression.

The bottom line: Anyone who is withdrawing socially, having suicidal thoughts, or experiencing changes in normal energy levels should see a doctor to be evaluated for depression. Offer to accompany the person to lend support.

with mild depression. Don't take St. John's wort in combination with SSRIs or tranquilizers; it could cause a dangerous rise in blood pressure. It can also blunt the effects of HIV drugs, medications that prevent rejection of organ transplants, blood thinners, and birth control pills.

Another supplement called SAM-e (S-adenosyl-methionine) may prove helpful, but further study is needed before it can be recommended.

SHEDDING SOME LIGHT ON SAD

Seasonal affective disorder (SAD) is a depression that hits in the late fall and winter, when daylight hours are short. It is more common in latitudes distant from the equator. SAD reflects a malfunction in the way the brain handles the hormone melatonin, which helps regulate wakefulness and sleeping. You can minimize symptoms by getting as much natural sunlight as possible. Also, paint the walls of your bedroom and other rooms white, keep blinds and curtains open, sit near windows, and take an hour-long midday walk. Many people benefit from phototherapy, which exposes you to bright nonultraviolet light from a light box for several hours daily.

WARNING

The herb ginkgo biloba may reduce the mental sluggishness that can accompany depression. But because ginkgo has blood-thinning properties, don't take it with aspirin or prescription blood-thinning medications.

Your Prevention Plan

Diet ▪ **Eat right.** Eat a well-balanced diet with lots of vegetables, fruits, and other complex carbohydrates—whole-wheat bread, cereal, pasta, and rice. Complex carbohydrates boost the brain's serotonin levels. Get enough protein in the form of dairy products, tofu, lean meats, and fish. Protein is essential for producing neurotransmitters.

▪ **Fish for dinner.** Researchers in Finland found that people who ate fish less than once a week had a 31 percent higher chance of mild to severe depression than those who ate fish more often. They think the beneficial component is the omega-3 polyunsaturated fatty acids in fish.

Exercise ▪ **Embrace exercise.** Aerobic exercise can boost your mood by stimulating the release of endorphins, chemicals that produce a natural "high" and reduce stress. Some studies have shown that regular aerobic exercise works as well as antidepressants to relieve mild depression. It may even help prevent depression in the first place. Work out 45 minutes to an hour five times a week or as near as you can manage. Good bets: brisk walking, swimming, running, dancing, and cycling.

You'll get the maximum mood-enhancing benefit if you exercise hard enough to feel out of breath.

Supplements ▪ **Vitamin B$_{12}$.** One study found that older women with vitamin B$_{12}$ deficiency were at higher risk for severe depression. To get enough B$_{12}$, consume plenty of milk, eggs, fish, and meat. If your diet is restricted or you are over age 70, consider taking a supplement of 5 mcg a day.

Natural Health ▪ **Stay in focus.** Yoga, tai chi, or meditation can help you relax, focus your thoughts, regulate breathing, and improve flexibility. Try 30 to 60 minutes a day to lift your mood.

Lifestyle ▪ **Sleep tight.** Get enough sleep. Avoid naps and try to go to sleep at the same time every night and wake up at the same time every morning.

▪ **Reach out.** Interacting with other people helps keep depression at bay. Stay active socially by doing volunteer work or joining a group.

▪ **Adopt a pet.** Caring for a dog, cat, or bird gives you another focus and provides companionship.

Diabetes

◀ There may be no symptoms until there is a complication, such as a heart attack, stroke, or kidney, nerve, or eye disease.

◀ Common complaints include frequent urination, unusual thirst or hunger, frequent infections (especially of the skin, gums, or bladder), slow-to-heal cuts and bruises, irritability, unusual weight loss, extreme fatigue, blurred vision, and tingling or numbness in the hands or feet.

What is it?

Approximately 2 million Canadians have diabetes, a group of diseases characterized by high blood-glucose levels. When you eat, your body metabolizes carbohydrates into glucose, which is then ushered out of the blood and into the body's cells by insulin, a hormone produced by the pancreas. If you have an insulin disorder, glucose remains in the blood and is unavailable to fuel the cells' activities. The result is elevated blood-sugar levels.

The most common form of diabetes is adult-onset, or type 2, diabetes (also called non-insulin-dependent diabetes). It's usually due to insulin resistance, in which your body's cells don't respond to the insulin produced by the pancreas. It may also involve low insulin production, but not the complete absence of insulin seen in type 1, or juvenile, diabetes (also called insulin-dependent diabetes).

Diabetes can lead to complications such as blindness, kidney disease, heart disease, and stroke. In fact, diabetics are two to four times more likely to suffer a stroke or have heart disease. Up to 50 percent of diabetics develop nerve damage, which can lead to leg or foot amputation. Diabetes is the seventh leading cause of death by disease in Canada.

How is it treated?

Serious complications can be prevented if treatment consistently lowers your blood-glucose levels to normal or close to normal. A healthy diet and regular exercise are the backbone of diabetes care—and they may be all you need, especially if you can stay at or near your ideal weight. Or you

SELF TEST
What Is Your Risk for Diabetes?

One of every three North Americans who has diabetes doesn't know it. But high blood-sugar levels may be secretly damaging organs throughout your body. Your odds of getting adult-onset diabetes increase if you:

◀ are over age 45
◀ are overweight, especially if you carry your weight around your middle
◀ get little or no regular exercise
◀ have higher-than-normal blood sugar levels

◀ have parents or siblings who have been diagnosed with diabetes
◀ are of Aboriginal, African, Latin American, or Asian descent
◀ are a woman who has given birth to a baby weighing more than

8.8 pounds or who developed diabetes during one or more pregnancies
◀ have low HDL ("good") cholesterol or high triglyceride levels
◀ have heart disease or high blood pressure.

may need to take one or more prescription drugs to help your body metabolize sugar more effectively.

If drugs are not enough, your doctor will prescribe insulin injections. (If you find out that you require insulin shots, don't fear. New superthin needles make them almost painless.) One or more insulin injections daily, either alone or in combination with oral drugs, can control diabetes. Your doctor may also prescribe drugs to control your blood pressure, cholesterol and triglyceride levels, if necessary, and to treat any nerve, kidney, or eye complications.

DRUG OPTIONS

Four types of oral drugs are available. Which one(s) you need depends on the severity of your diabetes, your lifestyle, and what (if any) other health problems you have. Sulfonylureas and repaglinide (GlucoNorm) help the body secrete more insulin. Sulfonylureas include tolbutamide (Orinase), chlorpropamide (Diabinese), gliclazide (Diamicron), and glyburide (DiaBeta). They are the most common drugs prescribed for type 2 diabetes. If one doesn't work for you or causes nausea or other side effects, another may be better.

Other drugs enhance insulin's effects. Metformin (Glucophage) reduces the liver's production of glucose. Acarbose (Prandase) blocks enzymes that break down foods into simple sugars. Taken before meals, it delays carbohydrate absorption, blunting postmeal glucose peaks. But it may cause flatulence, bloating, and diarrhea. Glitazones, including rosiglitazone (Avandia) and pioglitazone (Actos), reduce resistance to insulin.

If you take oral drugs or insulin shots to control your blood sugar, beware of overdoing it. Go too low and you could pass out. Hypoglycemia (low blood sugar) can occur if you take too much insulin, eat too little, skip a meal, drink alcohol on an empty stomach, or overdo exercise. You may feel shaky, tired, hungry, confused, or nervous. If this happens, check your blood-sugar level immediately. If it's too low—or if you can't check it—eat something sweet right away, such as a half cup of fruit juice or a few teaspoons of sugar.

If you have diabetes, remember that drugs aren't a substitute for a healthy diet and exercise. They are used only when self-care can't return your glucose levels to near normal.

SELF-CARE GUIDELINES

The following lifestyle measures can help control diabetes and improve the quality of life for people who have it.

- **Learn good self-care.** You are more or less in charge of your own care. So be sure to ask your doctor, nurse educator, or registered dietitian to teach you good diabetes-management skills.
- **Test yourself.** Check your blood-sugar levels daily with a simple finger-stick test and a monitoring device. Depending on how severe your disease is and whether or not you take insulin, you may need to self-test up to several times a day. Stay on top of your glucose fluctuations so

Fast Fact

As North Americans get heavier, diabetes is starting to be seen in younger people. The average age of baby boomers initially diagnosed with diabetes is 37, versus 54 for their parents' generation.

WARNING

If you have diabetes, your risk of heart disease is higher than average. There are three reasons. First, you are more prone to the buildup of fatty deposits in your arteries. Second, your blood clots more easily. And third, you are more likely to have high blood pressure. To help prevent heart disease, make sure your total cholesterol level stays below 5.2 mmol/L and your blood pressure below 130/85, and maintain a healthy weight. Most important of all, if you smoke, quit. (See pages 168-173 for advice on how to stop.)

you can modify your diet/exercise/drug regimen in order to maintain as normal a glucose level as possible.

- **Drink lots of water.** Since diabetes can cause excess urination, it can dehydrate you. So drink at least eight glasses of water daily—more when you're sick or have high glucose levels.

- **Watch your sugar intake.** Doctors have long believed that diabetics should avoid simple carbohydrates (sugars) and replace them with complex carbohydrates such as vegetables, breads, cereals, and pasta. But recent research has shown that people with diabetes *can* eat sugar. In fact, if the total carbohydrate value is the same, mashed potatoes can have the same effect on blood glucose levels as a cookie. That's why you need to monitor your total intake of carbohydrates, not just their source.

- **Investigate the glycemic index.** Debate continues over the use of the glycemic index, a rating of how quickly particular foods are broken down into glucose, raising your blood sugar. Starchy carbohydrates such as potatoes and tropical fruits such as bananas have a higher glycemic index rating than foods such as apples, pears, whole grain breads, and oats. Advocates including the World Health Organization (WHO) say that eating foods with a low glycemic index can help prevent type 2 diabetes. Critics like the National Institutes of Health and the American Diabetes Association say the index makes meal planning even more complicated, especially since a food's score changes depending on what it's eaten with. If you're willing to do the extra homework, ask your doctor or dietitian about the glycemic index.

- **See a dietitian.** A personal meal plan can help you address other health concerns, such as your cholesterol level. Meet with a registered dietitian to tailor a food plan that takes into consideration your age, weight, work schedule, lifestyle, medications, and tastes. Make sure your favorite foods are included or you won't stick with the plan.

- **Pamper your feet.** Wash, dry, and powder your feet carefully every night if you have diabetes. Because the blood vessels in a diabetic's legs narrow, foot injuries or infections can turn into serious ulcers that can lead to gangrene if you have poorly controlled diabetes. Wear shoes that fit properly to prevent blisters, corns, ingrown toenails, and other foot problems. See a podiatrist if any problems arise.

- **Get annual eye checkups.** Have your doctor examine your eyes every year. Careful monitoring can detect signs of diabetic retinopathy, in which many of the small blood vessels of the retina (at the back of the eyeball) become damaged and die. Prompt treatment of this condition can prevent blindness.

- **Be a smart exerciser.** If you have diabetes, talk to your doctor about what precautions you need to take during exercise. You may be advised to avoid certain types of exercise altogether. For example, people with eye complications should steer clear of jumping activities and weight-lifting. And if your blood-glucose level tends to drop and rise suddenly, you may have to eat just prior to exercising and self-test your blood-sugar level periodically during your workout.

Your Prevention Plan

Diet ■ **Doctor your diet.** For most people, carbohydrates (especially complex carbohydrates that are high in fiber) should form the bulk of the diet. Protein foods (meat, soy foods, and dairy) should make up 10 to 20 percent of daily calories. Choose protein foods that are lower in fat, especially saturated fat. That means emphasizing fish, poultry, beans, and low-fat or no-fat dairy products.

■ **Stick to a schedule.** Avoid delaying or skipping meals and binge eating, all of which can play havoc with blood-sugar levels.

■ **Shed some pounds.** At least 80 percent of people who develop type 2 diabetes are overweight. Slim down and you may avoid the disease. Even if you can't get to your ideal weight, a 10-pound loss can dramatically lower blood-sugar levels. (See Chapter 2 for weight-loss tips.)

Exercise ■ **Move it.** Exercise improves your body's sensitivity to insulin, aids glucose control, and can help you lose weight. Brisk walking an hour a day could cut your risk of developing diabetes in half.

Medical Options ■ **Get a diabetes test.** A simple blood test called a random plasma glucose test should be part of your regular health checkup. It can even be done shortly after eating. If the result is 11.1 mmol/L or higher, you may have diabetes and your doctor will order additional tests. If your blood-sugar level isn't high enough to classify you as diabetic, you still should take precautions if you have one of two forms of higher-than-normal levels: impaired fasting glucose (IFG), when results of a standard blood test, after an 8-hour fast, are between 6.1 and 6.9 mmol/L; or impaired glucose tolerance (IGT), when results of a 2-hour oral glucose tolerance test are greater than 7.0 mmol/L. These readings indicate that your body isn't using and/or secreting insulin properly, increasing your risk of diabetes, cardiovascular disease, and premature death. For either condition, follow the diet and exercise recommendations for people who already have diabetes; taking these steps may help prevent you from developing the disease.

Natural Health ■ **Protect yourself with E.** In one Finnish study, men with the lowest blood levels of vitamin E were found to be about four times more likely to develop diabetes than men with the highest levels. Some experts recommend taking a supplement of 200 to 400 mg of vitamin E daily.

Lifestyle ■ **Lower your stress.** Excess stress, in combination with poor coping skills, can raise your blood-sugar levels. See pages 200-203 for relaxation techniques that can help.

SimpleSolution

Ask your doctor about taking supplements of chromium, a trace mineral that plays a major role in cells' sensitivity to insulin. At least one study showed that taking 100 mcg of chromium picolinate twice daily helps lower blood-glucose levels.

Diarrhea

◀ Watery or loose stools passed more than three times a day

◀ Stomach cramping or pain, bloating, nausea, or fever

◀ Bloody stools, which may signal a serious infection

What is it?

Diarrhea is usually caused by a viral or bacterial infection of the small intestine. It can also be caused by certain medications (such as antibiotics, blood pressure drugs, and magnesium-containing antacids), certain medical conditions, and food poisoning.

Food poisoning occurs when you eat food contaminated with bacteria (often *Salmonella*) or parasites. Undercooked food and food that has been standing at room temperature are common culprits. You probably know someone who developed traveler's diarrhea after eating contaminated food outside Canada, but food poisoning is common here as well.

Intolerance to wheat, lactose (the sugar found in milk), or fructose (the sugar in fruits) is another cause. Diarrhea may also accompany inflammatory bowel disease and irritable bowel syndrome.

Diarrhea usually lasts a day or two and ends on its own with home treatment. See your doctor if you have a fever of 102° F or higher, if you have bloody or unusually dark stools, or if your diarrhea lasts for more than four days. Also call your doctor if you feel light-headed, weak, or listless, have pain in your stomach or rectum, or have symptoms of dehydration (strong thirst, dry mouth, dry skin, infrequent urination).

Because the causes of diarrhea are so wide-ranging, your doctor will ask you a variety of questions, including what you've been eating and drinking, whether you've been outside Canada recently, and what medications you take regularly. She may advise you to avoid certain foods for a week or to follow a bland diet to see if the problem clears up. If you've had diarrhea for more than three weeks and the common causes have been ruled out, your doctor may want to examine a stool sample under the microscope to check for parasites.

How is it treated?

The most important step you can take while you have diarrhea is to replace the fluids you're losing. Drink plenty of water, apple juice, cola drinks, electrolyte replacement drinks such as Gatorade, or chicken or beef broth. Stay away from milk, acidic fruit juices, and foods you suspect you can't digest properly. As your diarrhea eases, add bulk to loose stools by following the BRATT diet: bananas, rice, applesauce, tea, and toast.

DRUGS

Prescription or over-the-counter (OTC) drugs that stop diarrhea sometimes help, but they're not recommended for diarrhea caused by bacteria or parasites. Why? Because the drugs that stop diarrhea also prevent the

Fast Fact

Taking more than 1,000 milligrams of vitamin C a day can cause diarrhea.

intestines from expelling the organisms causing it, prolonging the problem. Antibiotics may help in these cases. Diarrhea caused by a virus is often allowed to run its course. Or you may wish to try one of these popular OTC antidiarrheal drugs.

- Loperamide (Imodium) slows the movement of stools through the intestines.
- Attapulgite (Kaopectate) absorbs diarrhea-causing irritants from the digestive tract.
- Bismuth subsalicylate (Pepto-Bismol) works by coating your intestine to protect it from irritants and reducing the fluid buildup that can contribute to a bout of diarrhea.

NATURAL REMEDIES

Astringent teas such as those made from agrimony, raspberry leaf, and blackberry leaf may reduce intestinal inflammation. And taking 5,000 mcg of folic acid three times daily for several days can cut bouts of infectious diarrhea nearly in half. Psyllium seed, available in most health-food stores, provides soluble fiber that adds bulk to stools.

Your Prevention Plan

Diet ▪ **Rinse your produce.** Wash all fruits and vegetables before eating them to remove bacteria.

▪ **Cook it well.** Rare meat can cause food poisoning. Always use a meat thermometer to make sure it's safe.

▪ **Use kitchen caution.** Always keep hot foods hot and cold foods cold. Throw out eggs that are cracked, as well as cans that are swollen or dented at the rim or seam. Defrost foods in the refrigerator, not on the counter. Make sure that raw meat juices don't come into contact with other foods in your refrigerator or on the cutting board.

▪ **Test the water.** If you have chronic diarrhea, have your tap water tested for bacteria or install a purification filter.

▪ **Say "yes" to yogurt.** Yogurt that contains live cultures helps restore beneficial bacteria to the intestines, keeping "bad" bacteria from thriving.

Supplements ▪ **Look to lactase.** If you are lactose intolerant, head off potential digestive problems, including diarrhea, by taking lactase (Lactaid) before eating foods that contain dairy products.

▪ **Consider acidophilus.** If you're taking antibiotics for a bacterial infection, consider taking acidophilus supplements to restore to your digestive tract the beneficial bacteria that antibiotics kill.

Lifestyle ▪ **Hygiene helps.** Always wash your hands before preparing foods or eating, after using the toilet, and in between handling cooked and raw foods, especially meats.

▪ **Travel smart.** When visiting other countries, take care to prevent traveler's diarrhea. Don't drink the tap water or even brush your teeth with it, and avoid ice made from it. Pass up raw fruits and vegetables (including lettuce), unless they can be peeled and you peel them yourself. Avoid unpasteurized milk or dairy products, and don't eat raw or rare meat or fish.

▪ **Keep stress under control.** Intense stress can disrupt the digestive system and cause diarrhea. See Chapter 7, *Giving Stress the Boot*, for ways to keep your cool.

Diverticular Disease

◆ SYMPTOMS ◆

◀ Diverticulosis: mild cramps, bloating, constipation, and lower abdominal pain, but often no symptoms

◀ Diverticulitis: fever, nausea, vomiting, chills, severe lower-left abdominal pain, constipation, rectal bleeding

Nutrition Note

Doctors once recommended that people with diverticular disease avoid high-fiber foods, believing the roughage could make the condition worse. Today they know that a high-fiber diet can prevent and help treat diverticular disease. During an attack, however, avoid seedy foods, such as berries.

What is it?

Diverticular disease can take two forms: diverticulosis and diverticulitis. In diverticulosis, grape-sized pouches called diverticula bulge out through weak spots in the walls of your colon (large intestine). About half of all North Americans age 60 to 80 have these pouches, the result of a low-fiber diet. Diverticulosis is rarely found in Asia and Africa, where people eat mostly high-fiber foods and little meat. Fiber makes stools soft and easier to pass, reducing pressure in the colon. Doctors believe that straining to have a bowel movement encourages diverticula to form—the reason constipation can cause diverticulosis.

In diverticulitis, the pouches become inflamed or infected, possibly because stools or food get caught in them. About 10 to 25 percent of people with diverticulosis develop diverticulitis, which can lead to tearing, blockage, or bleeding of the colon. If an abscess (a localized collection of pus) forms, it can cause swelling, tissue damage, and the spread of infection to other parts of the body. Sometimes the pus leaks out of the colon into the abdominal cavity. This can lead to an infection called peritonitis, a medical emergency requiring surgery to clean out and disinfect the cavity and remove damaged portions of the colon.

Most people with diverticulosis have no symptoms. The condition is often diagnosed during tests being performed for another reason. Sometimes doctors discover diverticulosis during an X ray of your colon in which barium (which outlines the colon) is used. If your doctor suspects diverticulosis, he may request a stool sample to test it for blood.

Your doctor may be able to diagnose diverticulitis from your symptoms. He will examine your abdomen for tenderness and take blood to check for signs of infection. An endoscope (a lighted, flexible tube with a tiny camera at its tip) may be used to view the inside of your colon.

How is it treated?

Most people can control mild diverticular disease with the recommendations in *Your Prevention Plan* (opposite). For more serious disease, the goals are to treat any infection, reduce inflammation, rest the colon, and prevent complications such as bleeding or perforation. Drugs and surgery are sometimes necessary.

DRUGS

Anti-inflammatory medication (such as ibuprofen) can ease the cramps, bloating, and constipation of diverticulosis. To allow your colon to rest, your doctor may prescribe a liquid diet and the drug propantheline bromide (Pro-Banthine), which helps control intestinal spasms. If you've had rectal bleeding, an artery-constricting drug such as vasopressin may be injected into the affected area to stop the bleeding and ease symptoms. An abscess requires treatment with antibiotics. If the drugs don't work, however, the abscess may need to be drained. Your doctor will insert a needle and a catheter (small tube) into the abscess to remove the fluid.

SURGERY

For serious diverticulitis, your doctor may recommend surgery to remove the troublesome portion of your colon. The healthy sections of the colon are then reconnected.

NATURAL MEDICINE

Visit your health-food store and ask about marshmallow root, slippery elm bark, licorice root, and aloe vera juice, all of which can soothe and protect inflamed intestines. Chamomile, goldenseal, red clover, and yarrow may also help. And fiber supplements in the form of psyllium or flaxseed can help ease flare-ups.

Fast Fact

A new treatment may cut the need for diverticular surgery, reports The New England Journal of Medicine. *An endoscope (a lighted, flexible tube with a camera at its tip) is guided into the large intestine and used to deliver drugs and perform tiny repairs on bleeding diverticula without full-scale surgery.*

Your Prevention Plan

Diet ■ **Go for bulk.** Increasing the amount of fiber in your diet can reduce diverticulosis symptoms and prevent diverticulitis. Be sure to consume at least 30 grams of fiber each day—but increase your intake slowly. Good sources include fresh fruits and vegetables, beans and legumes, and whole-grain breads and cereals. If you are unable to get sufficient fiber through diet alone, your doctor may recommend a daily dose of Citrucel or Metamucil. When mixed with water, these products provide about 4 to 6 grams of fiber in an 8-ounce glass.

■ **Drink up.** Make sure you drink at least eight 8-ounce glasses of water daily. This can help prevent the constipation that can result when you increase your fiber intake.

■ **Spoon up some yogurt.** Beneficial bacteria normally live in the colon, where they fight disease-causing bacteria. If you are taking an antibiotic drug (which can kill the good bacteria along with the bad), eat yogurt that contains active cultures every day to help restore the beneficial bacteria.

■ **Send garlic to the scene.** Use lots of garlic in your cooking to help fight harmful bacteria.

Exercise ■ **Move things along.** Exercise helps prevent constipation by keeping stools moving through the digestive system. Get 30 minutes of moderate activity each day, such as brisk walking, jogging, swimming, or biking.

Supplements ■ **Welcome "good" bacteria.** Take an acidophilus supplement to help restore the favorable bacteria in your colon—especially if you are on antibiotics.

■ **Take your vitamins.** Help keep your immune system in top shape by taking a daily multivitamin and mineral supplement that contains the immune boosters and infection fighters vitamin E, vitamin C, and zinc.

■ **Try cat's claw.** This herb, from the inner bark of the cat's claw vine, is valued for a variety of healing properties, including its ability to boost immunity and soothe inflammation.

Emphysema

◄ Early stages: shortness of breath when exercising and a chronic, mild cough with scant mucus

◄ Later stages: shortness of breath with little or no exertion and a chronic cough that produces thick, clear mucus. Also, an enlarged, barrel-shaped chest; wheezing; bulging eyes; bluish skin color; weight loss; headache; dizziness; irritability; and insomnia

SimpleSolution

Inhaling the aromatherapy oils eucalyptus, hyssop, pine, or rosemary may ease your breathing. Also try teas made from elecampane, which acts as an expectorant to help clear the lungs of mucus.

What is it?

Emphysema is an irreversible disease in which the walls between the alveoli (tiny air sacs) in your lungs are destroyed. The condition causes individual alveoli to merge with neighboring air sacs, leaving fewer, larger air sacs with less surface area. Less surface area means the air sacs are less efficient at exchanging carbon dioxide for life-giving oxygen. The sacs also become less elastic, so they can't completely deflate to force carbon dioxide out of your lungs. As a result of this damage, breathing—especially exhaling—becomes difficult.

Long-term cigarette smoking is by far the most common cause of emphysema, but air pollution and workplace exposure to fumes and dust can also contribute to it. Your risk also rises with a family history of chronic obstructive lung disease, which is emphysema that occurs with chronic bronchitis. In 2 out of 1,000 people, an inherited deficiency in the protein alpha-1-antitrypsin (AAT) causes the disease. While emphysema usually is diagnosed after age 50, the inherited form can surface 20 years earlier.

Emphysema is 22 percent more common in men than in women, but the numbers are changing as more women smoke. If you have emphysema, you have a higher risk of other medical problems, including repeated lung infections, pulmonary hypertension (high blood pressure in the arteries in the lungs), and heart failure.

To diagnose emphysema, your doctor will use a stethoscope to listen to your breathing and may tap on your chest in various places. A hollow sound indicates emphysema. She may also take an X ray of your chest. In a test called spirometry, the amount of air you can exhale is measured. A blood test may be performed to determine the amount of oxygen in your blood, which helps your doctor understand how much oxygen you're taking in through your damaged lungs.

How is it treated?

Emphysema is incurable. But if you smoke—and most people with emphysema do—quitting is your most important treatment. For advice on how to break the nicotine habit, see Chapter 6, *Avoiding Common Health Traps*. Your doctor may also recommend one or more of the following treatments.

OXYGEN

Inhaling supplemental oxygen eases breathing and improves the function of your heart. The oxygen comes in portable tanks, and you inhale it through a plastic tube with special openings that fit into your nostrils. While some people with emphysema use oxygen only at night, it's more effective when taken 24 hours a day. But it can seriously limit your mobility. Never smoke while using supplemental oxygen, and keep the tank away from open flames.

DRUGS

Inhaled corticosteroid drugs such as budesonide (Pulmicort) help heal the lining of your breathing passages. For people with the inherited form of emphysema, an alpha-1 proteinase inhibitor (Prolastin) may be given intravenously once a week to raise the blood level of AAT. Antibiotics are used to treat chronic lung infections such as bronchitis or pneumonia. Bronchodilators such as salbutamol (Ventolin) relax the muscles of your airways, which helps open breathing passages. You inhale these drugs through your mouth or nose, and they start to work in minutes.

SURGERY

Lung reduction surgery (still experimental) cuts away diseased lung sections, giving healthy parts more room to expand. It is usually reserved for severe cases.

WARNING

Think twice about taking Ephedra sinica (Ma huang), a Chinese herb sometimes used to treat upper respiratory problems. One of its ingredients is similar to amphetamine (a stimulant) and can raise your blood pressure and heart rate. If used improperly, it can cause seizures, psychosis, and even death. Hundreds of cases of adverse reactions have been reported.

Your Prevention Plan

Diet ■ **Eat your antioxidants.** Cornell researchers studying more than 18,000 people found that those with a high antioxidant intake had better lung function than those with a low intake. Be sure to get plenty of foods rich in vitamins A, C, and E, selenium, and beta-carotene. Good sources include dark-colored vegetables and fruits, whole grains and nuts, wheat germ, and vegetable oils.

Exercise ■ **Shake a leg.** Regular aerobic exercise such as walking helps clear mucus from the lungs and increases your lung capacity, boosting your endurance and decreasing breathlessness. Aim for at least 20 minutes of exercise daily.

Medical Options ■ **Build your defenses.** Get a flu shot every fall and a pneumonia shot at least one time.

Supplements ■ **Consider N-acetyl cysteine (NAC).** This antioxidant thins mucus and may also protect lung tissue.

Take 200 mg twice a day—but be sure to tell your doctor you're taking it.

■ **Give yourself a C.** Vitamin C thins mucus, may help prevent bronchitis, and may increase the amount of air you can exhale from your lungs. Ask your doctor about a safe dosage.

Lifestyle ■ **Stop smoking.** Quitting is the most important step in treating emphysema and preventing it from getting worse. Talk to your doctor about nicotine replacement, the drug bupropion (Zyban, which cuts cigarette cravings and is also marketed as an antidepressant under the name Wellbutrin), and group therapy. Many hospitals and local lung associations offer support groups. Acupuncture may also help.

■ **Watch what you breathe.** Avoid secondhand smoke, smog, car exhaust, fumes, dust, and chemical irritants. If smog levels are high, stay inside except in the early morning or evening. Keep your house well ventilated, use a humidifier if the air is too dry, and get rid of mold and mildew.

Fatigue

SYMPTOMS

◀ Lingering tiredness
◀ Diminished energy
◀ Feelings of indifference
◀ Difficulty concentrating

WARNING

If you wake up exhausted and you snore, you may have sleep apnea, a breathing disorder that can interrupt your sleep as many as 100 times an hour. See page 265 for more information.

What is it?

Short-term fatigue, that weary feeling you get after a stressful day or a long trip, is normal. But long-term, constant fatigue—the kind you feel every day, no matter what you've been doing—is not.

Fatigue is one of the most common complaints of people who visit a doctor. It can be a side effect of prescription drugs. It can also be caused by conditions such as depression, diabetes, multiple sclerosis, ulcers, gastroesophageal reflux, or sleep apnea (a breathing disorder that causes frequent awakening during the night). Thyroid disease affects 15 percent or more of adults and is a common cause of tiredness. About 10 to 15 percent of women in North America have iron-deficiency anemia, which causes fatigue. (Causes of iron-deficiency anemia include a heavy menstrual flow or blood loss from a bleeding ulcer.) A simple blood test can help your doctor diagnose both conditions. Some older adults lose the ability to absorb vitamin B_{12} from food, which also causes anemia. Vitamin B_{12} deficiency can be detected by a blood test and is treated by injections or by giving high oral doses of the vitamin.

In most cases, however, fatigue is caused by the lifestyle choices we make—smoking, drinking, a poor diet, too little exercise, overeating, and plain old lack of sleep. Fatigue may also accompany loneliness or boredom.

How is it treated?

If you are often tired for reasons you can't explain, see your doctor, who can determine whether there is a medical explanation and suggest an appropriate course of treatment. If your fatigue is not due to an underlying illness or condition, adopting certain changes in your lifestyle, diet, and exercise habits can make a significant difference. See *Your Prevention Plan* (opposite) for advice.

Recognizing Chronic Fatigue Syndrome (CFS)

CFS is an illness marked by intense exhaustion and flulike symptoms. Long-term fatigue could be CFS if the condition lasts at least six months and is accompanied by some of the following symptoms: severe fatigue unrelated to a medical cause, loss of short-term memory and concentration, sore throat, tender lymph glands, fever, muscle pain, joint pain without swelling or redness, severe headaches, and sleep disturbances. If you experience these symptoms, see your doctor. There is no cure for CFS, but there are ways to manage the symptoms.

Your Prevention Plan

Diet

Get complex. Complex carbohydrates such as whole-grain foods, fruits, and vegetables provide lasting energy because they take a long time to digest. Many also provide B vitamins needed for energy.

Make like a sheep and graze. Eating multiple small meals throughout the day helps stabilize your blood-sugar levels, preventing the lows that can make some people feel tired.

Skip the sweets. Sugar provides a quick pick-me-up, but that brief energy burst is usually followed by a bust that leaves you more tired than you were before.

Cut down on caffeine. If you're hooked on caffeine, you have to consume more and more of it to get a stimulating effect. Cutting down will reduce your tolerance, so a cup of joe will perk you up again. Note that, especially in older people, caffeine's effects can last as long as 10 hours, so make your noontime fix your last of the day.

Get enough magnesium. Many people don't get enough magnesium, a mineral essential for energy production. Good food sources include whole grains, green vegetables, avocados, bananas, legumes, nuts, and seeds.

Exercise

Make fitness a habit. When you exercise, your body releases energizing neurotransmitters called endorphins. Exercise also increases the amount of oxygen-rich blood reaching your brain and muscles and increases the number of blood cells in the body. And it makes you sleep better, too. Moreover, if you're in shape, everyday activities such as hauling groceries are less tiring.

Energize your inner self. Try yoga, meditation, or qigong (ancient Chinese breathing and meditation exercises) to revitalize yourself.

Medical Options

Check your meds. Certain medications, including some beta-blockers, the antidepressants paroxetine (Paxil) and sertraline (Zoloft), and the antianxiety drug alprazolam (Xanax), can produce fatigue as a side effect. Some over-the-counter pain medicines may interfere with your sleep because they contain caffeine—more than you'd find in a cup of coffee. Check with your doctor to determine if your medications might be contributing to your fatigue.

Switch your allergy medicine. All over-the-counter antihistamines may cause fatigue. Ask your doctor about prescription allergy drugs; they are less sedating.

Supplements

Do it daily. Take a multivitamin with minerals every day to make sure you get enough B vitamins (which aid carbohydrate and protein metabolism and blood cell formation), magnesium (critical to energy production), and other important nutrients.

Energize with ginseng. Consider taking either Panax ginseng (100 to 250 mg) or Siberian ginseng (100 to 300 mg) twice day. Both of these herbs have been shown to help fight fatigue.

Natural Health

Stimulate your senses. Some people find the scent of essential oils such as sandalwood and lemon invigorating. Use them in a diffuser or place a few drops on a handkerchief. Add a couple of drops of lavender oil to a prebedtime bath to help you sleep.

Lifestyle

Get enough rest. Only 35 percent of people sleep the recommended eight hours per night during the week. Make sleep time a priority. And remember, you can't "catch up" for lost sleep on weekends. For tips on more restful slumber, see Chapter 11, *Getting Enough Sleep*.

Stay connected. Avoid isolation, which can lead to boredom and depression, both of which can cause fatigue. Stay involved by joining a club or community association, or become a volunteer.

Nix nicotine. Like caffeine, nicotine is a stimulant, so you'd think it would give you more energy. But the opposite is true. Smoking lowers the oxygen levels in your blood, and since the muscles and tissues need oxygen for energy, the result is fatigue.

Fibromyalgia

SYMPTOMS

◄ Aching and pain in at least 11 of 18 recognized "tender point" sites found in muscles and other soft tissue of the neck, shoulders, back, hips, thighs, and arms

◄ Moderate to severe fatigue is common, and so is unproductive sleep that leaves you tired and listless during the day.

◄ Other complaints include headaches, high anxiety levels, trouble concentrating, and irritable bowel symptoms such as abdominal pain, bloating, and alternating constipation and diarrhea.

What is it?

Fibromyalgia is a painful rheumatic condition of the muscles, tendons, and ligaments (but not joints) that affects nearly 900,000 Canadians. Discomfort, ranging from flulike achiness to severe pain, may vary by time of day or in response to stress, amount of sleep, or activity levels. More common in women than in men, fibromyalgia may occur alone or develop as a result of another rheumatic disease, such as rheumatoid arthritis, osteoarthritis, or lupus. It may go away by itself, recur at intervals, or become chronic.

How is it treated?

No medical tests can confirm fibromyalgia, but they can rule out other conditions that cause similar symptoms. While no fully satisfactory therapy is available yet, treatment can ease symptoms. Research has shown that the best benefits come from a combination of exercise and psychological approaches, such as relaxation training, hypnotherapy, biofeedback, and cognitive therapy.

Although some drugs are useful, traditional painkillers—aspirin, NSAIDs, and narcotics—don't help most people with fibromyalgia. Injecting lidocaine into tender points offers temporary relief. Your doctor may recommend antidepressants, not for their mood-boosting benefits but for their ability to promote sleep and alter pain perception. Tricyclic antidepressants such as amitriptyline (Elavil) or imipramine (Tofranil) can offer relief. But if side effects occur—such as daytime drowsiness, constipation, dry mouth, and increased appetite—your doctor may try a different class of antidepressant: selective serotonin reuptake inhibitors (SSRIs), including paroxetine (Paxil), sertraline (Zoloft), or fluoxetine (Prozac). SSRIs may work because people with fibromyalgia seem to have lower levels of serotonin, a brain chemical related to sleep, mood, and pain sensitivity. But SSRIs may interfere with sexual response. If this becomes a problem, ask your doctor about taking medication-free weekends.

THE NATURAL WAY

A University of Maryland study showed that qigong (an ancient Chinese system of meditation, breathing exercises, and slow, graceful movements) may benefit fibromyalgia sufferers. Participants reported relief of depression and pain, improved ability to carry out daily activities, and more success in coping with ailment symptoms.

Your Prevention Plan

Exercise

Work out your pain. Regular exercise can produce dramatic relief. Studies have shown an average 30 percent reduction in achiness and a 40 percent drop in tender point pain after six weeks of exercise three times a week. Try walking, cycling, swimming, or low-impact aerobics. Exercise helps by toning muscles and increasing aerobic fitness so that day-to-day physical tasks require less energy. It also improves blood circulation and triggers the brain's release of endorphins (our feel-good hormones). Stick with it: For the first three weeks, you may feel worse as unused muscles learn to work again. But extra achiness dissipates with time.

Supplements

Consider magnesium and malic acid. Some doctors think low levels of magnesium, critical to muscle metabolism, contribute to fibromyalgia. Other researchers think boosting malic acid, which helps energize muscles, can help. A study in which participants took 300 to 600 mg of magnesium and 1,800 to 2,400 mg of malic acid daily, in divided doses, produced improvements after a few months. Get your doctor's advice. But don't take extra magnesium if you have kidney problems or take high blood pressure medication. And cut your dose if you develop diarrhea.

Improve your sleep. Although studies have yielded conflicting results, 2 mg of melatonin at bedtime may help you sleep better. But don't take it if you also have an autoimmune disease such as lupus or rheumatoid arthritis.

Natural Health

Get a massage. Twice-weekly Swedish massage provided more relief from symptoms than TENS (a transcutaneous electrical nerve stimulator, an electronic anti-pain device) in a Miami study. Recipients not only were happier and more relaxed after treatments but also had less pain, stiffness, depression, insomnia, and fatigue after five weeks. Massage helps raise brain levels of serotonin, the body's natural painkiller. Can't afford it? Ask your partner to massage you with your favorite moisturizing cream, or massage yourself.

Try acupuncture. In one study, six weekly acupuncture treatments cut pain by almost half and reduced tender points by about a third.

Heat it up. Hot compresses, showers, and baths can relax sore muscles.

Take tea. Chamomile or valerian tea before bedtime may help relax you and ease you into a sounder sleep.

Lifestyle

Learn to relax. Take a class or see a counselor for relaxation training to reduce your anxiety. Other useful techniques include hypnotherapy, biofeedback, and cognitive behavior therapy, as well as prayer and meditation.

Use positive self-talk. Be reassured that fibromyalgia is a benign condition and you won't become deformed or disabled. Most people get better, so try not to worry. Studies show that believing you'll feel better increases the odds that you will.

WARNING

Don't believe claims for guaifenesin (a common ingredient in cough medicine) that have spread on the Internet. A year-long study sponsored by the National Fibromyalgia Research Association found it no better than a placebo at easing symptoms.

Gallstones

◀ Intense pain in your upper-right abdomen —often after you eat— that may radiate to your right shoulder, back, or chest. Pain may last from a half hour to several hours.

◀ Nausea and vomiting

◀ Belching, passing gas, bloating, and indigestion

◀ Jaundice—yellowing of your skin and the whites of your eyes

What is it?

Gallstones form in the gallbladder, a pear-shaped organ located behind the liver. The gallbladder is a storage tank for bile, a substance made in the liver and released to help digest fat. Bile contains water, salts, cholesterol, and the pigment bilirubin, which gives stools their brown color. After you eat, your gallbladder contracts and releases bile through a narrow tube-like duct to your small intestine.

Gallstones are made up of a hard material that forms when the bile contains too much of one component. Three-quarters of all gallstones develop because the bile contains too much cholesterol. The stones can also form when the gallbladder doesn't empty completely. Other gallstones are pigment stones composed mostly of bilirubin. Although scientists aren't certain, they think this type develops in people who have cirrhosis of the liver, a gallbladder infection, or hereditary blood disorders.

About 80 percent of people who have gallstones don't have symptoms and don't need treatment. Pain starts when gallstones inflame the gall-bladder or become lodged in one of the nearby ducts. Gallstone attacks often follow a high-fat meal and frequently occur at night.

If your doctor suspects gallstones, he may order one of these tests to confirm the diagnosis:

- **Ultrasound** sends into your abdomen painless sound waves that bounce off your gallbladder and create a picture showing any stones.
- **Cholecystogram** involves taking several pills containing dye the night before the test so that your gallbladder—and any obstructions—can be seen on X rays the next day.

SELF TEST

What Is Your Risk for Gallstones?

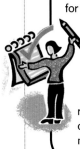

You are at greater risk for gallstones if you:

◀ are over age 60

◀ are a woman. Estrogen raises cholesterol levels in the bile. Estrogen from hormone replacement and oral contraceptives may also raise risk.

◀ are an obese woman. Overweight women have low levels of bile salts and elevated cholesterol, putting them at greater risk.

◀ have diabetes. High levels of triglycerides (fatty acids) in the blood may encourage gallstones to develop.

◀ fast or go on a crash diet. Fasting causes cholesterol to remain in the gallbladder. When you lose weight quickly, your liver responds by releasing extra cholesterol into the bile. In both situa-tions, excess choles-terol creates ideal

conditions for the for-mation of gallstones.

◀ take cholesterol-lower-ing drugs, some of which elevate bile and may lead to gallstones

◀ have ulcerative colitis or Crohn's disease, or have had surgery on your intestines

◀ have constipation.

- **Endoscopic retrograde cholangiopancreatography (ERCP)** uses a flexible tube guided down the throat to the small intestine. Your doctor locates the bile duct, injects dye, and looks for blockages on an X ray.
- **Blood tests** screen for infection and elevated bilirubin.

How is it treated?

SURGERY

Removing the gallbladder is the most common treatment. "Keyhole" surgery makes this procedure much less risky than it once was. The surgeon makes several small incisions in your abdomen and inserts, through one incision, a lighted flexible tube with a tiny camera so he can view the operation. Instruments are inserted through the other incisions to cut around the gallbladder and remove it.

EXTRACORPOREAL SHOCK-WAVE LITHOTRIPSY (ESWL)

Shock waves are used to smash gallstones into tiny pieces so they can flow out through the bile ducts. ESWL isn't nearly as successful as a similar treatment used to break up kidney stones.

DRUGS

Medications may dissolve small stones over 18 months to 2 years. But they work in only 1 in 10 people, and stones return in up to half of them.

SimpleSolution

Take a capsule of peppermint oil with meals to help dissolve gall-stones. Be sure to take coated pills, which don't dissolve until they reach your intestines, where they do their best work.

Your Prevention Plan

Diet ■ **Eat right.** A low-fat, high-fiber diet offers several benefits that may lower your risk of gallstones. First, it helps keep your weight in check. It also helps you avoid constipation. (Aim to get at least 25 to 30 grams of fiber a day, and increase your intake slowly, not all at once.) And cutting down on animal fats lowers your cholesterol levels and decreases the risk of a gallstone attack.

■ **Fill your tank.** Drink at least eight 8-ounce glasses of water daily. If you're boosting your fiber intake, drinking extra water is essential to prevent constipation.

■ **Favor fish.** Researchers have found that people who eat plenty of fish and monounsaturated fats found in olive and canola oils seem to have a lower risk of gallstones.

■ **Don't crash and burn.** Crash diets and rapid weight loss increase your risk.

Exercise ■ **Get moving.** Regular exercise helps control your weight and lowers cholesterol, reducing two gall-stone risk factors. It may also help correct abnormal blood-sugar levels, another risk factor.

Supplements ■ **Add psyllium.** This supplement helps prevent constipation and attaches to the cholesterol in bile, helping prevent gallstones from forming.

■ **Get more C.** New research shows that women with high blood levels of vitamin C may be less likely to experience gallstones. Vitamin C seems to lower bile cholesterol levels.

Natural Health ■ **Go herbal.** Try milk thistle and dandelion. These herbs, taken as pills, are thought to change the composition of bile and reduce its cholesterol content.

Gastroesophageal Reflux Disease (Heartburn)

◀ Heartburn, a fiery feeling in your chest or upper abdomen after you eat or lie down

◀ Chest pain so strong you may think you're having a heart attack

◀ Throat burning, tightness, soreness, or hoarseness (especially when you wake up)

What is it?

Gastroesophageal reflux disease (GERD) occurs when stomach acid (and sometimes food and liquid) backs up into your esophagus, the muscular tube that connects your throat and stomach. Normally, the lower esophageal sphincter (LES), a ringlike muscular valve located at the bottom of your esophagus, keeps acid and other substances in your stomach. The sphincter relaxes only when you swallow to permit food and liquids to pass into your stomach.

With GERD, the sphincter malfunctions, relaxing when it shouldn't and allowing acid to reflux (move up) into your esophagus. Because the tender lining of your esophagus doesn't protect against stomach acid, you suffer heartburn or indigestion. A serious complication of GERD is Barrett's esophagus, a precancerous condition in which the normally gray-pink tissue of your esophagus becomes inflamed and salmon-colored like the stomach lining. Persistent GERD can also lead to scarring of the esophagus. Pneumonia or bronchitis may occur as stomach acid refluxes and seeps into your lungs through the trachea (windpipe), usually while you're sleeping. GERD also destroys tooth enamel when stomach acid backs up into your mouth.

Some people experience GERD because they have a hiatal hernia. In this disorder, the upper portion of the stomach moves into the chest by way of an opening in the diaphragm, the band of muscle that separates the chest and stomach. A hiatal hernia impairs the functioning of the LES, allowing acid and other stomach contents to reflux into the esophagus, causing the symptoms of GERD.

DIAGNOSTIC TESTS

GERD is usually identified by its symptoms, but certain tests can help your doctor confirm the diagnosis or check for complications.

- **Barium esophagram or X ray** helps your doctor see the upper part of your digestive tract. You'll need to drink a barium solution (a chalky liquid that shows up on X rays) before this procedure so your organs can be visualized.
- **Endoscopy** involves inserting a small, lighted, flexible tube through your mouth and into your esophagus and stomach so your doctor can check for abnormalities.
- **Esophageal manometry** tests the pressure of your esophagus and LES, while **esophageal pH** confirms or rules out the presence of excess acid reflux. For both tests, a small flexible tube is inserted through your nose and into the esophagus.

Fast Fact

Scientists estimate that half of all people with asthma also have GERD, but they are not sure how the two conditions are related.

How is it treated?

Most people can control moderate GERD by avoiding foods that trigger it, making certain lifestyle modifications (see *Your Prevention Plan*, page 342), and taking over-the-counter (OTC) drugs. If these steps aren't enough, see your doctor. You may need to take a prescription drug. Severe cases may require surgery.

DRUGS

Both over-the-counter and prescription drugs are used to treat GERD. OTC antacids neutralize stomach acid and ease an attack that's already started. They include Maalox, Mylanta, Rolaids, and Tums. H2 blockers block the action of histamine, a chemical that encourages stomach-acid production. They can actually help prevent an attack if you take them before eating (how long before eating varies from drug to drug). H2 blockers include cimetidine (Tagamet), famotidine (Pepcid), nizatidine (Axid), and ranitidine (Zantac). If you find yourself taking these drugs often, see your doctor.

Prescription drugs called proton pump inhibitors, such as lansoprazole (Prevacid), omeprazole (Losec), and pantoprazole (Pantoloc), disable the cell-level pumps that move acid into the stomach. Another prescription drug, metoclopramide (Reglan), increases pressure on the LES to decrease acid reflux. Metoclopramide also helps move food out of the stomach, easing pressure.

SURGERY

In the past, if lifestyle changes and drug therapy were not effective, surgery (called fundoplication) was performed to tighten the LES muscle between the stomach and the esophagus. In this procedure, the surgeon folds and secures a portion of the stomach to establish a tighter sphincter. In a less invasive type of fundoplication the surgeon uses miniature instruments and a camera—inserted through small incisions in the abdomen—to perform the surgery.

Recently the U.S. Food and Drug Administration approved two new ways to treat GERD. Both methods involve inserting an endoscope (a slender, flexible, lighted tube) down the throat and into the esophagus to repair the faulty sphincter.

In the first method, electrodes on the end of the endoscope burn the muscle that opens and closes the LES, creating scar tissue. The scar tissue either calms the nerves that make the sphincter malfunction or tightens the sphincter itself—doctors aren't sure yet how it works. The second procedure uses a tiny stitching device—like a sewing machine—to gather up and tighten the valve.

Each of these new outpatient procedures takes only about an hour, and the side effects are minor: You may feel a little pain in your stomach or chest for a few hours after the surgery. Ask your doctor whether one of the new procedures might work for you.

DRUG CAPSULE

Which drugs work better? Proton pump inhibitors have been found to heal and cure erosive esophagitis, a serious form of GERD, more quickly than H2 blockers.

WARNING

If you are taking cisapride (Prepulsid), call your doctor now. The drug was taken off the market because of its link to dangerous cardiac side effects and more than 70 deaths.

Your Prevention Plan

Diet

Avoid trigger foods. Certain foods and beverages can trigger GERD, either by promoting stomach acid secretion or relaxing the LES. Stay away from alcoholic beverages, chocolate, citrus fruits and juices, caffeinated drinks, carbonated drinks, fatty and fried foods (French fries, hamburgers, eggs, whole milk, doughnuts), peppermint and spearmint (including breath mints and mint-flavored toothpaste), spicy foods, garlic, onions, peppers, and tomatoes and tomato-based foods (tomato juice, ketchup, spaghetti sauce, chili, and pizza).

Get lean. Extra weight can make it more difficult for the LES to stay closed, contributing to acid reflux. Start a sensible diet and exercise program to shed any extra pounds.

Start grazing. Eat smaller meals more frequently—perhaps five times a day—and eat them slowly to help avoid stomach bloating and pressure. Sit down and relax at each meal.

Timing is everything. Eat and drink at least three hours before going to bed, and don't snack at bedtime.

Lay off liquor. Alcohol aggravates GERD symptoms, and beer can bloat the stomach, driving stomach acid into the esophagus.

Stay upright. You have a greater risk of GERD when you lie on your back after a meal, so sit up for several hours after eating.

Wash it down. Drink plenty of water—eight 8-ounce glasses a day—to wash stomach acid down to the stomach where it belongs.

Exercise

Move things along. Exercise keeps the gastrointestinal system working normally. And gentle exercise done regularly can help ease GERD by reducing stress. But avoid exercises that involve bending over, because this can aggravate heartburn.

Medical Options

Avoid certain drugs. Some over-the-counter drugs, including ibuprofen and aspirin, may lead to the burning of GERD. Prescription drugs that can cause heartburn include some tricyclic antidepressants, some calcium channel blockers, and some bronchodilators (such as theophylline). Ask your doctor if one of your prescription drugs might be contributing to your GERD.

Natural Health

Try tea. Drinking chamomile tea between meals three to four times a day may relieve inflamed or irritated mucous membranes in your digestive tract and helps promote normal digestion. Ginger tea may also provide relief. Boil 1$\frac{1}{2}$ teaspoons of fresh ginger (or $\frac{1}{2}$ teaspoon of powdered ginger) in one cup of water for about 10 minutes before drinking.

Look to licorice. Licorice protects the esophagus by boosting production of mucin, a substance that forms a protective barrier against stomach acid. Before meals, chew licorice-root tablets in deglycyrrhizinated form (which doesn't increase blood pressure or cause water retention as licorice does).

■ **Look for herbal relief.** Mix ½ teaspoon of goldenseal extract with 3 table-spoons water and drink the mixture at the first sign of burning to soothe the membranes that line the gastrointestinal tract. Also, try drinking ½ cup aloe vera juice three times a day between meals. If indigestion is your main problem, several herbs can help, including fennel, yarrow, and barberry.

■ **Drink cabbage juice.** Visit a health food store to find cabbage juice, whose glutamine content may calm the burning of GERD.

■ **Sip a baking-soda cocktail.** Baking soda can help neutralize stomach acid. Mix 1 teaspoon baking soda in a glass of room-temperature water and sip at the first sign of burning pain. Baking soda is high in salt, so check with your doctor before using it if you're reducing your salt intake.

■ **Chew on this.** One study found that chewing a stick of sugarless gum provided heartburn relief in 70 percent of participants. The chewing action stimulates the production of saliva, which helps wash stomach acid back down the esophagus.

Lifestyle ■ **Stay loose.** Wear loose-fitting clothes. Tight belts, panty hose, and pants put pressure on the stomach and may force stomach acid upward.

■ **Douse the flame.** Don't smoke. Nicotine stimulates stomach-acid production and relaxes the muscle between the esophagus and the stomach, allowing acid to reflux.

■ **Say no to stress.** Stress reduction may help some people with GERD. Take up meditation, yoga, or deep breathing, and engage in regular exercise, such as brisk walking, swimming, or cycling.

WARNING

Frequent heartburn or indigestion may signal a more serious condition—such as ulcers or bleeding in the esophagus—that could worsen if not diagnosed and treated early. If you use OTC drugs to quell your symptoms more than twice a week, see your doctor.

Glaucoma

◆ **SYMPTOMS** ◆

◀ Glaucoma usually has no warning signs.

◀ In *open-angle glaucoma*, peripheral (side) vision gradually declines, and tiny blind spots slowly enlarge. Driving at night or going from bright to dim light is difficult. Eventually, you lose central vision.

◀ In *closed-angle glaucoma*, eye pain with nausea, vomiting, and vision loss occurs suddenly. Seek immediate medical care if this happens.

Fast Fact

About 3 million North Americans have open-angle glaucoma—and half don't know it.

What is it?

Glaucoma is the leading cause of preventable blindness in Canada. It occurs when high intraocular pressure (fluid pressure within the eyeball) cuts blood flow to your optic nerve, causing the nerve to deteriorate. Blind spots, blurry vision, poor peripheral vision, and, sometimes, headaches occur as the damage progresses.

Your eye has two fluid-filled chambers. The optic nerve is located in the retina behind the posterior (rear) chamber, which is filled with a jellylike fluid called vitreous humor. The anterior (front) chamber is filled with a fluid called aqueous humor. Normally, your eye continually produces aqueous humor and drains it away through an outlet, or angle, between the iris and cornea. But if you have glaucoma, the aqueous humor builds up within the anterior chamber, putting pressure on the posterior chamber and your optic nerve. The fluid buildup is caused either by too much fluid production or by inadequate fluid drainage.

As we age, we become more susceptible to two types of glaucoma:

- **Open-angle glaucoma,** which accounts for 90 percent of all cases of glaucoma, occurs when the drainage angle remains open, but excess fluid production causes increased pressure. It usually goes unnoticed because damage occurs so slowly.
- **Closed-angle glaucoma** occurs when the drainage angle becomes blocked, preventing sufficient fluid outflow. It may be gradual or sudden (acute glaucoma), with pain and vision loss. Sudden onset signals an emergency—the pressure must be released right away to prevent blindness.

Your ophthalmologist will measure your intraocular pressure with a tonometer, a small device that uses a jet of compressed air to press on the outside of your eyeball. The exam is painless and takes only a few seconds.

SELF TEST

What Is Your Risk for Glaucoma?

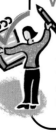

Doctors don't know exactly what causes glaucoma, but several factors put you at greater risk. You're more likely to develop glaucoma if you:

◀ are over age 40
◀ are of African descent
◀ have diabetes
◀ use corticosteroids

◀ have a family history of the disease
◀ are under stress
◀ have a blood vessel disease (which disrupts blood flow).

Glaucoma is diagnosed when your intraocular pressure is above 21 mmHg. At the same time, your retina and optic nerve can be examined. A visual field test, which checks both your peripheral and central vision, may also be performed.

How is it treated?

Glaucoma can't be cured, but treatment can lower your intraocular pressure to prevent optic nerve damage. Prescription eyedrops either decrease the amount of aqueous humor produced or increase its outflow. The most commonly used drugs are the beta-blockers levobunolol (Betagan) and timolol (Timoptic). Sometimes dipivefrin (Propine) or pilo-carpine (Isopto Carpine) are prescribed. Use these eyedrops every day and instill them properly. Here's how: First, wash your hands thoroughly. Tilt your head back and pull down your lower eyelid. Holding the drop-per, release one drop of medication into your eye. (Avoid touching the dropper to your eye to prevent contamination.) Release your lower lid and close your eye. Press your finger against the inside corner for one minute to keep your tear duct closed. This prevents side effects that can result when the drops are absorbed into your bloodstream too quickly.

If the medications don't work and surgery is needed, a tiny hole is made in your iris to drain the fluid (iridectomy). Or a laser is used to punch tiny holes in the trabecular network, the drainage system near the angle (laser trabeculoplasty). For acute closed-angle glaucoma, emergency reduction of eyeball pressure is done either with surgery (iridectomy) or drugs.

WARNING

Glaucoma can lead to driving accidents. Limited peripheral vision prevents you from seeing vehicles coming from the side. And poor night vision hinders your ability to adjust to oncoming headlights.

Your Prevention Plan

Diet ■ **Curb caffeine.** Caffeine may contribute to excess fluid pressure in the eye. Avoid drinking more than two cups of coffee, four cups of tea, or four caffeinated soft drinks a day.

Exercise ■ **Exert yourself.** Aero-bic and strength-training exercises can help decrease intraocular pressure. Some studies have found that people with glaucoma who exercise three times a week or more can lower their pressure by about 20 percent. But you'll still need to take your glaucoma medications. Ask your doctor to recommend a long-term exercise plan that's right for you.

Medical Options ■ **Schedule an exam.** Untreated glaucoma leads to blindness. But because it takes years to happen, early diagnosis and treatment can save your sight. Starting at age 40, have a complete ophthalmologic exam every year or two. After age 45, have a tonometry test every two years. If you're at high risk for glaucoma, have a complete eye exam every one to two years after age 35, and a tonometry test every year after age 45.

Lifestyle ■ **Butt out.** Nicotine constricts blood vessels, and smoking increases intraocular pressure. See pages 166-173 for advice on how to quit.

Gout

◀ Intense, often excruci-
ating pain and tender-
ness that occurs in one
or two hot, red, swollen
joints. It starts sud-
denly, often at night,
and gets worse over
several days.

◀ The big toe is the most
typical site (75 percent
of patients), but the
heel, ankle, instep, or
knee, and fingers and
knuckles, may be
affected.

◀ "Pseudogout" symp-
toms, typically in the
knee or wrist, may be
milder or resemble
rheumatoid arthritis or
osteoarthritis.

What is it?

Gout, one of the most painful forms of arthritis, typically occurs in joints already affected by osteoarthritis. It's caused by an inherited disorder that slows the kidney's ability to excrete uric acid (a by-product of digestion and cellular regeneration) or causes your body to make too much. The excess accumulates in the form of crystals that settle into one or more joints, eventually causing severe inflammation. Gout is diagnosed when these crystals are spotted in an X ray or in fluid extracted from the joint.

The disorder is more common in men than in women, most often striking men over age 45 who are overweight and heavy drinkers.

Gout can take three forms:

● Acute gout develops when uric-acid crystals form in the joint fluid. Left untreated, attacks may last days or weeks and become increasingly frequent and painful.

● Chronic gout leads to lumpy uric-acid deposits, called tophi, near the affected joints, at the elbows, and even under the skin of the ears. Some people never experience an acute attack, but eventually develop kidney problems, including kidney stones, as a result of the excess uric acid.

● "Pseudogout" also involves crystal deposits in and around the joints, but these crystals are made of calcium pyrophosphate dihydrate (CPPD), not uric acid.

How is it treated?

Gout can't be cured, but drug therapy offers relief, easing acute attacks and preventing flare-ups. Pseudogout is difficult to treat, however, because there are no drugs that prevent CPPD crystal buildup.

The drug colchicine can abort an acute gout attack within 12 hours, although the dose that is necessary often causes nausea and diarrhea. Non-steroidal anti-inflammatory drugs (NSAIDs), such as aspirin, ibuprofen, or naproxen, also can ease pain. To prevent recurrent gout attacks, your doctor may prescribe daily colchicine or, if side effects are a problem, drugs that lower uric-acid levels. These include allopurinol (Zyloprim), which blocks uric-acid production, and others that promote its excretion, such as probenecid (Benemid) and sulfinpyrazone (Anturan). Some people need both types. While colchicine may help prevent attacks of pseudogout, it's more effective against true gout. NSAIDs and shots of cortisone injected into the affected joint often ease the pain.

Smart dietary choices are a cornerstone of care, especially if you also have other medical conditions (such as heart disease, diabetes, and hypertension) that affect your meal planning. Nutritional counseling is a must.

Fast Fact

Gout is more likely to occur in spring and summer. Why? The dehydrating effects of warm weather may promote uric acid buildup. So drink up!

Your Prevention Plan

Diet ▪ **Slim down.** About half of gout sufferers are over-weight. Shedding excess pounds may normalize uric-acid levels, easing or banishing gout. But do it slowly; never skip meals or crash diet. Sudden weight loss can trigger an attack.

▪ **Watch your purines.** Foods rich in purines may contribute to gout because purine breaks down into uric acid. If you have gout and aren't tak-ing a medication to lower uric acid, avoid purine-rich foods. These include meat and poultry, especially organ meats such as liver; cured or smoked meat and fish; other seafood, especially scallops, sardines, anchovies, her-ring, and mackerel; chocolate; some vegetables, such as asparagus, cauli-flower, spinach, mushrooms, dried beans, and peas; dry cereals; and foods made with baking powder. Even if your gout is controlled, you may need to be cautious, limiting yourself to one high-purine food a day.

Medical Options ▪ **Get checked.** A blood test for uric-acid levels should be part of your periodic health exam. High levels don't necessarily lead to gout, but can be a warning sign of this or other problems. Sometimes other drugs (even daily aspirin or diuretics for hypertension) may compromise your kidneys' ability to excrete uric acid. You might need to change these drugs.

▪ **Monitor your blood sugar and heart health.** Diabetes, high triglyceride levels, and atherosclerosis of blood vessels supplying the heart and brain occur more commonly in people with gout.

Supplements ▪ **Steer clear.** Avoid supplements that contain niacin and nicotinamide. High doses may increase your uric-acid levels.

Natural Health ▪ **Berry, berry good.** Cherries, hawthorn berries, blueberries, and other dark red-blue berries contain substances that can help lower uric-acid levels. If you can't find cherries, try taking 1,000 mg daily of cherry-fruit-extract pills, available in some health food stores.

Lifestyle ▪ **Go easy on the alcohol.** Wine, beer, and hard liquor in large amounts decrease the kidneys' ability to clear uric acid, which can trigger a gout attack. Wine and beer are also high in purines. If you have gout, drink only moderately—no more than one drink a day for women and two drinks for men—especially if you are not taking drugs that lower uric acid.

▪ **Drink lots of water.** Two to three quarts of water daily can help you excrete uric acid and will dilute your urine, thereby discouraging the formation of kidney stones.

WARNING

If you have gout, get your thyroid checked. Hypothyroidism is more common among people with gout. The connection? Low levels of thyroid hormone may slow the excretion of uric acid. Taking thyroid pills can solve the problem.

Gum Disease

◀ Gingivitis: swollen, tender, red gums that bleed easily, bad breath

◀ Periodontitis: painful gums that pull away from teeth, pus in the pockets formed, bad breath, painful chewing

WARNING

Gum disease is linked to an increased heart-attack risk. Once the bacteria from gum disease enters your bloodstream, it causes your white blood cells to release clotting factors that contribute to both heart attacks and strokes.

What is it?

Gum disease, also called periodontal disease, occurs when plaque—a sticky substance composed of bacteria and other matter—collects in the gaps between your teeth and gums.

Mild gum disease, called gingivitis, is a common infection that causes swelling at the gum line. It can develop at any age and can lead to periodontitis (advanced gum disease). Periodontitis occurs when accumulated plaque creates tiny pockets at the gum edge, causing gum tissue to pull away from the teeth. The plaque can eventually destroy your jawbone and loosen your teeth.

Advanced gum disease is the primary cause of tooth loss in older people. As you age, your risk for gum disease increases. This is because even healthy gums gradually pull away from teeth, leaving the roots exposed. And roots that aren't protected are more easily damaged by plaque. Several drugs commonly taken by older people, such as diuretics and high blood pressure medications, reduce saliva production. That's a problem because saliva plays a key role in protecting your teeth by flushing away food and neutralizing the acids in plaque.

Some illnesses can also affect dental health. Arthritis may make it challenging for you to brush and floss properly, and diabetes hinders wound healing, leading to infection. Many older people don't eat a balanced diet, which decreases the body's ability to fight infection.

Gum disease may present another problem: Studies suggest that bacteria spread from infected gum pockets to saliva can be transmitted from one person to another through kissing or sharing a drinking glass.

How is it treated?

Gingivitis can be eliminated with scrupulous brushing, flossing, and regular professional cleaning. If you're in generally poor health, you're more prone to gum disease, so follow the wellness strategy outlined in *Your Prevention Plan* (opposite). And ask your dentist about protective fluoride treatments—they're not just for kids. Unlike gingivitis, periodontitis requires drugs and surgery.

DRUGS

Various anti-infective medications are available and can be prescribed by your periodontist for oral use or local application inside the periodontal pocket. Atridox, a controlled-release doxycycline gel, is used for seven days. The gel solidifies when applied inside the periodontal pocket.

349

SURGERY

Tooth scaling and root planing remove plaque and smooth the diseased root surface so your gums can reattach. If the pockets are very deep, flap surgery is used to cut your gums to the bone so the entire root can be scraped and planed. The gums are then sewn back in place. If periodontal disease has spread to your jawbone, tissue regeneration or bone grafting can save your teeth.

Fast Fact

People with periodontitis are twice as likely to have a fatal heart attack and 4.5 times more likely to have chronic lung disease than those with healthy gums.

Your Prevention Plan

Diet ▪ **Break the sugar habit.** Sugar provides a breeding ground for bacteria. If you do indulge, brush your teeth afterward or rinse your mouth with water or mouthwash.

▪ **Favor fruits and vegetables.** They contain antioxidants that help repair tissues. Bonus: Eating them raw helps clean your teeth.

Medical Options ▪ **See your dentist.** Have a cleaning and checkup every six months—every three months if you're susceptible to gum disease.

Supplements ▪ **C yourself healthy.** Taking up to 1,000 mg of vitamin C every day may help keep gums healthy by supporting the immune system, making the gums more resistant to bacteria. Vitamin C also strengthens weak gum tissue.

▪ **Bone up on calcium.** Calcium boosts bone and tooth formation. The current Dietary Reference Intake (DRI) is 1,300 mg (or the amount found in 4 cups of milk) for preteens and teens age 9 to 18, 1,000 mg for men and women age 19 to 50, and 1,200 mg for men and women age 51 and older.

▪ **Consider coenzyme Q10.** Found in all human cells, this substance increases tissue oxygenation. Taking 60 to 100 mg per day may help decrease bleeding and inflammation. For best absorption, take it in gelcap form.

▪ **Multiple choice.** Take a multivitamin that contains vitamin C and calcium. You may still need to take a separate calcium pill, however.

Natural Health ▪ **Different dentistry.** Holistic dentists have the same training as traditional dentists, but they're apt to use acupuncture for pain relief and to recommend supplements and stress reduction techniques (stress weakens the immune system, increasing the risk for gum disease). For a referral, check out www.holisticdental.org.

Lifestyle ▪ **Stop smoking.** A study of 12,000 adults showed that smoking quadruples the risk of periodontal disease. And smokers don't heal as quickly after gum surgery.

▪ **Brush up.** Brush your teeth at least twice a day with a soft-bristled brush. Spend about two to three minutes on the task—not 45 to 60 seconds, which is the average. Brush your tongue, too, since it's another breeding ground for bacteria.

▪ **Don't forget to floss.** Floss daily. Insert floss between your teeth, making a "C" at the side of each tooth and gently moving the floss up and down. Pull the floss across your back teeth, using the same up-and-down motion.

Hearing Loss

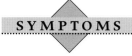

SYMPTOMS

◄ Inability to hear or understand sounds

◄ Sensitivity to loud sounds

◄ Hissing or ringing in your ears

◄ Difficulty following conversations because words seem slurred or mumbled, especially when there's background noise

What is it?

Age-related hearing loss, or presbycusis, affects about one-third of North Americans between age 65 and 74, and one-half of those over age 85. This progressive problem actually starts around age 20, then accelerates after age 50. At first, you have trouble hearing high-pitched sounds, then later, lower-pitched sounds. Hearing loss occurs as the tiny hair cells that act as sound receptors in your inner ear are gradually destroyed. Associated factors include repeated exposure to loud noises, heredity, and changes in the blood supply to the ear caused by heart disease or other circulatory problems. Presbycusis affects both ears equally but doesn't lead to total deafness. It occurs earlier in men than in women.

A sign of hearing loss, tinnitus is identified by a ringing, roaring, or hissing sound in your ears. It can be constant, frequent, or occasional. If you've experienced it (or any other sign of hearing loss), see your doctor.

If your hearing loss is accompanied by pain or discharge from your ear, see your doctor; you may have an ear infection.

How is it treated?

Your doctor will prescribe a hearing aid or suggest other assistive devices. A hearing aid is made up of a microphone, which changes sound waves into electrical signals; an amplifier, which makes the signals louder; a receiver, which changes the electrical signals back into sound waves and

A Guide to Hearing Aids

Here's what you need to know about some common types of hearing aids:

- **Behind-the-Ear (BTE).** In this device, the microphone is located at the opening of your ear, while the battery, amplifier, and receiver are tucked behind. It works well for all degrees of hearing loss. If your earpiece doesn't fit properly or is damaged, the device will start squealing, so have the mold remade periodically.
- **In-the-Ear (ITE).** Made of a hard plastic, this fits completely in the outer ear. It's appealing because it's hidden and simulates natural sound reception, but it can become clogged with ear wax and need cleaning, and the volume is more difficult to adjust.

- **In-the-Canal (ITC).** While similar to the ITE, this device is so small it actually fits in your ear canal. It's used only in cases of mild hearing loss and needs to be repaired more often than other devices because of where it's worn. Good manual dexterity is required to insert it.
- **Body-Style.** Worn on your body and attached to an earpiece, this device provides powerful amplification. The controls are easy to use, but because the microphone isn't at ear level, the sound reception isn't natural. And because it's generally worn under clothing, the microphone will also pick up the sound of rustling fabric whenever you move.

channels them into your ear; and a battery. Keep your expectations in check: A hearing aid won't bring your hearing back to normal. But it will certainly improve it. Don't feel discouraged if yours isn't working the way you want it to at first. Make regular appointments with your audiologist until it feels right to you.

Other assistive devices can be purchased through your audiologist or a medical supply store. They include:

- **Amplifying devices** used for watching TV or listening to the radio. An amplifier transmits sound to headphones that you wear. You can adjust your own volume without interfering with other people's hearing of the TV or radio. These devices are also available for telephones.
- **Alerting devices** that use loud noises, flashing lights, or a vibrator to alert you to certain sounds. They can be used with your telephone, doorbell, alarm clock, smoke detector, or anything else you need to hear. You can attach them to the specific appliance or to your bed or a chair. Many are portable so you can use them away from home.
- **Decoding devices** such as closed-captioning devices you can hook up to your TV, which convert audio transmission into text that appears onscreen, and teletypewriters (TTYs), specialized telephone systems that convert audio signals into text that is displayed on a monitor.

WARNING

High doses of certain medications—aspirin, quinine, and powerful antibiotics and diuretics—can diminish your hearing temporarily or lead to hearing loss.

Your Prevention Plan

Diet ■ **Cut down on salt.** Reducing your salt intake may help improve hearing. Salt causes the body to retain fluid, which may swell the functional organs of the ear. Canned soups and other processed foods often contain large of amounts of salt, so read labels.

Medical Options ■ **Now hear this.** If you suspect hearing loss or your loved ones have hinted at it, schedule a checkup with an otolaryngologist, a doctor who specializes in diseases of the ears, nose, and throat. If you are over age 65, you may want to have an audiologist test your hearing every 3 years—or every 6 to 12 months if you have a family history of hearing loss.

Natural Health ■ **Go with ginkgo.** By improving blood flow to the brain and the ears, this herb may help ringing in the ears (tinnitus), though noticeable benefits may take weeks or months of use. Some studies suggest ginkgo may be useful in treating some types of hearing loss. Take up to 240 mg of the extract a day, but check with your doctor first, since ginkgo can interact with other drugs.

Lifestyle ■ **Tune out.** Try to avoid situations that expose you to loud noise. If that's not possible, wear earplugs or ear protectors when shooting a gun or using lawn mowers, other noisy garden equipment, or power carpentry tools.

Heart Disease

◀ Angina: pressure or pain in the chest when you exert yourself or when you are at rest

◀ Heart attack: squeezing chest pain; chest pressure that comes and goes; constant chest pain that may spread to your jaw, neck, left shoulder, or left arm; anxiety with a sense of impending doom

◀ Shortness of breath, rapid heartbeat, profuse sweating, nausea, and light-headedness

What is it?

Heart disease, also called coronary artery disease, is the number one killer of Canadians. It causes more than 50,000 deaths every year.

The basic mechanism of heart disease is a buildup of cholesterol-laden plaque (a fatty deposit) inside the coronary arteries, the blood vessels that carry oxygen-rich blood to the heart. Plaque narrows the inner channel of the vessels and makes them less flexible. This process is called atherosclerosis, or hardening of the arteries.

As normal blood flow to your heart is restricted, you may experience angina (chest pain). If a clot forms or lodges inside a narrowed artery, it can completely cut off blood flow and cause a heart attack. Heart disease is often "silent"—producing no symptoms—until it causes a heart attack.

More than 85 percent of people who die from heart attacks are age 65 or older. The risk of having a heart attack is higher among some ethnic groups, and many other risk factors come into play as well. Take the self-test below to gauge your risk. A diagnosis of heart disease is usually based on your symptoms, medical history, and the presence of risk factors. Your doctor may also want you to have certain tests:

● **Electrocardiography (ECG)** records your heart's electrical activity and shows any abnormalities, such as disturbances in your heart rate or

SELF TEST

What Is Your Risk for Heart Disease?

Both your genes and your lifestyle habits contribute to heart disease. To calculate your risk, give yourself 1 point for each of the following risk factors:

What you can't control:

◀ **Age.** Over age 45 for men and over age 55 for women

◀ **Gender.** Men are more vulnerable than women.

◀ **Postmenopausal status.** Women's risk increases sharply after menopause.

◀ **Family history** of heart disease

◀ **Personal history** of a heart attack

◀ **Ethnicity.** people of African, Latin American, or Asian descent

What you can control:

◀ **Smoking** or regular exposure to second-hand smoke

◀ **Low-density lipoprotein,** or LDL ("bad" cholesterol), above 4.2 mmol/L

◀ **High-density lipoprotein,** or HDL, below 0.9 mmol/L

◀ **High blood pressure** (over 140/90 mmHg)

◀ **High triglyceride level** (over 5.2 mmol/L)

◀ **Diabetes**

◀ **Chronic stress or depression**

◀ **Physical inactivity**

◀ **Obesity**

◀ High intake of **saturated fat**

◀ Low intake of **heart-smart foods** (see *Your Prevention Plan,* page 354).

Subtract 1 point if you have high levels of HDL cholesterol (over 0.9 mmol/L). Then add up your total score. **A score of 0 to 2 points** puts you at low to moderate risk of heart disease. See page 354 for tips on keeping your risk low. **A score of 3 or more points** means you're at high risk. See your doctor now for an evaluation. And start making some lifestyle changes.

heart rhythm. An ECG can also help determine if your heart is getting enough blood and oxygen. And it can reveal thin or absent heart muscle tissue—a sign that a heart attack may have occurred.

- **An exercise tolerance test** (stress test) records how well your heart functions while you exercise (walking on a treadmill) to help detect any abnormal changes that occur when your heart is pumping hard.
- **Coronary angiography** may be used if your doctor suspects narrowing or blockage of your coronary arteries. In angiography, a dye that shows up on X rays is injected into the bloodstream, usually through a thin tube threaded up through an artery in the arm or groin. X-ray pictures are taken after the dye travels to the coronary arteries. If any of the arteries are blocked or narrowed, the flow of dye-treated blood will be visibly blocked or restricted.

How is it treated?

Many people can control early-stage heart disease by making lifestyle changes (see *Your Prevention Plan,* page 354) and taking certain drugs. Sometimes surgery is necessary.

DRUGS

To lower your cholesterol, a class of prescription drugs called statins may help. Statins can cut blood levels of cholesterol by up to 60 points and lower your risk of heart attack by one-third. They work by blocking an enzyme your body needs to manufacture cholesterol. The most commonly prescribed statins are simvastatin (Zocor), pravastatin (Pravachol), atorvastatin (Lipitor), cerivastatin (Baycol), fluvastatin (Lescol), and lovastatin (Mevacor).

For angina symptoms, three different classes of prescription drugs can alleviate pain. They can be used alone or in combination. Beta-blockers such as atenolol (Tenormin) and metoprolol (Lopresor) lower your heart rate and blood pressure to decrease your heart's workload. Nitrates (nitroglycerin) open up your blood vessels, increasing blood flow to the heart. Calcium channel blockers such as diltiazem (Tiazac) and verapamil (Chronovera) also dilate blood vessels and lower blood pressure.

After a heart attack, you'll receive clot-dissolving drugs or undergo immediate surgery.

SURGERY

In coronary bypass surgery, a healthy blood vessel—usually from your leg—is removed and stitched into place to bypass the diseased artery (or arteries) in your heart.

In coronary angioplasty, a catheter (a thin, flexible tube) with a tiny balloon on its tip is inserted into an artery and guided toward the blocked artery near your heart. The balloon is inflated to stretch open the blood vessel and is then removed. In some forms of angioplasty, a stent (a wire mesh device) is placed inside your artery to keep it open after surgery.

Your Prevention Plan

Diet

■ **Think international.** People who eat a traditional Mediterranean or Asian diet appear to have lower rates of heart disease than those who eat a typical Canadian diet. Incorporate elements of these diets into your healthy eating plan (see Chapter 1, *Eating to Age Well*, page 30).

■ **Eat heart-smart foods.** Choose foods that can reduce cholesterol and improve heart health, such as fruits (apples, avocados, dried fruits, grapefruit, oranges, strawberries), vegetables (broccoli, carrots, corn, lima beans, onions), seafood (clams, mussels, oysters), fish containing omega-3 fatty acids (salmon and bluefish), soy, nuts, and whole-grain breads and cereals.

■ **Cut the fat.** To keep your cholesterol level down, limit the amount of fat you eat, especially saturated fat. Your total fat intake should be no more than 30 percent of your daily calories. Focus on low-fat alternatives to red meat, such as fish or skinless chicken or turkey. Eating fish several times a week can cut your risk of heart attack by as much as half. Lower your intake of dairy fats by switching to low-fat or skim varieties. Or try soy milk—soy protein can lower cholesterol.

■ **Spice it up.** If you have high blood pressure, cut your sodium intake. In fact, researchers now think that even people whose blood pressure is within normal range should cut back on sodium. Avoid processed foods, which contain a lot of sodium, and ease up on salt at mealtime. But don't settle for bland fare. Add flavor with salsa, curry, peppers, or garlic. Eating one to three cloves of garlic a day has been shown to reduce blood pressure and possibly lower cholesterol.

■ **Add rough stuff.** Soluble fiber, plentiful in fresh fruits, vegetables, legumes, and whole grains, prevents plaque buildup in your arteries. Studies show that eating three or more servings of fruits and vegetables daily can lower the risk of heart attack and stroke by 25 percent or more. In one study, eating cooked dried beans daily lowered "bad" cholesterol by 20 percent in just three weeks. Other research showed that a diet high in whole grains can cut a woman's risk of dying from heart disease by up to 15 percent. And dozens of studies confirm that eating oats has a cholesterol-lowering effect.

■ **Seeing red.** Drinking alcohol in moderation raises HDL, or "good," cholesterol and "thins" the blood, reducing the likelihood of clots that can cause heart attack and stroke. Red wine offers additional benefits. Its dark pigments are rich in bioflavonoids that prevent the oxidation of LDL, or "bad," cholesterol, making it less likely to stick to artery walls. Research showed that people who drank two 8-ounce glasses of red wine a day were 40 percent less likely to have a heart attack than those who didn't imbibe. But don't overdo it—too much alcohol raises your triglyceride level. And if you have an alcohol problem, the harm far outweighs any potential benefit. Instead of drinking alcohol, you can get bioflavonoids from black and green tea, onions, kale, and apples.

Exercise

■ **Work your heart.** The best preventive medicine for your heart is aerobic exercise. It reduces high blood pressure and atherosclerosis by widening the blood vessels. Plus, it raises "good" cholesterol levels. Choose an activity that works the large muscles of your legs and buttocks (like brisk walking or bicycling), and strive to reach your target heart rate (see page 118) for at least 15 to 20 minutes, three or four times a week.

■ **An (up)lifting idea.** An American Heart Association (AHA) survey found that lifting weights a few times a week can improve heart health in some people. That's because stronger muscles can lower your heart rate and blood pressure. Having more muscle tissue also raises your metabolism, which helps control your weight. See pages 128-133 for strength-training exercises. But don't skip the brisk walk. The AHA recommends pumping iron in addition to aerobic exercise (and the Heart and Stroke Foundation of Canada concurs).

■ **Be flexible.** Flexibility exercises like yoga not only help keep your joints limber but also help cut the production of stress hormones that can contribute to heart disease.

Medical Options

■ **Schedule a checkup.** Until age 65, you should have your blood pressure checked at least every other year. At age 65, you should have it checked at least annually. Most doctors also recommend a yearly cholesterol screening if you have high cholesterol or other heart-disease risk factors. Your doctor may also recommend electrocardiography (an ECG) to evaluate your heart health. While you're there, ask about a simple blood test for a substance called C-reactive protein. According to Harvard researchers studying 28,000 healthy women, this test helped predict heart attack risk better than cholesterol tests.

■ **An aspirin a day?** People with existing heart disease may benefit from low-dose aspirin therapy, which may prevent heart attacks. The dosage ranges from part of an aspirin (80 mg) to one aspirin (325 mg) daily. Ask your doctor what's right for you.

■ **Depressurize.** High blood pressure can lead to heart disease. If diet and exercise can't control it, blood-pressure medication can help.

■ **Deal with diabetes.** People with diabetes, most of whom are adults with the type 2 form of the disease, are two to four times more likely to have heart disease or stroke. Controlling the disease is often just a matter of losing extra pounds, exercising regularly, and following a heart-healthy diet.

■ **Don't ignore depression.** One study found that depressed people were 1.7 times more likely to develop heart disease and that depressed men were nearly three times as likely to die from it. See your doctor for help.

Supplements

■ **Consider folate and vitamin B6.** These vitamins lower elevated levels of homocysteine, a substance in the blood that may raise your risk of heart disease. A daily intake of more than 400 mcg of folate and 3 mg of B6 appears to reduce the risk of heart disease in women.

■ **Go fish.** Fish oil capsules contain omega-3 fatty acids, which act as anticlotting agents. Check with your doctor before taking them to avoid interactions with other medications.

■ **Get garlic.** Garlic capsules offer the health benefits of garlic without odor. Choose pills that supply 4,000 mcg of allicin and take 400 to 600 mg a day.

Natural Health

■ **Time out.** Minimize stress, a risk factor for heart disease. Try meditation or visualization (see pages 201-202) or yoga. Prayer may also help. Take brisk walks with a friend; your conversation may add extra stress relief.

Lifestyle

■ **Rein in your rage.** Don't get mad—it's bad for your heart. A study of nearly 13,000 people found that those who were quick to anger were almost three times more likely to have heart attacks than their cooler-headed peers.

■ **Stay trim.** Being even slightly overweight can increase your blood pressure and put you at greater risk for heart disease. Follow a heart-smart diet and make exercise a priority.

■ **No ifs, ands, or butts.** According to the Heart and Stroke Foundation of Canada, smoking is the single most preventable cause of heart disease. Thirty percent of all coronary-related deaths each year are from smoking. After five smoke-free years, you run the same risk for heart disease as nonsmokers.

■ **Getting away is good for your heart.** Researchers found that men age 35 to 57 who took a yearly vacation were one-third less likely to die from heart disease than their stay-at-work colleagues.

Hepatitis

◄ Often, no symptoms

◄ Sometimes, flulike symptoms including appetite loss, nausea, vomiting, diarrhea, headache, fever, fatigue, weakness, and muscle or joint pain

◄ In severe cases, jaundice (yellow discoloration of your skin and the whites of your eyes), dark brown urine, clay-colored stools, itching, and pain in the upper right portion of your abdomen (where your liver is located)

What is it?

Hepatitis is inflammation of the liver, an organ that performs many vital functions. Your liver not only produces bile to help digest fats, it also stores nutrients and filters toxic substances (such as alcohol and other drugs and digestive by-products) out of your blood.

Hepatitis damages liver cells. As a result, the liver can't do its filtering job properly and toxins can build up. The disease can occur suddenly and last only weeks (called acute hepatitis) or persist for several months or even years (known as chronic hepatitis). You may not know you're infected because symptoms may not appear for years.

VIRAL CAUSES

Hepatitis is usually caused by a virus. There are five different hepatitis viruses, but the most common are hepatitis A, B, and C.

Hepatitis A (the most common type) can spread when you eat food or drink water contaminated with feces. This may occur when food preparers don't follow proper sanitary practices such as washing hands after using the toilet and before preparing food. Consuming contaminated raw or undercooked shellfish, contaminated fruits and vegetables, and contaminated drinking water or ice cubes can also lead to infection.

Once you're infected with hepatitis A you can transmit it to others for a period of time ranging from a week to more than a month. If you're

SELF TEST

What Is Your Risk for Hepatitis?

You're more likely to get hepatitis if you:

◄ had a blood transfusion before 1990

◄ have unprotected vaginal or anal sex with an infected person

◄ use intravenous drugs

◄ get a tattoo or body piercing

◄ share a razor or toothbrush with an infected person

◄ have a family member who has had liver disease

◄ abuse alcohol

◄ take large amounts of acetaminophen (such as Tylenol)

◄ travel to high-risk areas of the world; these include Mexico, Central or South America, the Caribbean, Asia (except Japan), Africa, southern or eastern Europe, or Pacific Islander communities.

Alcohol and Liver Failure

Alcohol is a known liver toxin. Some people can drink alcohol without any apparent ill effects while others, particularly women, can suffer permanent liver damage from even moderate amounts. Experts aren't sure why this happens, but genes seem to play a role. If someone in your family has had liver disease (caused or not caused by alcohol consumption), you may be more susceptible to liver failure.

infected, you must be scrupulous about hygiene, because exposing others to your blood or stools can infect them. North Americans are more likely to get hepatitis A when traveling abroad, but up to 50 percent of all North Americans have had the virus and, as a result, are now immune to it. Recovery is usually quick—most people are back to normal within one week and have no permanent liver damage.

Hepatitis B is transmitted through blood and other infected body fluids, including semen. You can contract it through unprotected sex (sex without a condom), infected needles, or blood transfusions. Unlike hepatitis A, this virus can turn into a chronic infection (in up to 10 percent of people), leading to liver disease and liver cancer.

Hepatitis C is spread through infected blood, either by transfusions given before 1990 (when blood was first screened for hepatitis C) or by contaminated needles. Doctors aren't sure if hepatitis C can be transmitted during sexual intercourse. For now, it's safest to always use a condom. This virus affects people in a variety of ways. Some develop a severe (acute) form of hepatitis but recover in several months with no liver failure. But up to 60 percent of those infected with hepatitis C go on to have chronic hepatitis. Some even develop liver failure and liver cancer. Hepatitis C kills some 10,000 people in North America every year.

NONVIRAL CAUSES

Hepatitis can also have nonviral causes including excessive alcohol consumption, certain medications, toxins (arsenic or poisonous mushrooms), and some herbal remedies (comfrey and chaparral leaf).

Alcohol poisons the liver and over time causes cirrhosis (scarring), which cannot be reversed. Prescription drugs that can lead to liver failure include the antibiotic trimethoprim/sulfamethoxazole (Septra), the heart drug amiodarone (Cordarone), the tuberculosis drug isoniazid (INH), and anabolic steroids (in overdoses). Talk to your doctor before you stop taking any drug.

Another cause of hepatitis is the over-the-counter pain reliever acetaminophen (Tylenol). When taken in overdoses (more than twenty 500 mg pills per day) or with alcohol, acetaminophen can cause sudden and severe hepatitis and rapid death if not treated.

If you have symptoms of hepatitis, your doctor will ask about your medical history and perform a physical exam, checking the area near your liver for tenderness and your skin for the telltale yellowing of jaundice. Your doctor might also use one of the following tests to confirm a diagnosis of hepatitis:

- **Blood tests** check for specific markers that can reveal if you've had the disease in the past and if you have an acute or chronic infection now.
- **Liver function tests (LFTs)** help your doctor evaluate how well your liver is operating. The tests can confirm the presence of jaundice and may be used to monitor your condition. LFTs aren't done routinely as part of a physical exam. If you have any hepatitis risk factors, ask your doctor whether it makes sense to order LFTs.
- **Computed tomography (CT)** scan of your abdominal area lets your doctor see a picture of your liver.
- **Liver biopsy** is a procedure in which a tiny piece of liver tissue is removed and studied under the microscope. For a liver biopsy, your skin is numbed with an anesthetic and a needle is guided into your liver to take the tissue sample.

How is it treated?

There is no medication to cure viral hepatitis; your body's immune system has to battle it on its own. If your hepatitis was caused by something other than a virus, your doctor will recommend that you stop using the causative substance to speed your recovery. Hospitalization is rarely needed for hepatitis, but for several months after you are diagnosed, blood tests may be done periodically to check how your liver is functioning. Your doctor may also recommend the following treatments.

LIFESTYLE MODIFICATIONS

Drink plenty of fluids, get lots of rest, and limit your activities until you feel better. Don't use alcohol or acetaminophen until you are completely recovered. To prevent spreading the disease, be scrupulous about hygiene and always use a condom during sex.

DRUGS

Therapy with high-dose interferon and ribavirin (Virazole) has helped some people with hepatitis C. Discuss this therapy with your doctor.

Canada's Blood Supply

Canadian Blood Services has 14 blood centers and 2 plasma centers across Canada. Héma-Quebec is responsible for blood management in Quebec. The CBS has put in place a rigorous screening system. Every potential donor must answer questions concerning high-risk activities, travels, and sexual behavior to determine whether he or she may give blood.

Your Prevention Plan

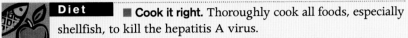

Diet ■ **Cook it right.** Thoroughly cook all foods, especially shellfish, to kill the hepatitis A virus.

■ **Please peel.** Peel all fruits and vegetables imported from countries where sanitary conditions are poor. Washing produce will not remove the hepatitis A virus.

■ **Water warning.** When traveling abroad, buy bottled water or make sure tap water has been boiled before you drink it or use it to brush your teeth, and ask for drinks without ice.

Medical Options ■ **Get vaccinated.** Vaccines are available for hepatitis A and B. Three doses provide full and lasting protection. If you are traveling to high-risk areas, start the hepatitis A vaccine at least one month before your trip. Get the hepatitis B vaccine if you might be exposed to infected blood or body fluids or if you are at high risk. People at high risk include health care workers, acupuncturists, tattoo artists, and people with multiple sex partners.

■ **Boost your immunity.** If you think you've eaten contaminated food, or if someone in your household has been diagnosed with hepatitis, ask your doctor for a shot of immune globulin (if you haven't had the hepatitis vaccine). It offers short-term protection against the virus.

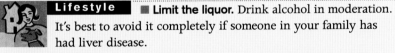

Supplements ■ **Helpful herb.** Milk thistle (Silybum marianum) improves the liver's ability to function in people with hepatitis, although it won't reverse liver damage. It's available in capsules, or the crushed seeds can be brewed as a tea. Take 200 mg two or three times a day.

Lifestyle ■ **Limit the liquor.** Drink alcohol in moderation. It's best to avoid it completely if someone in your family has had liver disease.

■ **Play it safe.** Practice safe sex and always use a condom. Be especially careful if your partner has been diagnosed with the disease.

■ **Wash up.** Wash your hands with soap and hot water before preparing food and after using the toilet and changing diapers to help prevent the spread of infection.

■ **Skip the needle.** Contaminated needles can spread hepatitis A and B. Avoid tattoos and body piercings, and don't inject illegal drugs.

■ **Don't share.** Don't share a razor or toothbrush with someone who's infected with hepatitis B or C, because the virus is spread through blood and body fluids.

WARNING

Taking even twelve 500 mg pills of acetaminophen (Tylenol) a day increases your risk of liver damage. And if you drink alcohol while you're taking it, as few as 4 pills can be toxic.

Hypertension

What is it?

Blood pressure is the force the blood exerts against vessel walls when your heart contracts (systolic pressure) and expands again as it fills with blood (diastolic pressure). It's measured in millimeters (mm) of mercury (Hg), with the systolic number given before the diastolic. Optimal blood pressure is 120/80 mmHg. Sustaining a higher level over time can damage blood vessels throughout your body and cause a cascade of complications, including heart attack, stroke, and kidney failure. Nearly 90 percent of people with the disease have primary or essential hypertension, in which the cause is unknown. The rest have secondary hypertension, which is caused by an underlying disorder such as kidney disease.

How is it treated?

It's treated first with a variety of lifestyle measures, including reducing the amount of salt and fat in your diet, getting regular exercise, and losing excess weight. If these measures haven't worked after six months, the doctor will prescribe antihypertensive medication. The choice of drug depends on your age, race, and medical history; finding the best medication or combination of medications may take some trial and error. These are the main types of antihypertensive drugs:

● **Angiotensin-converting enzyme (ACE) inhibitors** affect angiotensin I, a substance that indirectly raises blood pressure. A catalyst called angiotensin-converting enzyme turns angiotensin I into angiotensin II, a related substance that acts directly on the blood vessels, making them narrow and stiff, and thus pushing blood pressure upward. Angiotensin II also increases salt and water retention in the body. The four most

Fast Fact

More than 1 in 5 adult Canadians (close to 5 million people) have high blood pressure, or hypertension.

SELF TEST

Are You at Risk for Hypertension?

Blood pressure often rises with age. Diastolic pressure increases until about age 60, while systolic pressure can keep rising up to age 80. Doctors still don't know exactly why some people become hypertensive, but you may be at higher risk if you:
◀ have a family history of the disease
◀ have diabetes
◀ are chronically stressed
◀ are sedentary or overweight
◀ eat heavily salted food
◀ drink more than two alcoholic beverages a day
◀ smoke.

How High Is Too High?

One high blood pressure reading isn't enough to diagnose hypertension. You need at least two readings done on separate days. You might even need at-home checks to rule out "white coat hypertension," a high reading due to the stress that sometimes attends a visit to the doctor.

CLASSIFICATION	SYSTOLIC (mmHg)	DIASTOLIC (mmHg)
Optimal	120 or less	80 or less
Normal	up to 130	up to 85
High-normal	130 to 139	85 to 89
Stage 1 (mild) hypertension	140 to 159	90 to 99
Stage 2 (moderate) hypertension	160 to 179	100 to 109
Stage 3 (severe) hypertension	180 or over	110 or over

SimpleSolution

If you're taking an ACE inhibitor and develop a cough (the most common side effect), check your other medications. Are you using an antiarthritis skin rub containing capsaicin? Stop the rub and the cough may vanish.

widely tested ACE inhibitors are ramipril (Altace), enalapril (Vasotec), lisinopril (Prinivil or Zestril), and captopril (Capoten). Many doctors prescribe one of these drugs as initial therapy. The international Heart Outcomes Prevention Evaluation (HOPE) trial showed that ramipril can cut the threat of cardiovascular death, nonfatal heart attacks, and strokes by 22 percent in people at high risk of such crises, such as those with hypertension.

- **Angiotensin II receptor blockers** are similar to ACE inhibitors but don't cause the cough that's sometimes a side effect of those drugs. While angiotensin II receptor blockers reduce blood pressure, it's not known whether they provide the extensive heart and kidney protection of ACE inhibitors. They include losartan (Cozaar) and valsartan (Diovan).
- **Diuretics,** commonly called water pills, flush excess fluid and sodium from the body, decreasing the total blood volume so less pressure is exerted on the arteries. Thiazides, such as hydrochlorothiazide, also increase the amount of potassium your body excretes, so you may need a potassium supplement, although potassium-sparing diuretics, including spironolactone (Aldactone) and triamterene (Dyrenium), are available. Loop diuretics such as furosemide (Lasix) are the most powerful drugs in this class; they are often prescribed for hypertensives who also retain fluid due to heart failure or kidney disease. For Stage 1 hypertension (see box above), diuretics are often the drugs of first choice.
- **Beta-blockers** slow your heart and reduce its force and workload. They include propranolol (Inderal), timolol (Blocadren), metoprolol (Lopresor), and atenolol (Tenormin).
- **Calcium channel blockers** prevent calcium, which causes blood-vessel constriction, from entering the muscles that surround the arteries. They

include diltiazem (Tiazac) and verapamil (Chronovera). Because these drugs may trigger heart problems in some patients, they are rarely used as first-line therapy.

- **Alpha-blockers** work on the nervous system to relax blood vessels. They include prazosin (Minipress), terazosin (Hytrin), and doxazosin (Cardura). Unlike diuretics and beta-blockers, they don't raise cholesterol levels.
- **Vasodilators** relax the muscle in blood-vessel walls. They include hydralazine (Apresoline) and minoxidil (Loniten).
- **Centrally acting drugs,** which work in the nervous system and affect the circulatory system indirectly, include alpha-adrenergic antagonists, such as clonidine (Catapres) and methyldopa (Aldomet), and peripheral-adrenergic-neuron antagonists, such as guanethidine (Ismelin). In some cases, these drugs may be prescribed with a thiazide diuretic.

Nutrition Note

Here's a diet that works. Dietary Approaches to Stop Hypertension— the DASH diet—can lower systolic pressure by up to 11.4 points and diastolic by 5.5 points. It's low in saturated fat and high in fruits, vegetables, whole grains, and low-fat dairy products. For a copy and sample menu, call the National Institutes of Health at 301-592-8573, or go to http://www.dash.bwh.harvard.edu.

Your Prevention Plan

Diet

■ **If you're overweight, reduce.** Obesity stresses the heart, which raises blood pressure. Getting close to your ideal weight, with no other change, may return blood pressure to normal. Even slight weight loss helps. Boston University researchers found that middle-aged people who lost a pound a year—and kept it off—cut their risk of hypertension by about 25 percent over 40 years.

■ **Pass up the salt.** Cutting back to a teaspoonful daily (about half of what most North Americans eat) reduces your risk of hypertension. The Dietary Approaches to Stop Hypertension (DASH) Sodium trial showed that either the DASH diet (see *Nutrition Note*) or a reduced-sodium diet lowered blood pressure in people with and without hypertension. The DASH and low-salt combination produced even more dramatic reductions in blood pressure.

■ **Get fresh.** In addition to having no added salt, fresh fruits and vegetables contain scores of health-enhancing substances such as phytochemicals. When the fresh produce you want isn't available, choose frozen over canned—it's less likely to be salt- or sugar-laden.

■ **Trim fat.** Diets low in total fat and high in the ratio of unsaturated to saturated fat can help reduce blood pressure. Olive oil is your best bet and may even help lower systolic pressure.

■ **Up your garlic, onion, and celery intake.** All have been shown to help lower blood pressure.

■ **Eat cold-water fish.** The omega-3 fatty acids in salmon, mackerel, herring, sardines, and tuna can help lower blood pressure.

Exercise

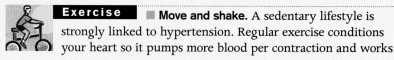

■ **Move and shake.** A sedentary lifestyle is strongly linked to hypertension. Regular exercise conditions your heart so it pumps more blood per contraction and works more efficiently, which helps lower your blood pressure. Aim for at least 30 minutes of aerobic exercise—brisk walking, running, swimming, tennis, or biking—three times a week.

Medical Options

■ **Get tested.** Know your usual blood pressure and have it checked yearly.

■ **Control diabetes, if you have it.** High blood-sugar levels, over time, can damage blood vessels, increasing your risk of heart complications.

■ **Beware of other medications.** Corticosteroids, which are often prescribed for arthritis, asthma, and other inflammatory problems, as well as over-the-counter decongestants taken for colds and allergies can elevate your blood pressure. Talk to your doctor before taking anything new.

Supplements

■ **Reach for C.** Researchers at Boston University School of Medicine have found that taking 500 mg of vitamin C daily lowered blood pressure in up to 9 percent of hypertensive patients. Though formal trials are still needed, it looks like a promising treatment.

■ **Consider calcium.** Some people with hypertension are calcium deficient. If you are not in the habit of consuming two to four servings of low-fat milk products a day, consider supplements.

■ **Ask about potassium.** It's an electrolyte that helps maintain salt and fluid balance, which affects your blood pressure. If you don't get enough in your diet, try eating a banana a day.

Lifestyle

■ **Quit smoking.** Nicotine constricts blood vessels, raising blood pressure. Quitting can lower diastolic pressure by 10 points.

■ **Calm down.** Stress leads to a temporary rise in blood pressure, and chronic stress may contribute to hypertension. Your response to stress may be the key. If you carry around a hostile outlook, it can raise your blood pressure even in nonthreatening situations. Learn to relax. Try meditation, yoga, or deep breathing.

■ **Don't give up hope.** A recent University of Michigan study showed that middle-aged men who felt utterly hopeless about their futures were three times more likely to develop hypertension than men who suffered from such feelings little or not at all. If this describes you, consider counseling to help build a sense of personal control and self-esteem.

■ **Avoid excessive alcohol.** Chronic drinking can raise blood pressure. Cutting back to no more than one alcoholic drink a day can lower diastolic pressure by about 10 points.

■ **Adopt a furry friend.** People with pets have lower blood pressure, probably because pets help us relax. Researchers found that hypertensive people who took blood pressure drugs—and owned a pet—experienced half the rise in stress-related blood pressure surges as nonpet owners who also took antihypertensive drugs.

SimpleSolution

New digital testing devices make it easy to check your blood pressure at home. Get to know your normal variations. Blood pressure is usually highest in the morning, lower in the afternoon, and very low during sleep. Eating, drinking, and exercise temporarily send diastolic pressure down and systolic pressure up. Keep a twice-a-day record so you can spot trends.

Incontinence

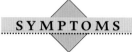

SYMPTOMS

◀ Uncontrollable leakage
of urine

◀ A constant feeling that
you have to urinate,
even when your blad-
der is empty

► What is it?

Urinary incontinence, or inability to control the passage of urine, affects
more than 13 million North Americans, 85 percent of whom are women. At
least 1 in 10 people over age 65 suffers from it. But there's good news:
More than 90 percent of cases are curable if treated promptly. Incontinence
may occur suddenly, indicating an acute condition such as bladder infection or inflammation of the prostate, urethra, or vagina, or it may develop
over time. The two most common types are stress and urge incontinence.

Stress incontinence occurs when pressure on the bladder increases
abruptly. It may be prompted by coughing, sneezing, lifting a heavy
object, or exercising. In women, it usually results from weakened muscles
in the pelvic floor that support the bladder and urethra. This weakening
may be caused by pregnancy and childbirth or by postmenopausal
estrogen deficiency. In men, it may result from an injury to the bladder
or urethra during prostate surgery.

Urge incontinence, sometimes called overactive bladder, occurs when
you feel a strong need to urinate, then immediately leak urine. It's associated with urinary tract infection, diabetes, stroke, dementia, Parkinson's
disease, multiple sclerosis, and prostate enlargement.

Other types of incontinence are overflow incontinence (when urine
leaks out of a full bladder), functional incontinence (when an illness prevents you from reaching the bathroom in time), and reflex incontinence
(due to neurological damage).

Your symptoms usually indicate which type of incontinence you have.
But you may also need a physical exam and tests to check for infection,
urine retention, bladder pressure problems, or reduced urine flow rate.

► How is it treated?

Treatment options depend on the type of incontinence and range from
easy behavioral changes to surgery.

BEHAVIORAL CHANGES

For women, Kegel exercises can strengthen the pelvic floor muscles that
support the uterus and bladder. You can do Kegels while urinating: Slowly
tighten your pelvic muscles to stop your urine stream, hold the muscles
tight for 10 seconds, then release. Repeat three or four times.

Bladder training—urinating at set times—works well for both men and
women with urge incontinence. Working urination into your eating schedule is often effective. Urinate 20 to 30 minutes after every meal and at least
twice between meals. (If you need a reminder, set your watch or alarm

clock.) Also urinate right before you go to bed. You should see results within a few weeks. Biofeedback is another method, one that uses computer technology to help you monitor your body's functions so you can learn how to regulate them.

DRUGS

Antibiotics are prescribed if your incontinence is caused by an infection. Tolterodine (Detrol) is effective for treating urge incontinence. Oxybutynin (Ditropan) relaxes your bladder muscles and blocks the contractions of urge incontinence. Imipramine (Tofranil) is a tricyclic antidepressant that decreases contractions and increases the urethra's resistance to urine leakage. Estrogen is prescribed for women to strengthen the pelvic floor.

MEDICAL DEVICES

A pessary, which fits over the cervix like the outer ring of a diaphragm, can be inserted into the vagina to support the pelvic muscles and prevent stress incontinence. An indwelling catheter (small tube) can be used to transfer urine from the bladder to an external container.

SURGERY

If other treatments fail, surgery may be performed to correct a misaligned bladder, enlarge a small bladder, or remove an enlarged prostate.

If incontinence can't be cured, special absorbent underclothing may be worn.

> **SimpleSolution**
>
> Women who suffer from stress incontinence should wear a tampon when exercising. The tampon helps support the urethra to prevent leakage.

Your Prevention Plan

Diet ■ **Drink up.** If you have reduced your fluid intake in order to avoid urination, you're only making matters worse. Urine becomes more acidic when it isn't expelled—and the acid causes spasms and even more leakage. Drink more than usual, especially water. Avoid alcohol, caffeine, carbonated beverages, and acidic fruit juices, all of which can irritate your bladder.

■ **Skip spicy foods.** These irritate your bladder and may lead to greater leakage.

■ **Shed some pounds.** Extra weight puts pressure on the bladder and may lead to stress incontinence.

■ **Favor fiber.** Constipation causes straining that can further weaken bladder muscles. To stay regular, eat plenty of fiber-rich fresh vegetables and fruits and whole-grain foods.

Exercise ■ **Keep up with Kegels.** Do Kegel exercises anytime—while sitting in a meeting, standing in a grocery line, or lying down reading a book.

Medical Options ■ **Read drug labels.** Incontinence is a possible side effect of certain drugs such as those used to treat heart disease, high blood pressure, depression, and insomnia. Changing a drug may prevent further problems.

Lifestyle ■ **Stop smoking.** A smoker's cough puts pressure on the bladder and can cause leakage. Nicotine also has other adverse effects on the bladder: Up to 40 percent of bladder cancer deaths are tobacco-related.

Irritable Bowel Syndrome

What is it?

Normally the intestines move food through the digestive system with smooth and steady contractions. But in irritable bowel syndrome— also called IBS or spastic colon—the intestines go into spasms that cause irregular bowel habits. IBS is the most common digestive complaint in Canada. About 10 to 20 percent of adults seek medical help for their symptoms, which can last for days or months. Some people have flare-ups throughout their lives. Women—who are three times more likely to suffer from IBS than men—report that symptoms typically are worse just before or during menstrual periods. While IBS is uncomfortable and unpredictable, it does not permanently harm the intestines or lead to more serious conditions like intestinal bleeding or cancer.

Stress, certain foods or drugs, and hormonal changes make the digestive tract contract more frequently, but none of these factors has been pin-pointed as the exact cause of IBS. Some doctors think it results from a nervous-system disorder that affects bowel contractions, a view supported by recent research demonstrating the activity of chemicals called neuro-transmitters, specifically serotonin, in the digestive tract.

No tests can diagnose IBS. But to rule out other conditions, your doctor may perform a blood test, a stool test (to check for parasites), and X rays, sigmoidoscopy, or anorectal manometry (to check the functioning of your anal sphincter).

How is it treated?

IBS symptoms vary, so treatment may require a combination of approaches:

DIETARY CHANGES

Adding fiber-rich foods to your diet will promote normal bowel function, which can ease both constipation and diarrhea. But don't overdo it, especially if your main symptom is diarrhea. Gradually increase your fiber intake to 30 grams a day. Good food sources include whole-grain breads and cereals and many fruits and vegetables. Drink 8 to 10 glasses of water a day, and avoid eating big meals, skipping meals, or eating too fast—all of which can play havoc with your digestive tract.

LIFESTYLE CHANGES

Because the colon is partly controlled by the nervous system, stress reduction and relaxation techniques may help. Also try to avoid medications that have digestive-system side effects, such as certain antibiotics (which

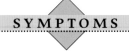

can cause diarrhea) and antihistamines and antacids that contain aluminum salts (which can cause constipation).

DRUGS

- **Antispasmodics** are used to treat intestinal spasms, cramping, constipation, and diarrhea. They include Propantheline bromide (Pro-Banthine), dicyclomine (Bentylol), and glycopyrrolate (Robinul).
- **Antidiarrheals or laxatives** can relieve severe diarrhea or constipation but should be used only on occasion.
- **Antidepressants** can help IBS sufferers who are overly sensitive to normal digestive contractions. Your doctor may prescribe low doses of tricyclic antidepressants such as amitriptyline (Elavil), desipramine (Norpramin), or imipramine (Tofranil), or selective serotonin reuptake inhibitors such as fluoxetine (Prozac), paroxetine (Paxil), or sertraline (Zoloft).

WARNING

Fever, bloody stools, and weight loss aren't typical IBS symptoms and may signal a more serious problem, such as ulcerative colitis, Crohn's disease, or cancer. Call your doctor right away if these symptoms occur.

A new drug appears to help women with IBS who suffer mainly from diarrhea. In a 12-week study, 41 percent of women taking 1 mg of alosetron (Lotronex) twice a day reported adequate pain and symptom relief compared with 29 percent of those taking a placebo. The most common side effect was constipation. The drug is now being tested in men. Two other experimental drugs, tegaserod (Zelmac) and prucalopride (Resolor) hold promise for IBS sufferers whose main symptom is constipation. All three drugs work by blocking intestinal cell receptors for the neurotransmitter serotonin.

Your Prevention Plan

Diet ■ **Don't pull the trigger.** Avoiding certain foods may help you dodge IBS attacks. Consider eliminating these potential triggers: alcohol, caffeine, carbonated beverages (with the possible exception of ginger ale), dairy products, gas-producing foods, high-fat foods, spicy foods, milk and fruit sugars (lactose and fructose), and artificial sweeteners (sorbitol and aspartame).

Exercise ■ **Work out your stress.** Exercise helps keep your digestive system healthy because it causes the release of brain chemicals called endorphins. Endorphins help buffer the body from the effects of stress, which in turn may help reduce IBS symptoms. Try 30-minute sessions of walking, swimming, bicycling, or other aerobic activities three to five times a week.

Supplements ■ **Faster fiber.** If you have trouble adding enough fiber-rich foods to your diet, consider supplementing with psyllium or methylcellulose. Both of these substances help soften stools and cleanse the intestinal tract.

Natural Health ■ **Pick peppermint.** A Welsh study found that four out of five IBS sufferers felt better after taking peppermint-oil capsules. Other herbals that may help reduce spasms or relax muscles in the digestive tract are ginger, chamomile, valerian root, rosemary, and cramp bark. Try them in brewed teas.

■ **Learn to relax.** Try reducing your stress through massage, meditation, yoga, or tai chi (a coordinated breathing and movement technique). Biofeedback and hypnosis can also help.

Kidney Stones

◀ Tiny stones may not cause symptoms.

◀ Larger stones cause excruciating pain in your back or side that may spread to your groin and inner thigh.

◀ Urine may be foul-smelling, cloudy, or bloody, and the flow may be reduced.

◀ Nausea, vomiting, fever, and chills can occur.

What is it?

One in 10 Canadians develops kidney stones, gravel-like masses that occur when a chemical imbalance causes minerals and proteins in your urine to crystallize. Stones may be smooth or jagged, as small as a grain of sand or large enough to cause pain. You may pass tiny stones in your urine without even knowing it. But larger stones cause intense pain as they pass through the ureter (the tube linking your bladder and kidney) or become stuck in the ureter, where they block urine flow.

Most kidney stones are caused by too much calcium in the urine. (This is not related to dietary calcium intake.) Calcium stones may also contain either oxalates or phosphates, salts found normally in the body. Less common types of stones are caused by urinary tract infections or by too much uric acid in urine. Researchers have discovered extremely small bacteria that live in some people's kidneys that may trigger the formation of stones.

How is it treated?

Most kidney stones leave the body on their own in the urine within six weeks. To help them along, drink two to three quarts of water a day. You may also need pain medication. If you can't pass the stone, your doctor may recommend:

● **Lithotripsy,** a nonsurgical procedure that uses sound waves to break up larger stones into smaller pieces that will flush out in the urine.

● **Ureteroscopic stone removal,** used for stones in the mid to lower ureter.

SELF TEST

What Is Your Risk for Kidney Stones?

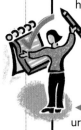

You're at greater risk for kidney stones if you:
◀ have a relative who has had them
  ◀ are male (two-thirds of people with stones are men)
  ◀ are Caucasian
  ◀ are between 20 and 40 years old
◀ don't pass much urine due to impaired kidney function, bowel

disease or surgery, or dehydration
◀ take drugs that form stones, such as the diuretic triamterene (Dyrenium), the AIDS drug indinavir (Crixivan), or the antibacterial drugs called sulfonamides. Glaucoma drugs called carbonic anhydrase inhibitors can cause stones by increasing the

pH of your urine and your body's production of calcium phosphate.
◀ have a condition that increases the amount of calcium in your urine, such as an overactive parathyroid gland
◀ consume large amounts of vitamin D or salt (calcium stones) or animal protein (calcium and uric-acid stones)

◀ live in a hot climate (for example, the south-western U.S.), probably because hot weather increases perspiration, which in turn decreases urine volume, and because sunlight stimulates the production of vitamin D, which increases the body's absorption of calcium from food.

A narrow instrument is passed into the urethra and up into the ureter to locate the stone, which is either grasped and removed or shattered so it can exit the body in the urine.

- **Tunnel surgery,** in which a small incision is made in your side, creating a tunnel to the kidney. A thin instrument is inserted to locate and remove the stone. This procedure is used for large stones or ones that lithotripsy can't reach and break up.

Your Prevention Plan

Diet ■ **Flush out with fluids.** Drink two to three quarts of water a day to dilute urine and flush out stones.

■ **Ask about oxalates.** Ask your doctor if you need to limit your consumption of high-oxalate foods, which can contribute to stone formation. Foods high in oxalates include coffee, beets, chocolate, nuts, spinach, rhubarb, cola, strawberries, tea, and wheat bran.

■ **Avoid grapefruit juice.** No one knows why, but drinking grapefruit juice can increase the risk of kidney stones in susceptible people by as much as 44 percent.

■ **Love your vegetables.** An Italian study found that eating lots of vegetables reduced the risk of kidney stones.

■ **Control uric acid.** If you have a uric-acid stone, eat less meat, fish, and poultry. Animal protein increases the amount of acid in your urine.

Medical Options ■ **Treat the cause.** Get prompt treatment for urinary-tract infections, an overactive parathyroid gland, gout, or other medical conditions that increase your risk of developing kidney stones.

■ **Avoid new stones.** Urinate through a strainer to catch a kidney stone, then take it to your doctor so its composition can be analyzed. The type of drug you take to prevent future stones is based on the components of the stone you pass. Diuretics prevent calcium stones by reducing the amount of calcium the kidneys release into the urine. Sodium cellulose phosphate binds calcium in the intestine so it doesn't leak into the urine and form stones. Potassium citrate raises urine levels of citrate, a salt that prevents calcium stone formation. It also prevents uric-acid stones by decreasing urine acidity. Allopurinol (Zyloprim) decreases uric acid in people with uric-acid stones and may prevent calcium stones.

Natural Health ■ **Consider aquaretics.** These plants improve blood flow to the kidneys and increase urine volume, flushing out bacteria and diluting calcium and oxalates. They are believed to ward off urinary-tract infections and may also help prevent kidney stones. Try brewing tea from goldenrod leaves and tops, parsley leaves and roots, birch leaves, lovage roots, and bearberry (also called uva ursi) or cranberry leaves.

Nutrition Note

For years, people with kidney stones were told to cut their calcium intake. But newer studies show that calcium-rich foods can actually help prevent some kidney stones. Calcium supplements (in pill form) also appear to be safe for people with kidney stones, but ask your doctor to recommend the right dose for you.

SimpleSolution

How can you tell if you are drinking enough fluids? Your urine should be light yellow— almost colorless.

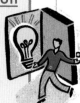

Lung Cancer

◀ Early stages:
no symptoms appear

◀ Later stages:
persistent cough that
may bring up phlegm,
blood, or blood-
streaked sputum;
chest pain; shortness
of breath; wheezing;
hoarseness; fatigue;
appetite loss or weight
loss; repeated bouts of
pneumonia, bronchitis,
other lung infections

What is it?

There are two types of lung cancer: small cell and non-small-cell. Small cell lung cancer is fast-growing, spreading quickly to other organs. It occurs almost exclusively in smokers and accounts for about 20 percent of lung cancers. In nearly two-thirds of people who have it, small-cell lung cancer has already spread to other parts of the body (such as the bones, brain, liver, or other lung) when it's diagnosed.

Non-small-cell lung cancers are usually linked to smoking, passive smoking, or radon exposure. They are slower to spread but are typically not curable by the time they're diagnosed.

Among all people with lung cancer, only about 14 percent live five years after being diagnosed. If detected before the disease has spread, the survival rate is 49 percent, but only 15 percent of lung cancers are discovered that early.

How is it treated?

Treatment depends on the size, location, and type of cancer, and on your overall health. Unfortunately, the standard therapies—radiation, chemotherapy, and surgery—don't cure many people, and the side effects can be difficult to tolerate. As a result, some people decide to participate

SELF TEST

What Is Your Risk for Lung Cancer?

You're more likely to develop lung cancer if you have one or more of these risk factors:

Factors you can't control:

◀ **Gender.** Women are more vulnerable. In one study, a gene linked to abnormal lung cell growth was found to be more active in women than in men, whether or not the women smoked. Research also shows that female smokers are more susceptible to the cancer-causing chemicals found in cigarettes.

Factors you can control:

◀ **Smoking.** As many as 9 out of 10 cases of lung cancer are caused by smoking. The more you smoke and the longer you've smoked, the higher your risk.

◀ **Secondhand smoke.** Even if you don't smoke, your risk rises as much as 30 percent from daily exposure to secondhand smoke.

◀ **Radon.** This odorless gas found in the ground and water is a distant second as a cause of lung cancer.

◀ **Workplace carcinogens.** In North America, some 9,000 men and 900 women develop lung cancer each year because of workplace exposure to such carcinogens as asbestos, arsenic, chloromethyl methyl ether, and chromium compounds. Risk is much higher among smokers.

◀ **Estrogen replacement.** According to University of Pittsburgh researchers, estrogen may fuel the growth of non-small-cell lung cancer.

in clinical trials that test new treatments and treatment protocols. Visit www.clinicaltrials.gov/ct/gui for details. One researcher is looking at a protein (called secondary lymphoid tissue chemokine, or SLC) produced in human lymph glands that killed lung cancer cells in 40 percent of laboratory mice injected with it and slowed tumor growth in the rest.

Small-cell lung cancer is treated with radiation (high-dose X rays) and chemotherapy (drugs) to kill cancer cells. Surgery is usually not an option because the disease has spread by the time it is discovered. Non-small-cell lung cancer is treated with surgery if it's confined to a limited area, such as one part of the lung. In surgery, the doctor may remove a portion of the lung, a complete lobe (section) of the lung, or the entire lung. Radiation therapy may be used alone or with surgery and chemotherapy.

Fast Fact

Call the Cancer Information Service at 1-888-939-3333 and ask for clinical trials. They will search for trials in both Canada and the U.S. Or visit www.ctg.queensu.ca and www.cancer trials.nci.nih.gov.

Your Prevention Plan

Follow the guidelines covered in *Cancer*, page 310, plus the ones below.

Diet

■ **An apple a day.** Lung cancer risk is lower among both smokers and nonsmokers who eat at least five servings of vegetables and fruits daily. Include apples and onions, which are rich in cancer-fighting flavonoids. In a Finnish study, people who ate the most apples were 58 percent less likely to develop lung cancer.

■ **Try tomato sauce.** Research indicates that tomatoes—particularly cooked ones—seem to protect against lung cancer.

■ **Bet on beta-carotene.** If you smoke, a high intake of carotenoid compounds found in certain produce (especially peaches, melons, mangoes, sweet potatoes, squash, pumpkins, and dark leafy greens) can cut your lung cancer risk. Avoid supplements of beta-carotene, however. A Finnish study reported 18 percent more lung cancer cases among heavy smokers who'd been taking beta-carotene supplements. And National Cancer Institute researchers halted a study on the effects of vitamin A and beta-carotene because smokers taking the supplements had 28 percent more lung cancer than those taking a placebo.

Medical Options

■ **Request an X ray.** Some doctors believe that smokers—especially those who are age 50 or older—should have an annual chest X ray to screen for lung cancer.

■ **Ask about aspirin.** Taking 81 to 325 mg of aspirin daily shows promise in warding off lung cancer, but check with your doctor before you start, since aspirin therapy is not without side effects.

Supplements

■ **Seek out selenium.** Selenium (found in many multivitamin/mineral supplements) shows promise in warding off cancer when taken over the long term. In one study, people taking 55 to 200 mcg of the mineral daily had a 46 percent lower rate of lung cancer.

■ **C is for cancer prevention.** Studies suggest that people who get less than 90 mg of vitamin C a day may have a 90 percent higher risk of lung cancer than those who get 140 mg or more.

Lifestyle

■ **Stop smoking.** When you quit smoking, your lung cancer risk drops by half in 10 years. While the addictive properties of nicotene make quitting difficult, many programs and products can help (see pages 166-173).

■ **Check for radon.** Use a kit (available in home-supply stores) to test your home, or hire a professional to do it.

Macular Degeneration

SYMPTOMS

◄ Common complaints include blind spots in the center of your visual field, blurry vision (especially when reading or looking at faces), and straight lines that appear wavy.

What is it?

Located in your retina, the light-sensitive macula provides sharp details and images in the center of your visual field. Age-related macular degeneration (ARMD) is a progressive, painless disease that causes you to lose your central vision. When the macula begins to fail, your central vision becomes blurry and distorted, and tiny blind spots appear. Your peripheral vision remains intact. ARMD affects 10 million North Americans and accounts for 35 percent of all cases of legal blindness. (Generally, you're considered legally blind if your vision is 20/200 to the best correction, which means you can see shapes and shadows but can't read, drive, or move around unassisted.)

Among people over age 65, ARMD is the most common cause of legal blindness. Incidence increases with age.

● **Dry ARMD** is the most prevalent form, accounting for 90 percent of all cases. Small, hard yellow spots called drusen form on the macula and then merge, forming larger spots and causing the macula to atrophy. Only a small percentage of people with drusen progress to have ARMD vision loss, however.

● **Wet ARMD** is so named because fluid or blood leaks from abnormal blood vessels in the macula. The leakage causes the macula to detach and form scar tissue in place of macular cells. Wet ARMD leads to rapid visual deterioration and can occur in addition to dry ARMD.

You'll need an eye exam if you've had central vision loss accompanied by blind spots or blurry vision. Your regular doctor can sometimes detect the drusen and macular atrophy using an ophthalmoscope (a lighted device used for seeing inside the eye). But you should see an ophthalmologist—a doctor specializing in the eyes—for visual acuity and Amsler Grid testing (see Chapter 5, page 151). If you have wet ARMD, the ophthalmologist can perform a test called fluorescein angiography (FANG) to see if you're a candidate for laser therapy. With FANG, an injected dye helps track the abnormal vessels' pattern of leakage.

How is it treated?

There's no cure for ARMD. Although your vision progressively declines, partial sight may remain for long periods. To help stem vision loss, there are several options:

● **Photodynamic therapy** uses strong dyes to plug up the leaky blood vessels. Health Canada recently approved a new drug called verteporfin

SimpleSolution

When outdoors, always wear UV-protective sunglasses to shield your eyes from excessive sun exposure.

(Visudyne), a dye that's injected into the blood vessels and activated by a laser to prevent abnormal blood-vessel growth. Multiple treatments are typically necessary.

- **Laser photocoagulation** destroys abnormal blood vessels and helps a small percentage of people with wet ARMD. But there's a high recurrence rate. Vision is lost again in three to five years, and additional treatments may or may not be successful.
- **Macular translocation** is a surgical procedure that repositions the retina. It is rarely used because it sometimes worsens vision.
- **Low vision aids** can greatly improve your vision. Bright lighting can help. So can large-print computer software, books, newspapers, games, and playing cards. Magnifying glasses that you can wear or hold in your hand come in various power levels to enlarge words or objects. Talking clocks, watches, and calculators can help you stay oriented and manage your finances. Audio books help educate and entertain. Computer magnification systems, such as video magnifiers, enlarge print material on television.

WARNING

If you have dry ARMD and experience a sudden change in vision, seek emergency care immediately—your disease may have progressed to wet ARMD. Laser treatment can be performed to stop the leakage and limit injury to your retina. Otherwise, you may suffer extensive and permanent retinal damage.

Your Prevention Plan

Diet ▓ **Greens and more.** Some foods contain high amounts of lutein and zeaxanthin, two antioxidants that figure prominently in eye health. Researchers at the Massachusetts Eye and Ear Infirmary in Boston found that people who ate antioxidant-rich kale, spinach, and broccoli once a day cut their risk of ARMD by 43 percent. Other good sources of lutein and zeaxanthin include collard greens, egg yolks, corn, orange peppers, kiwis, orange juice, and zucchini.

▓ **Favor fish.** Australian researchers who studied more than 3,500 adults over age 49 found that those who ate fish at least monthly had about half the risk of late-stage ARMD of those who didn't. People who ate fish once a week benefitted the most. Omega-3 fatty acids in fish—also found in the retina—may explain this phenomenon.

▓ **Think zinc.** Also important for retinal health, zinc may help slow the development of macular degeneration. Find it in pumpkin and sunflower seeds, barley, chicken, crab, and oysters.

Medical Options ▓ **Look out for yourself.** If you're over age 45, have your eyes examined every year or two—more often if you have a family history of the disease, other risk factors, or vision changes. Early diagnosis allows for as much intervention as possible to slow the disease's progression. Wet ARMD can quickly develop into an emergency. Your doctor can help you monitor your vision.

▓ **Check your pressure.** High blood pressure might increase your risk of ARMD. Researchers studying 1,200 people found that those with wet ARMD were four times more likely to register high blood pressure than those without either wet or dry ARMD.

Supplements ▓ **Consider antioxidants.** Additional lutein and zeaxanthin might offer some protection. If you don't get enough of these antioxidants in your diet (see *Greens and more*), improve your diet first, then ask your doctor about taking supplements.

Lifestyle ▓ **Kick the habit.** Here's yet another reason to quit smoking: As part of the large-scale, multiyear Nurses' Health Study, researchers found that those who smoked had over twice the risk of developing ARMD.

Osteoporosis

◀ In the early stages, osteoporosis causes no symptoms.

◀ Fractures of tiny vertebral bones in the back may cause mild to severe pain, loss of height, and spinal deformities such as "dowager's hump."

◀ Fractures of the back, hip, ribs, or wrist may occur as a result of a bump or a strain.

What is it?

Osteoporosis is a progressive disease that diminishes the mass (mineral content) of bones and weakens their structure, making them highly susceptible to fracture, especially of the back and hip. According to the Osteoporosis Society of Canada, 1.4 million Canadians have osteoporosis—one in four women and one in eight men over the age of 50 have the disease.

Bone cells are constantly dying and new ones being formed in a process known as remodeling. But once you start losing bone faster than you create it, as you do with age, your bones thin and become more brittle. Bone mass peaks when we're in our twenties or thirties, then slowly declines. After age 50, thin bones may present serious problems—particularly in postmenopausal women, since estrogen plays a pivotal role in bone density.

How is it treated?

Treatment starts with a bone-healthy lifestyle that includes calcium and vitamin D supplements. The first-line therapy for postmenopausal women is estrogen replacement. Although not as effective as estrogen, one or more other drugs may be added, or substituted, to help slow bone loss. No drugs are currently available to build bone, although several are under study. One of them, parathyroid hormone, is now being tested in humans.

DRUGS

● **Estrogen.** The rate of bone loss is greatest in women in the 5 to 10 years after menopause, with up to 50 percent of total bone loss occurring then. By slowing the rate of bone breakdown, estrogen replacement therapy (ERT) is the best way to prevent or halt this loss. It's available as a synthetic estrogen pill (such as Premarin, Ogen, Estrace) or as a transdermal patch (such as Climara and Estraderm). Drawback: ERT increases your risk of breast cancer by about 30 percent when it's taken for more than five years. It isn't advised in women who have a personal or family history of breast or endometrial cancer, or who have fibroids, endometriosis, thromboembolic disorders, or liver disease. It also may present problems for women with gallbladder disease and severe migraines. For women who prefer the idea of a plant-based estrogen, early studies suggest that Cenestin (made from soy) may have a positive impact. Cenestin is not yet available in Canada.

● **Progesterone.** Unless you've had a hysterectomy, adding a synthetic progestin (such as Provera) to your ERT regimen is essential to cut the risk of uterine cancer. However, progestin has now been linked to an

Fast Fact

Choosing a drug therapy approach to osteoporosis calls for a risk-benefit analysis based on your personal health profile. Keep in mind, however, that for most women, the risk of hip fracture is equal to the combined risk of breast, uterine, and ovarian cancer.

increased risk of breast cancer when combined with estrogen. For women who experience unpleasant side effects, such as symptoms similar to PMS, from the synthetics, natural progesterone is available (Prometrium). Estrogen and progestin combos (in medications such as Premplus or FemHRT) are also popular.

- **Selective estrogen receptor modulators (SERMs).** Raloxifene (Evista) can increase bone-mineral density in the spine and hip and cut the risk of vertebral fracture. Another SERM, tamoxifen (Nolvadex), also protects bones, but it's approved only for use in breast cancer patients.
- **Testosterone.** In men who don't produce adequate testosterone, replacement therapy may play a role in osteoporosis treatment. Available testosterone products include Andriol (oral capsules), Androderm (transdermal patch), and Delatestryl (injection).
- **Bisphosphonates.** These are nonhormonal alternatives to treat osteoporosis in men and women. Alendronate (Fosamax) and etidronate/calcium carbonate (Didrocal) are commonly prescribed. Risedronate (Actonel), approved for another bone disorder (Paget's disease), may have potential for osteoporosis. All of these drugs may have gastrointestinal side effects.
- **Calcitonin.** This is a synthetic hormone that regulates calcium metabolism and inhibits the loss of calcium from bones. Among osteoporosis drugs, it has the fewest unpleasant side effects (possible nasal irritation), but it's also the least potent. It's available as a nasal spray (Miacalcin) or an injection. A side benefit: It may help relieve bone pain.

A NEW DEVELOPMENT

Bone glue is an exciting experimental approach for treating spinal osteoporosis. Called vertebroplasty, doctors inject liquid cement into a recently fractured vertebra for faster healing. The long-term effects still aren't known, but the glue has been used in hip replacements for decades.

> **SimpleSolution**
>
> Having a small body frame increases your osteoporosis risk. Here's an easy way to size up yours. With your thumb and ring finger, encircle the wrist of your other hand. If your fingers overlap, you're small-framed.

SELF TEST

Are You at Risk for Osteoporosis?

You are at greater risk if you tick off one or more of the following factors.

For men and women, if you:
- have a family history of the disease
- are thin or small-framed
- are over age 50
- eat a diet low in calcium
- are sedentary
- smoke
- drink alcohol excessively
- have a malabsorption problem or a disease that can interfere with bone formation, such as kidney failure or certain cancers
- use drugs that promote bone loss, such as corticosteroids, anticonvulsants, heparin, thyroid supplements, and certain anticancer and immunosuppressant drugs
- are Caucasian or Asian.

For women, if you:
- are past menopause
- have had your ovaries surgically removed
- have gone extended periods without menstruating, owing to various factors: extreme exercise, an eating disorder, or other causes.

For men, if you:
- have a low testosterone level.

DRUG CAPSULE

Cholesterol-lowering drugs called statins provide an extra bonus: They may increase bone density as well.

Your Prevention Plan

Diet ■ **Drink your milk.** Low-fat and skim milk, nonfat yogurt, and reduced-fat cheeses (except cottage cheese) provide the calcium you need to build strong bones. Fortified milk products also have the vitamin D needed for proper calcium absorption.

■ **Go fish.** Canned sardines and salmon, eaten with their bones, are also rich in calcium. Mackerel and other oily fish are rich in vitamin D.

■ **Eat greens with gusto.** Leafy green vegetables have lots of calcium, plus the potassium and vitamin K you need to block calcium loss from bones. Fill up on broccoli, bok choy, kale, Swiss chard, and turnip greens. Bananas also supply a potassium boost.

■ **Serve yourself soy.** Soy contains not only calcium but also plant estrogens, and it seems to help maintain bone density. Substitute soy flour for regular flour in recipes from pancakes to cupcakes. Nibble on roasted soybean "nuts" instead of peanuts. Reach for soy cereal and soy cheeses. Make malts and smoothies with soy milk (see the recipes on pages 39 and 53).

■ **Don't overdo protein.** High protein intake can raise your excretion of calcium. Some experts recommend consuming no more than 50 grams daily for women, 63 grams for men. Many of us eat twice that much.

■ **Limit caffeine.** Limit your caffeine intake to the equivalent of three cups of coffee a day, since caffeine causes the body to excrete calcium more readily.

■ **Eat your onions.** In male rats, those fed one gram of dry onion daily experienced a 20 percent reduction in the bone breakdown process that can lead to osteoporosis—slightly more than with the drug calcitonin.

Exercise ■ **Get with the program.** A regular program of weight-bearing exercise helps stop further bone loss and may be one of the few ways to build bone as you age. By improving your posture, balance, and flexibility, it also reduces your risk of falls that can break fragile bones. Exercise for at least 30 minutes three times a week. Try walking, running, weight lifting, stair climbing, tennis, or volleyball. Swimming won't do; your bones and muscles must work against gravity for a bone-building effect.

Medical Options ■ **Test your bones.** Bone-density tests are the only way to predict your fracture risk and definitively nail down a diagnosis of osteoporosis. All women over 65 should be scanned, as well as younger postmenopausal women with one or more osteoporosis risk factors. Some doctors recommend that women have a baseline scan at menopause. When repeated at intervals of a year or more, the scans can determine your rate of bone loss and help monitor prevention and treatment efforts. Most experts recommend a dual energy X-ray absorptiometry (DEXA) test. For more about bone-density testing, see page 160.

■ **Get measured.** Ask your doctor to measure your height on an annual basis. A loss of one or two inches is an early sign of undiagnosed vertebral fractures and osteoporosis.

■ **Seek treatment.** Confer with your doctor about conditions that can threaten bone density and what countermeasures you may need. Conditions include hyperparathyroidism, hyperthyroidism, hypogonadism, certain intestinal and kidney disorders, and certain cancers.

Supplements

■ **Choose calcium.** The Dietary Reference Intakes for calcium are 1,300 mg for preteens and teens age 9 to 18 (the amount in 4 cups of milk), 1,000 mg for men and women age 19 to 50, 1,200 mg for men and women age 51 and older. Most people don't get enough calcium in their diets, so supplements are recommended. Because the body can absorb only a limited amount of calcium at once, take supplements in two or three doses during the day, preferably with meals. Make sure the supplement contains vitamin D, which facilitates the absorption of calcium. See page 94 for help in choosing a calcium supplement.

Lifestyle

■ **Quit smoking.** Among 80-year-olds, smokers have up to 10 percent lower bone-mineral density, which translates into twice the risk of spinal fractures and a 50 percent increase in risk of hip fracture. One in eight hip fractures in women is linked to long-term cigarette use. What's more, fractures heal slower in smokers, and are more apt to heal improperly.

■ **Avoid excessive alcohol.** Too much alcohol prevents your body from absorbing calcium properly. Limit yourself to one drink a day for women and two drinks a day for men.

■ **Don't let depression linger.** Depression causes your body to produce cortisol, a stress-related hormone that saps minerals from bones. One study showed that women with clinical depression had lower bone densities in their hips and spines. So see a doctor or therapist for treatment.

WARNING

Osteoporosis is not a form of arthritis, but if you have inflammatory arthritis (such as rheumatoid arthritis or lupus), you may be at greater risk for osteoporosis—even at a young age. Here's why:

- *You may take corticosteroid drugs, which increase the rate of bone loss. Have a baseline bone density test before starting long-term use of these drugs. Use the lowest possible dose for the shortest period of time, and have bone checkups every 6 to 12 months.*
- *Pain and disability may discourage you from exercising. But exercise helps ease arthritis and prevent bone loss. Ask your doctor or a physical therapist about a safe exercise regimen.*

Ovarian Cancer

What is it?

Ovarian cancer develops in one of the ovaries, the almond-size egg-producing reproductive organs on either side of the uterus. When a woman ovulates, an egg bursts through the wall of the ovary. To repair the hole, ovarian cells must divide and reproduce. As in all cancers, when cell division gets out of control, a tumor forms.

Ovarian cancer is hard to detect because there are no early symptoms, and later ones are vague and can mimic common disorders. Most cases occur in women over 50. Your risk is higher if a close relative has had ovarian cancer or if you have the BRCA1 gene (which also influences breast cancer risk). If you have the gene, you have about a 45 percent chance of getting ovarian cancer; women without the gene have a 2 percent lifetime risk.

In about 70 percent of cases, ovarian cancer is not diagnosed until it has spread to other parts of the body. At that stage, survival rates are between 20 and 25 percent. Women who are treated before the cancer has spread have an 85 to 90 percent chance of cure.

Unfortunately, there's no foolproof screening test for ovarian cancer. In the later stages, your doctor can feel a tumor during a pelvic exam or see it on an ultrasound. She may remove a tiny sample of cells to check them for cancer under the microscope.

SELF TEST

What Is Your Risk for Ovarian Cancer?

What you can't control:

◄ **Age.** Risk increases with age. The average ovarian cancer patient is 61.

◄ **Family history.** Most cases occur in women without a family history of the disease, but if you have a close relative with ovarian cancer, your risk nearly triples.

◄ **Disease history.** If you've had breast cancer, you're more susceptible to ovarian cancer.

◄ **Ethnicity.** You are at higher risk if you are of Western European or Jewish descent *and also* have a family history of breast cancer.

What you can control:

◄ **Previous surgery.** Having had a tubal ligation or hysterectomy during your reproductive years lowers your risk. Removal of the ovaries lowers risk but does not eliminate it, since cancer can still form in the cells that line the pelvic cavity where the ovaries were located.

◄ **Medications.** Hormone replacement therapy seems to increase risk for ovarian cancer in post-menopausal women.

◄ **Reproductive history.** Anything that prevents a woman from ovulating seems to protect against ovarian cancer. Taking birth control pills during your reproductive years reduces the risk because the drugs stop ovulation. A woman who takes the pill for 10 years cuts her risk by 70 percent. Each time a woman bears a child, her risk drops by 10 percent. Breast-feeding offers protection as well.

Be on the lookout for new screening tests to detect ovarian cancer early. A 1998 study published in the *Journal of the American Medical Association* reports that a substance in the blood called lysophosphatidic acid (LPA) appears to be consistently elevated in women with ovarian cancer. Another test being studied at the Mayo Clinic evaluates blood levels of an epidermal growth factor receptor called sErbB1.

How is it treated?

Treatment depends on the cancer's spread, as well as your overall health.

SURGERY

Surgery is always used to remove the cancerous ovary and other areas likely to be affected, including the fallopian tubes, uterus, and the other ovary. Most surgeons recommend an aggressive approach, since removing more tissue increases your chance for survival.

ANTICANCER DRUGS

Chemotherapy is usually necessary.

RADIATION

Radiation therapy may be used with surgery and chemotherapy.

TREATMENT DEVELOPMENTS

New combinations of anticancer drugs have improved survival rates. For many years, the standard treatment was cisplatin (Platinol-AQ) and cyclophosphamide (Cytoxan). But in 1995 trials showed that cisplatin and a new drug, paclitaxel (Taxol), improved the survival rate among women with advanced ovarian cancer.

Your Prevention Plan

Follow the guidelines in *Cancer*, pages 310–311, and the ones below.

Diet ■ **Eat cancer smart.** Follow the dietary guidelines in *Cancer*, page 310, and *Breast Cancer*, page 308.

Medical Options ■ **See your doctor.** Although there is no screening test that reliably detects ovarian cancer, reduce your risk by having an annual pelvic exam and Pap smear. If ovarian cancer runs in your family, have a yearly ultrasound scan of your ovaries. Also, ask your doctor about the CA125 blood test to screen for ovarian cancer. It's not a foolproof predictor, but it may be worthwhile.

■ **Medical measures.** If you are at high risk, ask your doctor about removing your ovaries, which provides some protection against ovarian cancer.

■ **Rethink hormones.** If you are at risk for ovarian cancer, ask your doctor about any additional risks associated with hormone replacement therapy.

Supplements ■ **Aspirin a day?** Aspirin shows promise in preventing ovarian cancer. Ask your doctor about taking a dose of 80 to 325 mg daily.

Parkinson's Disease

◀ Tremors of hands, arms, legs, or voice— especially when you're under stress

◀ Muscle rigidity, arm and leg stiffness, and a slowing of movements

◀ Loss of coordination and balance

◀ Walking in tiny shuffling steps

◀ Anxiety, depression, memory loss, and, in advanced disease, dementia

◀ Constipation and incontinence

◀ In later stages, a fixed facial expression, with unblinking eyes and open mouth

What is it?

Parkinson's disease, a nervous system disorder, is caused by a decrease in the brain's production of dopamine. Dopamine is an essential chemical that transports signals from one brain cell to another in order to produce smooth, coordinated muscle movements.

In Parkinson's disease, the dopamine-producing cells in the tiny area of the brain where they are produced—the substantia nigra—begin to die. Symptoms are mild in the early stages and are often attributed to the aging process. By the time most people are finally diagnosed, they've lost more than half their dopamine-producing cells and their symptoms have become more obvious.

Parkinson's disease grows progressively worse over time, which is why doctors call it a "degenerative disorder." It is most common in people over age 55, although it affects younger people, too.

Researchers don't know what causes the brain cells to stop producing dopamine and die, but environmental factors and genetic predisposition are possible causes. There is no cure for Parkinson's disease, and there is no way to screen for it before symptoms occur.

If you have symptoms, see your doctor. He may want you to have a CT scan or MRI to rule out other disorders, such as a brain tumor, that could cause similar symptoms. He will also review any medications you're taking to ensure that your symptoms aren't being caused by a drug side effect. A nonthreatening condition called "benign essential tremor" can also cause tremors, but is not related to Parkinson's disease.

How is it treated?

Lifestyle modifications (see *Your Prevention Plan,* opposite) play an essential role in controlling the symptoms of Parkinson's. But as the disease progresses, most people require drugs and some choose surgery.

DRUGS

In the past, Parkinson's disease was treated primarily with levodopa (L-dopa), a drug that helps brain cells manufacture dopamine. L-dopa reduces symptoms in at least three-quarters of the people who use it, but causes severe side effects including nausea, vomiting, low blood pressure, and restlessness. Over time, the body can grow accustomed to L-dopa, reducing the drug's beneficial effects. Today, when L-dopa is prescribed, it is generally given along with decarboxylase inhibitors such as benserazide (Prolopa) or carbidopa (Sinemet CR), substances that enhance the effects of L-dopa in the brain, allowing lower doses of L-dopa to be given. Other

Fast Fact

Cigarette smokers have a reduced risk of Parkinson's disease because nicotine stimulates the production of dopamine. But don't take up smoking. Scientists are developing a drug that will simulate the positive effects of nicotine for Parkinson's patients.

drugs used to treat Parkinson's include bromocriptine (Parlodel) and pergolide (Permax), which mimic the role of dopamine in the brain, and selegiline (Eldepryl), which helps protect dopamine-producing neurons and delays the need for levodopa therapy.

SURGERY

When drugs stop helping symptoms, many people consider surgery. In pallidotomy (also called thalamotomy), cells that have become overactive as a result of the disease are destroyed with a heat probe inserted into the brain. This helps stop tremors and reduces rigidity. Scientists are currently trying transplants of dopamine-producing cells into the brains of people with Parkinson's. The cells take over the job of producing dopamine, and results so far have been promising.

Your Prevention Plan

Diet

■ **Limit protein.** Avoid high-protein foods such as meats and fish if you're undergoing L-dopa therapy. Protein diminishes the effectiveness of L-dopa.

■ **Increase fiber.** Adding fiber to your diet can help control constipation related to Parkinson's. Eat five to 10 servings of fruits and vegetables daily.

■ **Soften up.** In the later stages of Parkinson's, difficulty chewing can make mealtime more aggravating than enjoyable. Choose soft foods including pasta, yogurt, and applesauce.

Exercise

■ **Get moving.** Make exercise, in the form of stretching and walking, a part of your daily routine. It will improve your strength, balance, and muscle coordination.

■ **Therapy helps.** A physical therapist can teach you how to move your body so you can reduce your chances of falling.

Supplements

■ **Nutrition is key.** Researchers suspect vitamin E (400 IU per day) may slow the progression of Parkinson's. Calcium (1,500 mg per day) aids in nerve impulse transmission. Vitamin B₆ (25 mg, three times daily) speeds the transmission of messages between brain cells, and omega-3 fatty acids, found in flaxseed oil, may reduce tremors (ask your doctor how much to take).

Natural Health

■ **Herbal help.** Visit your local health-food store for Tibetan saffron and tree peony formulations, which may help alleviate tremors. Polygaia can help enhance your mood.

Lifestyle

■ **Try alternatives.** Acupuncture has been used to control tremors and loosen rigidity as well as to ease depression.

■ **Dress accordingly.** Choose clothing you can put on and take off with ease. Zippers and Velcro are easier to maneuver than buttons, snaps, and laces.

■ **Keep it safe.** Install handrails in your home—especially in the shower and next to the toilet. Get rid of throw rugs and any loose cords, which are easy to trip over. Carpeting is best for cushioning a fall.

■ **Helping hands.** Parkinson's can take its toll on your emotional health. You may feel embarrassed or depressed by the symptoms. A support group can help ease the emotional burden. Sharing your concerns with others in the same situation can help you cope with the disease.

Prostate Cancer

◆ **SYMPTOMS**

◀ Usually none

◀ Frequent urination, especially at night

◀ Weak, interrupted, or painful urine stream

◀ Blood in the urine

◀ Pain in the pelvis, spine, hips, or ribs

◀ Loss of appetite and weight

Fast Fact

Having a vasectomy doesn't raise your risk of prostate cancer.

What is it?

Prostate cancer is a tumor that develops in the prostate, the walnut-size gland located below the bladder that produces the fluid portion of semen. Prostate cancer often grows very slowly over many years.

About 60 percent of prostate cancers are discovered before they have spread to surrounding tissue or other parts of the body. Finding them early offers your best chance for a cure. In fact, more than 93 percent of men who are treated at this stage are cured. Once the cancer begins to spread, however, it can be deadly.

Scientists know that prostate cancer is linked to male hormones but they are not sure exactly what triggers it. You can minimize its impact by detecting it early through screening—with a rectal exam and a blood test to measure prostate-specific antigen (PSA), a substance more abundant in men with prostate cancer.

To reach a definite diagnosis of prostate cancer if the rectal exam and PSA suggest abnormalities, your doctor may order X rays, blood and urine tests, or an ultrasound of the prostate. A small tissue sample will also be taken so it can be studied for cancer cells.

How is it treated?

Treatment depends on your age and the grade and stage of the cancer. Before making any treatment decisions, ask your doctor to explain every option along with its possible side effects. Take notes or ask if you may tape record the session so you'll remember the information later. As with any cancer treatment, consider getting a second opinion before proceeding. Here are the most common options:

SELF TEST

What Is Your Risk for Prostate Cancer?

You're more likely to develop prostate cancer if you have one or more of these risk factors:

What you can't control:

◀ **Age.** Your risk increases rapidly after age 50. More than 80 percent of prostate

cancers are diagnosed in men over age 60.

◀ **Family history.** Prostate cancer seems to run in families, particularly when it's diagnosed before age 60. Your risk

doubles if your father or brother has been diagnosed with it.

◀ **Ethnicity.** People of African descent have a 30 to 50 percent higher risk

than Caucasians and twice the death rate.

What you can control:

◀ **Alcohol and tobacco.** Smoking and heavy drinking increase your risk.

◀ **Diet.** A high-fat diet is a risk factor.

WATCHFUL WAITING

If your cancer is detected at an early stage, the side effects of aggressive treatment can outweigh the benefits. Many older men who monitor their condition carefully never need treatment because prostate cancer grows so slowly.

SURGERY

The prostate gland may be removed, especially if the cancer is confined to the gland itself. There is substantial risk for incontinence and impotence after this surgery. In some cases in which the cancer has spread, the testicles are removed in order to drastically diminish the production of testosterone. This can cause a marked decrease in sex drive.

RADIATION THERAPY

Uses high-dose X rays—directed toward the prostate from the outside of the body or embedded as seeds near the prostate—to kill cancer cells.

ANDROGEN-DEPRIVATION THERAPY

Drugs that inhibit the production of testosterone or block its effects include flutamide (Euflex) and leuprolide (Lupron).

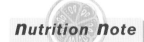

Nutrition Note

One study showed a 20 percent reduction in prostate cancer risk among men who ate cooked tomatoes or tomato sauce four times a week, and a 35 percent reduction among men who ate 10 servings a week.

Your Prevention Plan

Follow the guidelines in *Cancer*, pages 310-311, and the ones below.

 Diet ■ **Trim the fat.** Eat a low-fat diet consisting mainly of fish, skinless poultry, low-fat dairy products, and five to 10 daily servings of fruits and vegetables. Strictly limit foods high in saturated fats.

■ **Vital vegetables.** Lycopene, the red pigment in tomatoes, has protective properties. It is best absorbed when cooked. Green peas, baked beans, broccoli, and cabbage may also cut your risk.

■ **Fill up on fruits.** One study showed that men who ate five or more servings of fruit daily were about half as likely to develop advanced prostate cancer as those who averaged less than one serving daily.

■ **Sample some soy.** The low rates of prostate cancer in Japan may be linked to a soy-rich diet. Try eating tofu, tempeh, green soybeans, or soy burgers at least twice a week.

■ **Get enough zinc.** Foods high in zinc can promote prostate health. Good sources include whole grains, seafood, mushrooms, and pumpkin and sunflower seeds.

 Exercise ■ **Get moving.** Exercising regularly and maintaining a healthy weight helps reduce risk.

 Medical Options ■ **Be on the safe side.** Doctors differ on the type and frequency of screenings they recommend, but err on the safe side. The Canadian Cancer Society recommends that men over age 50 should discuss the benefits and risks of early detection testing using PSA and rectal exam with their doctor. Men in high-risk groups should discuss the need for testing at a younger age.

Supplements ■ **Boost C and E.** Taking 1,000 mg of vitamin C and 400 to 800 IU of vitamin E may offer protection. Talk to your doctor for advice.

■ **Consider selenium.** Harvard researchers found that men with the highest selenium levels were 65 percent less likely to develop advanced prostate cancer than those with the lowest levels. Consider taking 200 mcg daily, but ask your doctor first.

Shingles

What is it?

Shingles is an encore presentation of the chicken pox attack you had as a child. This very painful nerve condition is caused by the same varicella zoster virus that causes chicken pox.

If you ever had chicken pox, the varicella zoster virus is probably hibernating in your nerve cells. Although the virus remains dormant in most people, shingles can occur when the virus is reactivated in the nerve pathways. Although shingles is most common in people over 50, it can erupt in younger people, too.

Scientists don't know exactly what "wakes up" the hibernating shingles virus, but they believe advancing age, a weakened immune system, some medications (such as cortisone-type drugs or immune-suppressing medications), emotional stress, or recovery from surgery may trigger it. Shingles also affects some people who have cancer or AIDS. Skin injuries and sunburn may also trigger it.

In some people who have had shingles, the rash clears up, but numbness, tingling, or pain continues along the affected nerve pathways. This is called postherpetic neuralgia (PHN). (Neuralgia means "pain in the nerve.") PHN is most common in people over age 50 who have had a shingles outbreak. The painful condition can last for months or even years.

Your doctor can usually tell from the pattern of the blisters if you have shingles. To confirm the diagnosis, she may order lab tests to exam a sample of the fluid from your blisters. She may also recommend that you see a dermatologist to ensure the blisters don't scar your skin.

How is it treated?

Like most viruses, shingles has to run its course. Your doctor's goal is to thwart blister formation, hasten the end of the shingles attack, relieve your pain, and prevent chronic pain. There are some lifestyle efforts (see *Your Prevention Plan*, opposite) that can help speed your recovery. But most people also take some type of medication for shingles.

DRUGS

Over-the-counter pain relievers such as aspirin or acetaminophen can help ease the pain of shingles. For intense pain, your doctor can prescribe extra-strength painkillers. Also, ask your doctor about antiviral creams or ointments that can help prevent skin infection due to leaking blisters.

For people over 50, anti-inflammatory corticosteroid drugs (prednisone, methylprednisolone) are sometimes prescribed. Studies show that taking an antiviral drug such as acyclovir (Zovirax) within 72 hours of the appearance of the rash reduces the incidence of PHN six months after the initial outbreak by nearly 50 percent. A newer antiviral drug, famciclovir (Famvir), may also shorten the duration of your symptoms and limit your chances of getting PHN. Some studies show that combining antiviral therapy with antidepressants can shorten the duration of serious shingles pain.

Your Prevention Plan

 Diet ■ **Eat well.** Diets that are low in vitamins, minerals, and antioxidants can weaken your immune system, making you more vulnerable to infection. Strive for a low-fat diet rich in fruits, vegetables, and whole grains.

 Exercise ■ **Address your stress.** Stress can trigger shingles, and exercise can help reduce stress. Try walking briskly for half an hour a day or take up swimming, biking, or yoga.

 Medical Options ■ **Avoid chicken pox.** The best way to avoid shingles is to avoid chicken pox. A chicken pox vaccine (Varivax) is now available. If you've never had chicken pox and take the vaccine now, it might protect you from getting shingles, too, although doctors aren't yet certain if the vaccine works against both conditions.

 Supplements ■ **Take B₁₂.** For pain relief from PHN, ask your doctor about vitamin B₁₂ injections, which can strengthen the tissue that covers your nerves.

Natural Health ■ **Rub it in.** Applying a cream containing capsaicin (the heat in hot peppers) three or four times a day has reduced pain for many sufferers after a couple of weeks of use.

■ **Rub it on.** Gels containing glycyrrhizin, an active component of licorice, have been proven to block the shingles virus when rubbed into the affected areas three or four times a day.

■ **Sleep now.** Bed rest is recommended during the early stages of shingles, especially if you have a fever. Because open blisters can spread chicken pox to anyone who hasn't had it before, change bed linens frequently.

■ **Soothe your skin.** To promote healing (and relaxation), add a few drops of rose, lavender, bergamot, or tea tree oil to your warm bath. Mix them in a carrier oil, such as vegetable oil, first.

■ **Numb the pain.** Calendula lotion or ointment applied to blisters several times a day eases pain. Or apply a paste made of two crushed aspirin tablets and two tablespoons rubbing alcohol three times a day to soothe throbbing nerve endings.

■ **Itching for relief.** Ask your pharmacist to prepare a mixture with 75 percent calamine, 20 percent rubbing alcohol, and 1 percent each phenol and menthol. (Inert ingredients account for the remaining 2 percent.) Apply to blisters continuously until you're healed. Other itching remedies include vitamin E oil or aloe vera gel.

■ **Ice, ice, baby.** Apply ice packs for 10 minutes at a time to affected areas. Keep them off for at least five minutes between applications.

■ **Pack it on.** Compresses containing aluminum acetate solution, available over the counter in pharmacies, can help relieve the itching.

■ **Dust your skin.** To keep your clothes from rubbing against your blisters, dust yourself with colloidal oatmeal powder.

 Lifestyle ■ **Pins and needles.** There are reports that acupuncture is an effective treatment for shingles. It is especially helpful for easing the pain of PHN.

■ **Stress busters.** Try tai chi, meditation, and self-hypnosis techniques to help reduce your stress and manage pain. Even after your symptoms disappear, these techniques can help you cope with the day-to-day stress that can lead to shingles.

Skin Cancer

◄ Basal cell carcinoma: painless smooth bump that grows slowly, often on the face, ear, or neck

◄ Squamous cell carcinoma: painless reddish bump or patch that may form a crusted or scaly surface on the face, ears, neck, hands, or arms

◄ Melanoma: painless dark bump or spot, a mole with an irregular shape and border, or a sore that doesn't heal, located anywhere on the body

What is it?

There are three common types of skin cancer. If detected early, all of them can easily be treated and cured. About 80 percent of skin cancers are basal cell or squamous cell carcinomas. Basal cell carcinomas are rarely fatal, but they can be disfiguring if they're not treated. Squamous cell carcinomas are more likely to be life-threatening than basal cell carcinomas.

Melanoma is the most lethal form of skin cancer. It can spread quickly to other parts of your body through the blood or lymph system. The five-year survival rate is 95 percent if melanoma is found early, but in its later stages, the disease is difficult to cure.

Skin cancer rates are soaring. There are about 60,000 new cases of all skin cancers in Canada each year, of which 7 percent are malignant melanoma. In 2000, there were 3,700 new cases of melanoma, compared to 2,400 new cases in 1989. What's contributing to the increase? One possibility is that it's linked to the decline of outdoor occupations since the turn of the century. When people worked outdoors, they were continually exposed to the sun, so their skin was more accustomed to UV light and less susceptible to sunburn. Now people spend relatively little time in the sun. When they do, they tend to get sunburned, which increases their risk of skin cancer. Another theory is that more harmful solar radiation is reach-

SELF TEST

What Is Your Risk for Skin Cancer?

You're at increased risk for skin cancer if you have one or more of these risk factors:

What you can't control:

◄ **Skin type and body characteristics.** The most serious risks include having red or blond hair, light-colored eyes, fair skin that freckles or burns easily, and a large number of moles.

◄ **Ethnicity.** Caucasians are about 10 times more likely to develop skin cancer than people of African descent.

◄ **Age.** The older you are, the greater your chance of developing skin cancer. The risk of melanoma increases sharply after age 50.

◄ **Family history.** Your risk increases if you have a family history of the disease.

What you can control:

◄ **Exposure to ultraviolet (UV) rays.** Over 90 percent of skin cancers occur on skin that's regularly exposed to UV radiation from the sun or tanning lights.

◄ **Burns.** You're at higher risk if you've had severe or blistering burns from sunlight, tanning beds or lamps, X rays, or radiation. Having been sunburned more than once as a child increases your risk for developing skin cancer as an adult.

◄ **Geography.** If you winter in the U.S. Sun Belt or live at a high elevation.

◄ **Environmental factors.** Your risk increases if you've been exposed to chemicals such as coal, tar, pitch, creosote, arsenic compounds, radium, or some herbicides.

ing the earth today because of damage to the atmosphere's ozone layer.

If you notice a new growth, a change in your skin, or a sore that hasn't healed in two weeks, see your doctor.

How is it treated?

Treatment depends on the size, type, depth, and location of the cancer. Most people need surgery—usually minor—to remove skin cancers.

SURGERY
Types include cryosurgery (tissue destruction by freezing), laser therapy (destruction with laser light), and electrodesiccation (destruction by heat). Some people with melanoma must have nearby lymph glands and large areas of skin removed.

RADIATION THERAPY
Administration of high-dose, localized X rays to kill cancer cells.

CHEMOTHERAPY AND BIOLOGICAL THERAPY
Advanced melanoma is also treated with chemotherapy (anticancer drugs) or biological therapy (using the body's immune system to fight the cancer).

Your Prevention Plan

Follow the guidelines in *Cancer*, pages 310-311, and the ones below.

Medical Options ■ **Scan your skin.** If you have a family history of melanoma, if you have many moles (especially on your trunk), or if you were sunburned regularly as a youth, see a dermatologist for an annual screening.

Lifestyle ■ **Limit sun exposure.** Stay out of the sun between 10 A.M. and 3 P.M., when UV rays are strongest.

■ **Use sunscreen.** Whenever you're outside, liberally apply a sunscreen with a sun protection factor (SPF) of at least 15, which blocks 93 percent of UV rays. Be sure the product contains avobenzone (or Parsol 1789) so you'll be protected against both types of sunlight—UVA and UVB. Reapply every two hours to lips, bald spots, the part in your hair, and the tops of your ears—common sites for skin cancer.

■ **Cover up.** Wear tightly woven clothing outdoors, covering as much skin as possible. A broad-brimmed hat provides excellent protection. Be particularly careful if you're on snow, water, or ice, which intensify exposure.

■ **Check yourself.** Perform a monthly self-check, looking for new skin growths or changes in existing moles, freckles, or birthmarks. (For more details on how to check your skin, see page 155.) If you find any suspicious changes, see your doctor promptly.

SimpleSolution

These ABCDs describe suspicious moles:

• **Asymmetry:** The mole is oddly shaped —not symmetrical.

• **Border:** It has irregular, notched, scalloped, or vaguely defined edges.

• **Color:** Some areas may be darker than others, and more than one color may be present.

• **Diameter:** It's more than a quarter-inch in diameter (the size of a pencil eraser) or clearly becoming larger.

Stroke

◄ Sudden weakness, tingling, or numbness in your arm, leg, or face, especially on one side your body

◄ Sudden confusion, with trouble speaking (including slurred speech and drooling) or understanding speech

◄ Sudden vision loss in one or both eyes, or double vision

◄ Sudden dizziness, loss of balance or coordination, or fainting

◄ Sudden severe headache with nausea and vomiting

Call 911 or your local emergency number immediately if you have any of these symptoms. Prompt medical care can dramatically reduce stroke damage and save your life.

Fast Fact

Uncontrolled high blood pressure causes 80 percent of strokes.

What is it?

Stroke is the third leading cause of death in Canada, after heart attacks and cancer. The good news? Stroke rates have dropped dramatically over the last 10 years, and new treatments make nearly full recovery possible for many people.

Stroke is sometimes called a "brain attack" because blood flow to part of the brain is disrupted in a stroke, just as blood to part of the heart is disrupted in a heart attack. When oxygen-rich blood can't reach your brain cells, the cells die or are damaged. Oxygen must be restored quickly to save the damaged cells.

There are two main types of strokes:

● **Ischemic strokes** are caused by a blockage—usually a blood clot in your brain or the blood vessels in your neck. Ischemic strokes, which represent 80 percent of all strokes, are of two types. In an embolic stroke, a blood clot that formed in another part of your body travels to your brain and clogs a blood vessel there. The most common cause of embolic stroke is a clot released by atrial fibrillation, a type of irregular heartbeat that causes blood to pool in the atria, the two upper chambers of the heart (pooled blood tends to clot). In thrombotic stroke, a buildup of plaque due to atherosclerosis (narrowed arteries) cuts off the blood supply to the brain.

● **Hemorrhagic strokes** account for just 20 percent of all strokes, but they are more likely to be fatal. They are caused by bleeding in the brain, usually from a broken blood vessel or a burst aneurysm (a bulging sac in a weakened blood vessel).

If you suspect that you or someone else has had a stroke, call 911 or your local emergency number for an ambulance. Once at the hospital, the

Early Warning Sign of Stroke

Transient ischemic attacks (TIAs) are so-called "mini-strokes" because they produce the same symptoms as a full-blown stroke, but TIAs go away in a few hours with no aftereffects. Don't ignore them. TIAs can signal that a stroke will occur; they precede a stroke in about 40 percent of people who have them.

See your doctor if you suspect you have had a TIA. An ultrasound (a painless test using sound waves) or magnetic resonance imaging scan may be done to determine if plaque is clogging the arteries in your neck that carry blood to the brain. If they are over 70 percent blocked, you may need surgery to remove the plaque.

doctor will do a physical and neurological (brain) exam to assess the extent of any stroke damage.

It's critical to determine what type of stroke you've had in order to recommend the most appropriate treatment choices. As a result, your doctor may also order the following tests to get more information:

- **Computed tomography (CT)** scanning of your brain to help confirm the diagnosis of stroke
- **Magnetic resonance imaging (MRI)** to confirm that you've had a stroke and determine what type it was
- **Electrocardiogram (ECG)** to record your heartbeat and reveal an irregular heart rhythm.

> ### Nutrition Note
>
> Overweight people who eat lots of salty foods have a 32 percent higher risk of stroke, reports the *Journal of the American Medical Association.*

SELF TEST

What Is Your Risk for Stroke?

Your chances of having a stroke are greater if you have one or more of these risk factors:

What you can't control:

- ◀ **Ethnicity**. People of African descent have strokes at nearly twice the rate of whites.
- ◀ **Age**. After 55, your stroke risk doubles with each decade.
- ◀ **Gender**. Men have a 1.25 times greater risk of stroke than women.
- ◀ **Heredity**. Inherited blood-clotting disorders raise your risk of stroke. Protein C deficiency is more common in whites, while sickle-cell disease occurs primarily in people of African descent.
- ◀ **Family history** of TIA or stroke.
- ◀ **Diabetes**. If you have diabetes, you are at greater risk of having a stroke.

- ◀ **You've already had a TIA or stroke**. Men who've had one stroke have a 42 percent chance of having another within five years; women have a 24 percent chance of having another. And about 35 percent of all people who've had a TIA have a stroke within the following five years.

What you can control:

- ◀ **Hypertension**
- ◀ **Smoking**
- ◀ **Irregular heartbeat**. Atrial fibrillation, the most common irregular heartbeat, raises your risk of stroke sixfold.
- ◀ **Heart disease**. Atherosclerosis (narrowed arteries) and carotid stenosis (narrowed neck arteries) can increase your risk sixfold.
- ◀ **High cholesterol**. According to some studies (but not others), high total cholesterol levels may increase your risk of stroke. Some research indicates that low HDL levels may prove to be the real culprit.
- ◀ **Stress response**. Some studies suggest that your response to stressful situations may predict your risk of stroke. People who respond with anger or an increased heart rate are considered to be at higher risk.
- ◀ **Weight**. Being overweight makes you more susceptible to risk factors such as diabetes, high blood pressure, and elevated cholesterol.
- ◀ **Illegal drugs**. Using cocaine can narrow your arteries and cause your heart to beat erratically, which can cause

clots to form and lead to stroke. Smoking marijuana may also be a risk factor, since it can cause blood pressure to change rapidly. Using heroin, amphetamines, and anabolic steroids are also thought to increase your risk.

- ◀ **Excessive alcohol use**
- ◀ **Poor diet**. Limit salt, reduce fat, and boost fiber to keep your blood pressure and cholesterol levels in check.

For more information about strokes, log on to the Heart and Stroke Foundation of Canada's Web site at www.heartand stroke.ca, or in the U.S., the National Institute of Neurological Disorders and Stroke's Web site at www.ninds.nih.gov.

How is it treated?

DRUGS

Tissue-plasminogen activator (tPA) is a powerful drug that dissolves clots blocking the brain's arteries. To be effective, tPA must be given intravenously within three hours of the start of stroke symptoms. A study published in the *Journal of the American Medical Association* describes tPA's amazing results. Among stroke sufferers who received tPA, 35 percent had no lasting symptoms. And another 43 percent were able to go home and care for themselves with only mild symptoms. But tPA can be dangerous if given for a hemorrhagic stroke because it can increase bleeding or cause death. For a hemorrhagic stroke, treatment usually includes strict bedrest and medications to help lower blood pressure and brain swelling.

SURGERY

People who have had a hemorrhagic stroke often need surgery to repair a burst aneurysm or remove blood that's accumulated in the brain. Transplanting cells from embryos into stroke victims' brains to replace damaged cells has proved promising, but further studies are needed.

Your Prevention Plan

Diet ▪ **Eat for your health.** A healthy diet helps control stroke risk factors, such as high cholesterol, diabetes, and high blood pressure. Eat a low-fat, low-cholesterol, high-fiber diet, including at least five to 10 servings a day of fruits and vegetables, to keep cholesterol levels down. And stick to a low-salt diet to help manage high blood pressure.

▪ **Opt for omega-3s.** Omega-3 fatty acids help prevent blood clots that can lead to stroke. Eat foods containing these fatty acids two to three times a week. Good sources are salmon, sardines, trout, mackerel, wheat germ, and canola and soybean oils.

▪ **Drink within limits.** Drinking four ounces of alcohol a day (but no more) may protect against stroke by "thinning" the blood, reducing the risk of blood clots. A study published in a 1999 issue of *The New England Journal of Medicine* found that, among men, having just one drink a week offered protective effects against strokes. Binge drinking, on the other hand, actually increases your risk.

Exercise ▪ **Burn it up.** Daily aerobic exercise (activity that makes you slightly out of breath) can cut your stroke risk. A study reported in *The Journal of the American Heart Association* found that people who burn 2,000 calories a week through exercise cut their stroke risk by 46 percent. A brisk one-hour walk five days a week is ideal. People who walked for a half hour five days a week and burned 1,000 calories cut their stroke risk by 24 percent.

Medical Options ■ **Get checked.** If you're over age 55, have an annual checkup. Blood pressure readings over 140/90 and cholesterol readings over 5.2 mmol/L put you at higher risk.

■ **Pressure pills.** If your high blood pressure doesn't improve with diet and exercise, medications can help. Up to 90 percent of stroke sufferers had high blood pressure prior to their strokes. Research indicates that anti-hypertensive drugs can cut the incidence of stroke by 38 percent and the death rate by 40 percent.

■ **Cholesterol control.** If diet and exercise haven't worked, your doctor may prescribe cholesterol-lowering statin medications to help reduce your risk. Several studies show they cut stroke risk by about 30 percent.

■ **Half an aspirin a day.** Taking a low-dose aspirin every day can help reduce your risk of blood clots. If you can't tolerate aspirin, the prescription blood-thinning drugs ticlopidine (Ticlid) and clopidogrel (Plavix) can be used instead. Warfarin (Coumadin) helps high-risk people, such as those with atrial fibrillation. While aspirin may decrease your risk of ischemic stroke, it may increase your risk of hemorrhagic stroke. Talk to your doctor to weigh the risks and benefits.

■ **(Ultra)sound advice.** If you're over 60 and you smoke or have diabetes or heart disease, ask your doctor about having a carotid ultrasound (see *Early Warning Sign of Stroke,* page 388) to check for possible blockages.

■ **Say eye.** If you're over 50, see an ophthalmologist for an eye exam, which can detect damage to the arteries in your eyes—a precursor to stroke in some people.

■ **Sugar patrol.** If you have diabetes, keep tight control of your blood-sugar level and see your doctor regularly.

Supplements ■ **Consider antioxidants.** Vitamins C, E, and beta-carotene are antioxidants that can help reduce arterial damage caused by free radicals, unstable oxygen molecules. Recent studies have questioned their benefit in preventing stroke, but there is some evidence that they may help minimize damage once a stroke has occurred.

Natural Health ■ **Practice transcendental meditation.** Reducing stress may reduce plaque buildup in the arteries, suggests a study published in *Stroke,* an American Heart Association journal. See pages 201-202 for an easy way to meditate.

Lifestyle ■ **Just quit it.** Stroke risk is 50 percent greater for smokers (even higher for women) than nonsmokers. Quitting lowers your risk right away, but the greatest decrease comes two to four years down the road.

■ **Seek out serenity.** Stress management helps reduce high blood pressure, a major risk factor for stroke. Prayer, biofeedback, and visualization (see page 202) can lower your heart rate and blood pressure. Yoga, tai chi, and dance can calm you and elevate your mood. Learning how to express anger or frustration constructively can also reduce stress.

Thyroid Disorders

◄ Hypothyroidism: low energy, fatigue, weight gain, intolerance to cold, depression, slowed thinking, headaches, fluid retention, coarse skin, brittle nails, constipation, goiter (enlarged thyroid gland), and irregular menstrual periods

◄ Hyperthyroidism: increased pulse rate, weight loss despite an increased appetite, heat intolerance, tremor, irritability, insomnia, sweating, goiter, diarrhea, light menstrual periods, bulging eyes, and confusion or apathy (especially in older people)

◄ Thyroid nodules: often no symptoms, or a tiny lump on the thyroid gland

Fast Fact

In studying data from 25,000 adult patients in Oregon, researchers discovered nearly 10 percent had undiagnosed hypothyroidism or hyperthyroidism.

What is it?

The thyroid is a butterfly-shaped gland located at the front of your neck, around the voice box. It produces and releases hormones that regulate your metabolism, influencing strength, heart rate, energy level, bowel function, fat breakdown, hair growth, and mood.

The release of thyroid hormones is controlled partially by thyroid stimulating hormone (TSH), made in the pituitary gland, which releases more or less TSH according to your body's need for the hormone.

In hypothyroidism (underactive thyroid), not enough thyroid hormone is released and your metabolism slows, making you feel tired. Also, low levels of thyroid hormone cause cholesterol levels to rise. Women have about four times the rate of hypothyroidism as men, and women over 50 are especially vulnerable. Hypothyroidism is often caused by the autoimmune disorder Hashimoto's thyroiditis, in which thyroid cells are destroyed by a misdirected immune-system attack.

In hyperthyroidism (overactive thyroid), your thyroid releases too much thyroid hormone and your metabolism speeds up, making you feel jumpy. Hyperthyroidism is also more common in women, usually developing between the ages of 30 and 40. In many cases, it is caused by the autoimmune disorder Graves' disease, which triggers overproduction of thyroid hormone.

Sometimes one or more nodules grow on the thyroid gland. They're usually noncancerous, but your doctor may check them periodically to see if they're producing thyroid hormone, which can cause hyperthyroidism.

A goiter is an enlarged thyroid gland. Goiters can occur with either hypo- or hyperthyroidism. In some cases, goiters grow large enough to interfere with swallowing or breathing, although most don't cause problems and many go away on their own. Goiters are sometimes caused by insufficient iodine. (The thyroid gland absorbs iodine, which is used to make thyroid hormone.) Most people in Canada get enough iodine from their diets. Most salt has added iodine to prevent the iodine-deficiency goiter that was common in certain areas of North America before the 1950s. Conversely, too much iodine can cause improper thyroid function, especially if the gland is already being attacked by the immune system. In this case, extra iodine causes the levels of thyroid hormones in the blood to rise even higher.

Certain tests can help your doctor diagnose a thyroid problem.

● **Blood tests.** These measure the amount of TSH in your blood.
● **Radioactive iodine uptake tests.** You take a liquid or pill form of radioactive iodine, which is absorbed by the thyroid as iodine is. Within 24 hours, the radioactivity is measured to see how much iodine the gland has absorbed. Increased absorption points to Graves' disease.

- **Biopsy.** Your doctor removes a few cells through a fine needle. The cells are examined in a laboratory for cancer.
- **Ultrasound scanning.** Shows whether a nodule is fluid-filled or solid.

How is it treated?

DRUGS

For hypothyroidism, your doctor will prescribe a synthetic thyroid hormone replacement, adjusting your dosage as needed. For hyperthyroidism, your doctor may recommend an antithyroid drug, which you take every day to stop the gland from making hormones. Another option is to take a single dose of radioactive iodine, which destroys the thyroid cells that are making too much hormone. The substance is absorbed only by the thyroid and doesn't injure any other structure. Usually the radioactivity results in hypothyroidism, and you need to take thyroid replacement.

SURGERY

For hyperthyroidism that has not improved with drugs, a portion of the gland may be removed to limit hormone production. Many people must take thyroid drugs for life after surgery. For a thyroid nodule, your doctor may use a delicate needle to remove any fluid. If a nodule is cancerous, the thyroid gland is removed.

WARNING

Before using seaweed or kelp supplements, ask your doctor if they are safe for you. They contain iodine, which can worsen a thyroid condition.

Your Prevention Plan

Diet ■ **Watch your diet.** For hypothyroidism, get enough iodine (found in shellfish and iodized salt) and limit your fat intake, since the condition can elevate your cholesterol level. For hyperthyroidism, shun iodine-rich foods, and eat plenty of calcium-rich foods to offset the leaching of calcium from your bones by excess thyroid hormone. Include cruciferous vegetables such as broccoli in your diet; they curb thyroid production naturally.

■ **Savor spinach.** Many scientists believe iron is necessary for proper thyroid hormone production, so eat plenty of iron-rich foods. Because excess iron interferes with the absorption of thyroid medication, ask your doctor before taking a supplement.

Exercise ■ **Get moving.** Exercise helps control cholesterol, which hypothyroidism tends to elevate. Take brisk, half-hour walks most days to help get your level in the normal range.

Supplements ■ **Take your vitamins.** For any thyroid problem, be sure your daily multivitamin contains all the B vitamins and vitamin C, which boost the immune system and help the thyroid perform. If you have hyperthyroidism, take an extra 1,000 mg of calcium daily, in divided doses, to offset the calcium loss it can cause.

Ulcers

◄ Gnawing, aching, and/or burning pain in the upper abdomen or lower chest, often occurring between meals and during sleep and usually relieved by eating or taking antacids

◄ Anemia and fatigue

◄ Nausea, sometimes accompanied by vomiting a substance that looks like coffee grounds

◄ Black, tarry stools

What is it?

An ulcer is a hole or break in the mucous membrane that lines the esophagus, stomach, or duodenum (the uppermost section of the small intestine). Ulcers in the stomach or duodenum are called peptic ulcers. Because the lining must withstand constant contact with digestive juices and stomach acid, it is generally resistant to injury. But sometimes there is a breakdown in the mucous membrane, and a hole develops. Most ulcers are no larger than a pencil eraser, but they can be extremely painful and cause serious and life-threatening bleeding.

About 90 percent of ulcers are caused by an infection with bacteria called *Helicobacter pylori* (*H. pylori*). But because the organism also exists in the stomachs of people who do not develop ulcers, most scientists believe *H. pylori* infection leads to ulcer formation only in people genetically predisposed to ulcers.

Another cause of ulcers is the use of aspirin and pain medications called nonsteroidal anti-inflammatory drugs (NSAIDs), such as naproxen or ibuprofen. These drugs can weaken the mucous membrane that lines the stomach and cause ulcer development and massive intestinal bleeding.

You've probably heard people say, "Take it easy. You'll give yourself an ulcer." A laid-back personality is an admirable attribute, but it won't protect you from ulcers. In the past, medical experts thought ulcers were caused by stress. Doctors have now rejected that theory. The bottom line? Stress won't give you an ulcer, but the added stomach acid that stress generates can make your ulcer worse.

To help ease the pain, your doctor may recommend that you try an acid-blocking medication (see below) for two weeks. If that doesn't help, he may order one or more of the following tests:

● **Upper GI series,** in which you drink a barium liquid, then have an X ray of your digestive tract. The barium helps reveal any ulcer.
● **Endoscopy,** in which a narrow, flexible tube with a tiny camera on its tip is inserted through the mouth and into the esophagus and stomach to look for abnormalities and to collect some tissue for examination. This test is performed under light anesthesia.
● **Blood tests** or a **breath test** to determine if you have *H. pylori.*
● **Stool sample** to look for blood in your bowel movements.

How is it treated?

Your doctor may prescribe a three-part medication strategy. Acid control is achieved with over-the-counter antacids such as Mylanta and Tums, as well as H2 blockers like cimetidine (Tagamet), ranitidine (Zantac), and

Fast Fact

More than 20 million North Americans will have an ulcer in their lifetime. Duodenal ulcers are twice as common among men, often occurring between ages 30 and 50. Stomach ulcers are more common in women over age 60.

famotidine (Pepcid). A prescription drug such as omeprazole (Losec), which blocks all acid production, may be used instead. Antibiotics, prescribed to fight the infection, can cure 80 to 90 percent of ulcers. Bismuth subsalicylate (Pepto-Bismol) may also be prescribed to form a protective coating over the ulcer.

Your Prevention Plan

Diet ▪ **Graze like sheep.** Cut your usual meals in half to make six mini-meals, and eat them a couple of hours apart so you'll always have food in your stomach.

▪ **Know your triggers.** In the past, doctors advised ulcer patients to avoid spicy and fatty foods. They now know that diet has little to do with ulcer healing. Avoid only those foods that worsen your symptoms. For some people, this may include cow's milk, salt, chocolate, or mint.

▪ **Axe the acid.** Limit your consumption of alcohol, coffee, caffeinated tea, and caffeinated soft drinks, which can irritate the stomach lining.

▪ **Try the cabbage cure.** Cabbage juice has been shown to protect the gastrointestinal lining from stomach acid and speed ulcer healing. If you have a juicer, you can make your own. Drink a quart a day.

▪ **Go bananas.** Bananas help strengthen the protective barrier between the stomach lining and corrosive stomach acid. They have been shown to protect rats from ulcers in laboratory tests.

Medical Options ▪ **Avoid NSAIDs.** Ulcers caused by NSAIDs such as aspirin and ibuprofen are best avoided by replacing these drugs with acetaminophen or newer COX-2 inhibitors like Vioxx. Four grams of acetaminophen per day is comparable to painkilling doses of ibuprofen—without the gastrointestinal side effects.

Supplements ▪ **A to zinc.** Vitamin A and zinc are thought to be helpful in ulcer healing, although there is no firm evidence. Take a multivitamin that contains them.

Natural Health ▪ **Try licorice.** Ask your doctor if it's okay to chew a 380 mg tablet of deglycyrrhizinated licorice 20 minutes before you eat (four times a day) to soothe and heal broken mucous membranes.

▪ **Teatime.** Drinking teas brewed from marshmallow root or slippery elm bark several times a day helps form a protective layer over ulcers.

Lifestyle ▪ **Toss tobacco.** People with ulcers should not smoke or chew tobacco—it inhibits healing and is linked to ulcer recurrence.

▪ **Seek stress relief.** Stress can exacerbate ulcers and lower your immune system, possibly making you more susceptible to them. Practice stress-reducing techniques such as deep breathing, meditation, and yoga. Exercise also helps reduce stress.

Urinary Tract Infection

◀ Burning pain when you urinate

◀ Frequent need to urinate, although you pass very little urine

◀ Urine that is cloudy or tinged with blood

◀ Women may have an unusual vaginal discharge or odor.

◀ Along with the symptoms above, soreness in your back or lower abdomen, chills, fever, nausea, or vomiting can signal a kidney infection; call your doctor immediately.

WARNING

An untreated UTI can lead to a dangerous kidney infection. Even if you've had a UTI before and you think you know how to treat it, see your doctor. You probably need antibiotics to clear up the infection.

What is it?

A urinary tract infection (UTI) occurs when bacteria from the lower intestine colonize the bladder (the holding tank for urine) and urethra (the outlet for urine). An infection that spreads to the kidneys is called pyelonephritis and requires urgent medical attention.

Doctors treat more than 50 million UTIs each year in North America. The infection occurs about 20 times more often in women because they have a shorter urethra—about 2 inches compared with 10 inches in men. This means bacteria have easier access to a woman's urinary tract. Women who have gone through menopause and young sexually active women are especially susceptible to UTIs. But the infection is most common in the elderly—one-third of older individuals suffer from UTIs.

When bacteria—usually the *E. coli* strain—enter the urethra, they can move up the urinary tract into the bladder, causing infection along the way. *E coli* can be transferred from your hands, from your anal area after a bowel movement, or from the skin of your genitals. For women, sex is a major culprit, because bacteria that live in and around the vagina can be pushed up the opening to the urethra during sexual activity. Women who use a diaphragm are at slightly higher risk.

Having kidney stones or an enlarged prostate also raises your risk for UTIs. And if you've already had a UTI, you are more susceptible to having another than if you've never had one.

Most doctors are able to diagnose a UTI by the symptoms alone. But sometimes they ask for a urine sample so it can be tested for bacteria. This helps determine which antibiotic will be most helpful in killing the bug causing the infection.

How is it treated?

You can often prevent a UTI by making certain lifestyle changes (see *Your Prevention Plan,* opposite). Take a nonprescription painkiller (such as aspirin or Tylenol) to ease the pain of infection, but remember that only antibiotics can kill the bacteria that cause UTIs in the first place.

DRUGS

If you have uncomplicated cystitis, your doctor will probably prescribe the antibiotics sulfamethoxazole and trimethoprim for three days. In order to completely kill the bacteria, it's essential that you take the entire amount prescribed—even if you start to feel better. In the past, the antibiotic ampicillin was widely prescribed. As a result, more than a third of the *E. coli* bacteria that cause UTIs are resistant to that drug today.

If you are a sexually active woman with recurrent UTIs, ask your physician if you should take a single dose of antibiotic after sex to kill any bacteria that have entered your urinary tract. For stubborn infections that keep coming back, some doctors prescribe a strong course of antibiotics followed by a very low dose of the drug for as long as a year or two.

Your Prevention Plan

Diet ▇ **Flush with fluids.** Drink at least eight 8-ounce glasses of water every day, even when you don't have a UTI.

▇ **Sip cranberry.** If you are prone to repeat infections, drink up to a quart of unsweetened cranberry juice daily to make your urine more acidic, creating a hostile environment for bacteria.

▇ **Avoid alkalinity.** Stay away from alcohol, spicy foods, coffee, citrus juices, carbonated beverages, and dairy products, all of which make your urine more alkaline, creating a friendly environment for bacteria.

Supplements ▇ **Increase acidity.** Take 1,000 mg of vitamin C daily. It will make your urine inhospitable to bacteria by making it more acidic. Plus, vitamin C may help boost your immunity to help prevent infections in the first place.

Natural Health ▇ **Teatime.** Sip teas made of nettle, a natural diuretic, to help flush out bacteria. Use 1 teaspoon of dried herb per cup of hot water, and drink one cup a day.

▇ **Herbal prevention.** By promoting a healthy immune system, echinacea may help stave off recurrent urinary-tract infections. Take it for up to eight weeks, then take a two-week break. Goldenseal can help you fight an infection once you have one. Drink several cups of goldenseal tea (available commercially) a day at the first sign of a UTI.

▇ **Aromatherapy.** Blend essential oils of bergamot and lavender or chamomile with a carrier oil, like safflower oil, and massage into your lower abdomen to relieve discomfort.

Lifestyle ▇ **Hygiene first.** Keep your genital area clean and always wipe from front to back after a bowel movement. This prevents bacteria from contaminating the vagina and urethra.

▇ **Empty out.** Empty your bladder completely every time you urinate so bacteria don't have a chance to multiply in stagnant urine.

▇ **Choose cotton.** Wear cotton underpants. They "breathe" and are less likely to provide a friendly environment for bacteria, which thrive in warm, moist environments.

▇ **Don't douche.** Don't use feminine hygiene sprays or douches. They upset the pH balance of the vagina and make it more inviting to bacteria.

▇ **Speaking of sex.** Drink a large glass of water and urinate right after sex to help flush any bacteria from your urethra so they can't cause infection.

Varicose Veins

SYMPTOMS

◀ Prominent blue-purple swollen veins, usually on your legs

◀ Aching, throbbing, cramping, heaviness, or swelling in your legs or ankles, especially after a day on your feet

◀ Burning or itching skin on your legs

SimpleSolution

If you sit for much of the day, try this easy leg exercise under your desk several times daily:
1. Sit back in your chair with your heels on the ground and your toes pointed upward.
2. Raise your legs to about knee level (or as high as is comfortable).
3. Point your toes outward and then upward.
4. Lower your legs.

What is it?

Varicose veins are twisted swollen veins that are most often found in the legs. They develop when the one-way valves that allow blood to flow from the veins of the legs back to the heart don't close completely. This permits some of the blood to pool in the leg veins, causing them to bulge.

If you have varicose veins, you're not alone. Although women are more likely to get them than men, more than half of people over age 50 have them. After 50, the skin supporting the veins—and the veins themselves—lose their elasticity, contributing to the condition.

For most people, varicose veins are more a cosmetic concern than a serious medical problem. But in other people, weakness in the walls of the blood vessels—in addition to the faulty valves—causes blood to seep into nearby tissue. If the skin near a varicose vein becomes discolored or you have a sore that won't heal near one of them, see your doctor promptly.

Any condition that places additional pressure on the leg veins, including obesity, constipation (due to straining on the toilet), pregnancy, or standing for long periods, can contribute to varicose veins. Doctors aren't always certain what causes them, but they believe that some people inherit a tendency to the condition. Having a history of deep vein thrombosis (in which a blood clot forms in a large vein in the leg) may also be a cause of severe varicose veins.

How is it treated?

Many people with varicose veins make lifestyle modifications (see *Your Prevention Plan,* opposite) to ease discomfort. But others choose surgery.

SURGERY

There are several ways to surgically treat varicose veins. After these procedures, blood in the treated vein finds a healthier vein to flow through. In sclerotherapy (used for spider veins and small varicose veins), the doctor injects a salt solution into the affected vein, causing it to shrink and eventually be absorbed by your body. Sclerotherapy is an outpatient procedure. For more severely affected veins, a surgeon makes cuts near the affected veins and either ties them off (called ligation) or removes them altogether (called stripping). These surgeries are performed in a hospital.

WARNING

See your doctor if your veins are giving you trouble. Advanced varicose veins can lead to skin cancers, dangerous vein inflammation, and clotting problems. Rough contact with an affected vein can cause severe bleeding.

Your Prevention Plan

Diet
■ **Skip the salt.** Avoid salty foods. They cause your body to retain water, which can lead to swollen legs.

■ **Focus on fiber.** Eat high-fiber foods such as whole-grain breads, fruits, and vegetables every day to reduce your chances of constipation, which can contribute to varicose veins.

■ **Stay lean.** Obesity increases the pressure on the leg veins and slows the flow of blood from the legs back to the heart.

Exercise
■ **Walk, swim, bike.** These exercises, done 30 minutes a day several days a week, improve leg strength—and vein strength. They also keep blood pumping toward the heart.

■ **Stand up and move.** If you sit for extended periods, get up every 45 minutes and walk briskly for 5 minutes.

Supplements
■ **Strength in vitamins.** Vitamins E and C encourage the circulation of blood and strengthen blood-vessel walls. Take 500 mg of vitamin C and 400 international units (IU) of vitamin E every day.

Natural Health
■ **Smooth on relief.** Witch hazel (full-strength or as a cream) applied to varicose veins may help relieve soreness. Keep it in the refrigerator for cool relief.

■ **Herbal help.** Visit a health-food store to find a supplement containing bilberry and gotu kola. These herbs keep blood flowing and reinforce vein flexibility and strength. An alternative is a horse chestnut supplement, which some researchers believe can limit the swelling and fluid buildup of varicose veins as effectively as compression hose.

■ **Massage.** A leg massage can help alleviate the discomfort of swollen veins.

Lifestyle
■ **Hydrotherapy.** Sponge or spray your legs with cold water for relief. Or try alternating hot and cold sponge baths. Fill two basins with water: one warm and one cold. First, immerse your feet in the warm water for one minute, sponging your legs. Then switch to the cold water, keeping your feet immersed for half a minute and again sponging your legs. Return to the warm water for one to two minutes. Repeat five times.

■ **Support the cause.** Wear support stockings or compression hose at all times—even under your blue jeans. They give your leg veins added support and keep veins from bulging. It's not a good idea to wear knee-high stockings, which can cut off circulation below the knee.

■ **Elevate to relieve.** Put your feet up any time you can in order to reduce the workload of your leg veins. Elevating your feet eases the amount of pumping leg veins have to do.

■ **Ankles, not knees.** Crossing your legs at the knees impedes the circulation of blood through your veins. If you cross your legs regularly, cross them at your ankles, not your knees.

Resource Guide

Looking for more information on a particular subject? The organizations below can help. Log on to their web sites for instant access, or call or write to learn what materials are available through the mail.

Alternative Medicine

■ **Canadian Association of Herbal Practitioners**
1228 Kensington Road NW, Suite 400
Calgary, AB T2N 4P9
403-270-0936

■ **Canadian Federation of Aromatherapists**
868 Markham Road, Suite 109
Scarborough, ON M1H 2Y2
800-803-7668

■ **Canadian Massage Therapist Alliance**
365 Bloor Street East, Suite 1807
Toronto, ON M4W 3L4
416-968-2149
www.collinscan.com/~collins/clientspgs/cmtai.html

■ **Canadian Natural Health Association**
439 Wellington Street W, Suite 5
Toronto, ON M5V 1E7
416-322-4225

■ **The Chinese Medicine and Acupuncture Association of Canada (CMAAC)**
154 Wellington Street
London, ON N6B 2K8
519-642-1970
www.cmaac.ca

■ **Tzu Chi Institute for Complementary and Alternative Medicine**
715 West 12th Avenue
Health Centre, 4th Floor West
Vancouver, BC V5Z 1M9
604-875-4769
www.tzu-chi.bc.ca

Consumer

■ **Canadian Association of Retired Persons (CARP)**
27 Queen Street East, Suite 1304
Toronto, ON M5C 2M6
416-363-8748
www.fifty-plus.net

Drugs, Smoking, and Alcohol

■ **Canadian Centre on Substance Abuse**
75 Albert Street, Suite 300
Ottawa, ON K1P 5E7
613-235-4048
www.ccsa.ca

■ **Canadian Council for Tobacco Control**
170 Laurier Avenue West, Suite 1000
Ottawa, ON K1P 5V5
613-567-3050
www.cctc.ca

■ **General Service Office of Alcoholics Anonymous**
Grand Central Station
P.O. Box 459
New York, NY 10163 USA
212-870-3400
www.alcoholics-anonymous.org

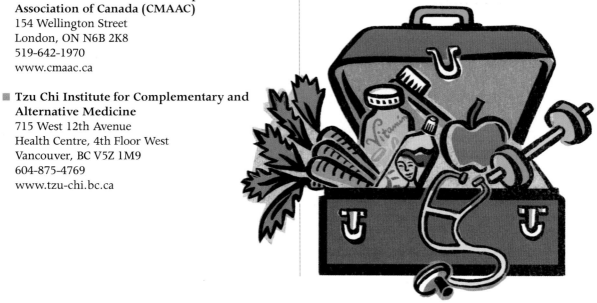

■ **Health Canada Tobacco Reduction**
www.hc-sc.gc.ca/hppb/tobaccoreduction

■ **Physicians for a Smoke-free Canada**
1226A Wellington Street
Ottawa, ON K1Y 3A1
613-233-4878
www.smoke-free.ca

Exercise

■ **Canadian Society for Exercise Physiology**
www.paguide.com

■ **Canadian Volkssport Federation**
P.O. Box 2668, Station D
Ottawa, ON K1P 5W7
www.chebucto.ns.ca/Recreation/CVF/

■ **Coalition for Active Living in Canada**
www.activeliving.ca

■ **ParticipACTION**
www.participaction.com

Food and Nutrition

■ **Centre for Science in the Public Interest (Canada)**
One Nicholas Street, Suite 412
Ottawa, ON K1N 7B7
613-565-2140
www.cspinet.org/canada/

■ **Dietitians of Canada**
480 University Avenue, Suite 604
Toronto, ON M5G 1V2
416-596-0857
www.dietitians.ca

■ **National Institute of Nutrition**
265 Carling Avenue, Suite 302
Ottawa, ON K1S 2E1
613-235-3355
www.nin.ca

Medical

■ **The Arthritis Society**
393 University Avenue, Suite 1700
Toronto, ON M5G 1E6
800-321-1433
www.arthritis.ca

■ **Asthma Society of Canada**
130 Bridgeland Avenue, Suite 425
Toronto, ON M6A 1Z4
800-787-3880
www.asthmasociety.com

■ **Alzheimer Society of Canada**
20 Eglinton Avenue West, Suite 1200
Toronto, ON M4R 1K8
800-616-8816
www.alzheimer.ca

■ **Breast Cancer Society of Canada**
401 St. Clair Street
Point Edward, ON N7V 1P2
800-567-8767
www.bcsc.ca

■ **Canadian Academy of Audiology**
250 Consumers Road, Suite 301
Willowdale, ON M2J 4V6
800-264-5106
www.canadianaudiology.ca

■ **Canadian Cancer Society**
10 Alcorn Avenue, Suite 200
Toronto, ON M4V 3B1
416-961-7223
cancer information line: 888-939-3333
www.cancer.ca

■ **Canadian Dental Association**
1815 Alta Vista
Ottawa, ON K1G 3Y6
613-523-1770
www.cda-adc.ca

■ **Canadian Diabetes Association**
15 Toronto Street, Suite 800
Toronto, ON M5C 2E3
800-BANTING (226-8464)
www.diabetes.ca

■ **Canadian Lung Association**
3 Raymond Street, Suite 300
Ottawa, ON K1R 1A3
613-569-6411
www.lung.ca

Crohn's and Colitis Foundation of Canada
21 St. Clair Avenue East, Suite 301
Toronto, ON M4T 1L9
800-387-1479
www.ccfc.ca

Heart and Stroke Foundation of Canada
222 Queen Street. Suite 1402
Ottawa, ON K1P 5V9
613-569-4361
www.na.heartandstroke.ca

Migraine Association of Canada
365 Bloor Street East, Suite 1912
Toronto, ON M4W 3L4
24-hour info line 416-920-4917
800-663-3557
www.migraine.ca

National Advisory Council on Aging
Postal Locator: 1908A1
Ottawa, ON K1A 1B4
613-957-1968
www.hc-sc.gc.ca/seniors-aines

National Cancer Institute of Canada
10 Alcorn Avenue, Suite 200
Toronto, ON M4V 3B1
416-961-7223
www.ncic.cancer.ca

National Cancer Institute of Canada
Clinical Trials Group
A cooperative oncology group that carries out
clinical trials in cancer therapy and supportive
care across Canada and internationally
www.ctg.queensu.ca

**North American Chronic Pain Association
of Canada**
150 Central Park Drive, Unit 105
Brampton, ON L6T 2T9
800-616-PAIN (7246)
www.chronicpaincanada.org

Osteoporosis Society of Canada
33 Laird Drive
Toronto, ON M4G 3S9
800-463-6842
www.osteoporosis.ca

Parkinson Foundation of Canada
4211 Yonge Street, Suite 316
Toronto, ON M2P 2A9
800-565-3000
www.parkinson.ca

Prostate Cancer Research Foundation
1262 Don Mills Road, Suite 1-F
Toronto, ON M3B 2W7
888-255-0333
www.prostatecancer.on.ca

Rosacea Awareness Program
368 Notre Dame Ouest, Suite 402
Montreal, QC H2Y 1T9
888-ROSACEA (767-2232)
www.rosaceainfo.com

Thyroid Foundation of Canada
P.O. Box 1919, Station Main
Kingston, ON K7L 5J7
800-267-8822
home.ican.net/~thyroid/Canada

Tinnitus Association of Canada
23 Ellis Park Road
Toronto, ON M6S 2V4
416-762-1490
www.kadis.com/ta/tinnitus_1.htm

Mental Health

Canadian Mental Health Association
2160 Yonge Street, 3rd Floor
Toronto, ON M4S 2Z3
416-484-7750
www.cmha.ca

Canadian Psychological Association
151 Slater Street, Suite 205
Ottawa, ON K1P 5H3
888-472-0657
www.cpa.ca

Centre for Addiction and Mental Health
33 Russell Street
Toronto, ON M5S 2S1
800-463-6273
www.camh.net

Sleep

■ **The Canadian Movement Disorder Group**
www.cmdg.org

■ **Canadian Sleep Society**
3080 Yonge Street, Suite 5055
Toronto, ON M4N 3N1
416-483-6260
www.css.to

■ **Sleep/Wake Disorders Canada**
3080 Yonge Street, Suite 5055
Toronto, ON M4N 3N1
416-483-9654
www.swdca.org

Travel and Volunteer Opportunities

■ **AmeriSpan Unlimited**
P.O. Box 40007
Philadelphia, PA 19106-0007
USA
215-751-1100
www.amerispan.com

■ **Elderhostel**
75 Federal Street
Boston, MA 02110-1941
USA
Toll-free in Canada 877-426-8056
www.elderhostel.org

■ **Habitat for Humanity International**
121 Habitat Street
Americus, GA 31709
USA
229-924-6935, ext. 2551
www.habitat.org

■ **Languages Abroad**
317 Adelaide Street West, Suite 900
Toronto, ON M5V 1P9
800-219-9924
www.languagesabroad.com

■ **Talking Traveler**
620 SW Fifth Avenue, Suite 610
Portland, OR 97204
USA
www.talkingtraveler.org

Women's Health

■ **The Canadian Women's Health Network**
419 Graham Avenue, Suite 203
Winnipeg, MB R3C 0M3
888-818-9172
www.cwhn.ca

■ **The North American Menopause Society**
P.O. Box 94527
Cleveland, OH 44101
USA
440-442-7550
800-774-5342
www.menopause.org

For additional information online

■ www.brain-teaser.com
■ www.canoe.ca/HealthReference/home.html
■ www.cfia-acia.agr.ca
■ www.hc-sc.gc.ca
■ www.logic.com
■ www.mayohealth.org
■ www.nlm.nih.gov/medlineplus
■ www.readersdigesthealth.com
■ www.webmd.ca

Credits

Illustrations

Calef Brown 11, 20, 22, 24, 25, 58, 85, 146, 150, 151, 166, 183, 191, 218, 231, 243, 261, 266

John Edwards & Associates 124, 125

Joel and Sharon Harris 18, 19, 159, 162, 272

Becky Heavner 1, 4, 13, 21, 26, 28, 34, 37, 40, 48, 52, 73, 74, 83, 88, 101, 110, 147, 155, 163, 167, 171, 178, 179, 181, 182, 185, 189, 196, 203, 209, 215, 223, 227, 229, 232, 249, 255, 262, 274, 279, 287, 288, 294, 295, 400, 416

Photographs

Cover *Front: top to bottom* Comstock; Augustus Butera; PhotoDisc (4); Augustus Butera. *Spine:* Comstock; *Back:* PhotoDisc. **2** *clockwise from top left* Augustus Butera; Mark Thomas; PhotoDisc; Jon Feingersh/The Stock Market. **8-9** Zefa Visual Media. **13** Peter Griffith/Masterfile. **14** *background* PhotoDisc; *top* PhotoDisc; *bottom* Michael A. Keller/The Stock Market. **15** *top* Reader's Digest Assoc. GID#2849; *middle* Charles Thatcher/Tony Stone Images; *bottom* PhotoDisc. **16** *top* C/B Productions/The Stock Market; *middle* PhotoDisc; *bottom* PhotoDisc. **17** ROB & SAS/The Stock Market. **23** *background* Gary Irving/PhotoDisc; *foreground* Beth Bischoff. **30-31** Mark Thomas. **34** PhotoDisc. **35** *all* PhotoDisc. **38-43** Mark Thomas. **46** Steven Needham/Envision. **47-55** Mark Thomas. **56** Susan Goldman. **57** Mark Thomas. **60** Digital Vision. **61** Mark Thomas. **62** *top* PhotoDisc; *top right* PhotoDisc; *bottom left* Digital Stock. **63** *top* PhotoDisc; *middle* Digital Stock; *bottom left* PhotoDisc; *bottom center* PhotoDisc. **64** *all* PhotoDisc. **65** *top* PhotoDisc; *middle* PhotoDisc; *bottom* Digital Stock. **66-67** Beth Bischoff. **68** PhotoDisc. **71** PhotoDisc. **75-81** Mark Thomas. **82** Stefan May/Tony Stone Images. **84** Mark Thomas. **86-87** Susan Goldman. **90** Lisa Koenig. **92** Susan Goldman. **94** Lisa Koenig. **95** Susan Goldman. **96** *top* Lisa Koenig; *bottom* Susan Goldman. **97** *top* Lisa Koenig; *middle* Lisa Koenig; *bottom* Susan Goldman. **98** *top and bottom* Lisa Koenig. **99** *top* Lisa Koenig. **100** Susan Goldman. **103** Susan Goldman. **105** Lisa Koenig. **106** Susan Goldman. **108-109** PhotoDisc. **111** PhotoDisc. **112** PhotoDisc. **113** Jack Star/PhotoLink/PhotoDisc. **114** Beth Bischoff. **117** Jon Feingersh/The Stock Market. **119** *top* Jon Feingersh/The Stock Market; *bottom* Richard Dunoff Stock. **120** Tom & Dee Anne McCarthy/The Stock Market. **121** Beth Bischoff. **126** Beth Bischoff. **128-140** Beth Bischoff. **141** *top left* Beth Bischoff; *top right* Beth Bischoff; *middle left* Beth Bischoff; *middle right* Beth Bischoff; *bottom* Jack Gescheidt/Index Stock Imagery. **144-145** PhotoDisc. **152** Simon Metz. **153** ATC Productions/The Stock Market. **158** Howard Socherek/The Stock Market. **160** *above* SPL/Photo Researchers, Inc. *below* Catherine Ursillo/Photo Researchers, Inc. **161** *top* Yoav Levy/Photo Take; *bottom* Photo Researchers, Inc. **164-165** *top left* PhotoDisc; *top right* Comstock; *bottom left* PhotoDisc; *bottom right* Comstock. **168** Bruce Ayers/Tony Stone Images. **171** Richard Dunoff. **173** David Madison/Tony Stone Images. **174** Larry Williams/Masterfile. **180** Photo Link/PhotoDisc. **184-185** Richard Dunoff. **186-187** PhotoDisc. **188** Claudia Kunin/Tony Stone Images. **193** PhotoDisc. **194** Dynamic Graphics. **197** Rob Lewine/The Stock Market. **198** *top* S. Pearce/PhotoLink/PhotoDisc; *middle* John Dowland/PhotoAlto; *bottom* Richard Dunoff. **199** *top* PhotoDisc; *bottom left* Richard Dunoff; *bottom right* Barbara Penoyar/PhotoDisc. **200** Beth Bischoff. **201** Maximilian Stock Ltd./SPL Photo Researchers, Inc. **203** *top* Aneal Vohra/Index Stock Imagery; *bottom* Richard Dunoff. **204** Ted Wood/Tony Stone Images. **207** Lori Adamski Peek/Tony Stone Images. **208** *top* Michelangelo Gratton/Tony Stone Images; *bottom* Digital Vision. **210** Pierre Dufour. **212** Francois Gohier/ Photo Researchers, Inc. **214** Robert Maass/Corbis. **216** Josh Pulman/Tony Stone Images. **217** PhotoDisc. **220-221** Masterfile. **222** Leo de Wys/Leo de Wys Stock Photo Agency/Germany IT International Ltd. **224** Michael A. Keller/The Stock Market. **225** Susan Goldman. **226** Christopher Bissell/Tony Stone Images. **235** *top* Susan Goldman; *middle* Lisa Koenig; *bottom* Jack Star/Photo Link/PhotoDisc. **236** PhotoDisc. **237** Bill Aron/PhotoEdit. **238** C. Bronico. **239** Lisa Koenig. **240-241** R. B. Studio/The Stock Market. **242** Dave Bartruff/Index Stock Imagery. **244** Lazlo Kubinyi. **246** David Young-Wolff/Tony Stone Images. **251** Lori Adamski Peek/Tony Stone Images. **252** Lonnie Duka/Index Stock Imagery. **254** NIH/Science Source/Photo Researchers, Inc. **256** PhotoDisc. **258-259** Ariel Skelley/Stock Market. **263** PhotoDisc. **265** Susan Goldman. **269** John Dowland/PhotoAlto. **270-271** *top left* Romilly Lockver/Image Bank; *top right* PhotoDisc; *bottom left* Benelux Press/Index Stock Imagery; *bottom right* Zefa Visual Media/Index Stock Imagery. **273** James Darell/Tony Stone Images. **276** Nicholas Eveleigh. **277** Susan Goldman. **278** Will & Demi McIntyre/Photo Researchers. **282** LWA-Dan Tardif/The Stock Market. **283** Susan Goldman. **284-285** American Academy of Cosmetic Dentistry. **286** Christian Peacock/Index Stock Imagery.

Index

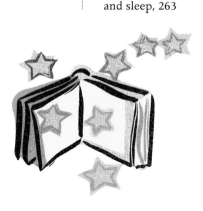